ACP | MKSAP® 17
Medical Knowledge Self-Assessment Program®

Gastroenterology and Hepatology

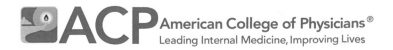

ACP American College of Physicians®
Leading Internal Medicine, Improving Lives

Welcome to the Gastroenterology and Hepatology Section of MKSAP 17!

In these pages, you will find updated information on gastroesophageal reflux disease, Barrett esophagus, *Helicobacter pylori* infection, gastrointestinal complications of NSAIDs, celiac disease, inflammatory bowel disease, liver disease, gallbladder disease, and other clinical challenges. All of these topics are uniquely focused on the needs of generalists and subspecialists *outside* of gastroenterology and hepatology.

The publication of the 17th edition of Medical Knowledge Self-Assessment Program (MKSAP) represents nearly a half-century of serving as the gold-standard resource for internal medicine education. It also marks its evolution into an innovative learning system to better meet the changing educational needs and learning styles of all internists.

The core content of MKSAP has been developed as in previous editions—newly generated, essential information in 11 topic areas of internal medicine created by dozens of leading generalists and subspecialists and guided by certification and recertification requirements, emerging knowledge in the field, and user feedback. MKSAP 17 also contains 1200 all-new, psychometrically validated, and peer-reviewed multiple-choice questions (MCQs) for self-assessment and study, including 96 in Gastroenterology and Hepatology. MKSAP 17 continues to include *High Value Care* (HVC) recommendations, based on the concept of balancing clinical benefit with costs and harms, with links to MCQs that illustrate these principles. In addition, HVC Key Points are highlighted in the text. Also highlighted, with blue text, are *Hospitalist*-focused content and MCQs that directly address the learning needs of internists who work in the hospital setting.

MKSAP 17 Digital provides access to additional tools allowing you to customize your learning experience, including regular text updates with practice-changing, new information and 200 new self-assessment questions; a board-style pretest to help direct your learning; and enhanced custom-quiz options. And, with MKSAP Complete, learners can access 1200 electronic flashcards for quick review of important concepts or review the updated and enhanced version of Virtual Dx, an image-based self-assessment tool.

As before, MKSAP 17 is optimized for use on your mobile devices, with iOS- and Android-based apps allowing you to sync your work between your apps and online account and submit for CME credits and MOC points online.

Please visit us at the MKSAP Resource Site (mksap.acponline.org) to find out how we can help you study, earn CME credit and MOC points, and stay up to date.

Whether you prefer to use the traditional print version or take advantage of the features available through the digital version, we hope you enjoy MKSAP 17 and that it meets and exceeds your personal learning needs.

On behalf of the many internists who have offered their time and expertise to create the content for MKSAP 17 and the editorial staff who work to bring this material to you in the best possible way, we are honored that you have chosen to use MKSAP 17 and appreciate any feedback about the program you may have. Please feel free to send us any comments to mksap_editors@acponline.org.

Sincerely,

Philip A. Masters, MD, FACP
Editor-in-Chief
Senior Physician Educator
Director, Content Development
Medical Education Division
American College of Physicians

Gastroenterology and Hepatology

Committee

Amy S. Oxentenko, MD, FACP, Section Editor[1]
Associate Professor of Medicine
Division of Gastroenterology and Hepatology
Mayo Clinic
Rochester, Minnesota

Allan R. Tunkel, MD, PhD, MACP, Associate Editor[2]
Professor of Medicine
Associate Dean for Medical Education
The Warren Alpert Medical School of Brown University
Providence, Rhode Island

Carol A. Burke, MD, FACP[2]
Director, Center for Colon Polyp and Cancer Prevention
Department of Gastroenterology and Hepatology
Cleveland Clinic
Cleveland, Ohio

Matthew J. DiMagno, MD[2]
Assistant Professor of Internal Medicine
Division of Gastroenterology and Hepatology
University of Michigan School of Medicine
Ann Arbor, Michigan

Seth A. Gross, MD[2]
Associate Professor of Clinical Medicine
NYU School of Medicine
NYU Langone Medical Center
New York, New York

Michael D. Leise, MD[2]
Assistant Professor of Medicine
Mayo Clinic
Division of Gastroenterology and Hepatology
Rochester, Minnesota

Darrell S. Pardi, MD, MS[2]
Professor of Medicine
Vice Chair, Division of Gastroenterology
   and Hepatology
Associate Chair for Fellowship Education
Department of Internal Medicine
Associate Dean of Medicine and Pediatrics
Mayo School of Graduate Medical Education
Mayo Clinic
Rochester, Minnesota

John Poterucha, MD[1]
Professor of Medicine
Mayo Clinic
Division of Gastroenterology and Hepatology
Rochester, Minnesota

Richard Saad, MD, MS[2]
Assistant Professor of Medicine
Division of Gastroenterology and Hepatology
University of Michigan
Ann Arbor, Michigan

Editor-in-Chief

Philip A. Masters, MD, FACP[1]
Director, Clinical Content Development
American College of Physicians
Philadelphia, Pennsylvania

Director, Clinical Program Development

Cynthia D. Smith, MD, FACP[2]
American College of Physicians
Philadelphia, Pennsylvania

Gastroenterology and Hepatology Reviewers

Amindra S. Arora, MD[1]
Frantz M. Duffoo, MD, FACP[1]
Rabeh M. Elzuway, MD[1]
Gloria T. Fioravanti, DO, FACP[1]
John D. Goldman, MD, FACP[2]

Gastroenterology and Hepatology ACP Editorial Staff

Katie Idell[1], Digital Content Associate/Editor
Margaret Wells[1], Director, Self-Assessment and Educational
   Programs
Becky Krumm[1], Managing Editor

ACP Principal Staff

Patrick C. Alguire, MD, FACP[2]
Senior Vice President, Medical Education

Sean McKinney[1]
Vice President, Medical Education

Margaret Wells[1]
Director, Self-Assessment and Educational Programs

Becky Krumm[1]
Managing Editor

Valerie A. Dangovetsky[1]
Administrator

Ellen McDonald, PhD[1]
Senior Staff Editor

Katie Idell[1]
Digital Content Associate/Editor

Megan Zborowski[1]
Senior Staff Editor

Randy Hendrickson[1]
Production Administrator/Editor

Linnea Donnarumma[1]
Staff Editor

Susan Galeone[1]
Staff Editor

Jackie Twomey[1]
Staff Editor

Kimberly Kerns[1]
Administrative Coordinator

---

1. Has no relationships with any entity producing, marketing, reselling, or distributing health care goods or services consumed by, or used on, patients.

2. Has disclosed relationship(s) with any entity producing, marketing, reselling, or distributing health care goods or services consumed by, or used on, patients.

Disclosure of Relationships with any entity producing, marketing, reselling, or distributing health care goods or services consumed by, or used on, patients:

Patrick C. Alguire, MD, FACP
Board Member
Teva Pharmaceuticals
Consultantship
National Board of Medical Examiners
Royalties
UpToDate
Stock Options/Holdings
Amgen Inc, Bristol-Myers Squibb, GlaxoSmithKline, Covidien, Stryker Corporation, Zimmer Orthopedics, Teva Pharmaceuticals, Express Scripts, Medtronic

Carol A. Burke, MD, FACP
Consultantship
Ferring
Other
Pfizer
Research Grants/Contracts
Pfizer, Salix, Cancer Prevention Pharmaceuticals, American College of Gastroenterology
Speakers Bureau
Salix, Takeda

Matthew J. DiMagno, MD
Board Member
British Medical Journal
Research Grants/Contracts
National Institutes of Health, University of Michigan Office of Vice President of Research
Honoraria
Lippincott Williams and Wilkins, Springer, Oakstone Publishing, LLC, American Gastroenterological Association Institute

John D. Goldman, MD, FACP
Employment
Pinnacle Health

Seth A. Gross, MD
Consultantship
EndoCDx, Given Imaging, Cook
Stock Options/Holdings
CSA Medical

Michael D. Leise, MD
Consultantship
Tranzyme Pharmaceuticals
Research Grants/Contracts
Bristol-Myers Squibb, Salix, Merck
Royalties
UpToDate

Darrell S. Pardi, MD, MS
Advisory Board Member
Cubist
Consultantship
Salix, Optimer, Seres Health
Research Grants/Contracts
Merck, ViroPharma, Cubist, Sanofi, Salix, Seres Health

Richard Saad, MD, MS
Consultantship
Ironwood Pharmaceuticals
Research Grants/Contracts
Takeda Pharmaceuticals, Tioga Pharmaceuticals, Salix, Sk Life Sciences

Cynthia D. Smith, MD, FACP
Stock Options/Holdings
Merck and Co., spousal employment at Merck

Allan R. Tunkel, MD, PhD, MACP
Employment
American College of Physicians
Other
Infectious Diseases Society of America
Research Grants/Contracts
UpToDate

Acknowledgments

The American College of Physicians (ACP) gratefully acknowledges the special contributions to the development and production of the 17th edition of the Medical Knowledge Self-Assessment Program® (MKSAP® 17) made by the following people:

Graphic Design: Michael Ripca (Graphics Technical Administrator) and WFGD Studio (Graphic Designers).

Production/Systems: Dan Hoffmann (Director, Web Services & Systems Development), Neil Kohl (Senior Architect), Chris Patterson (Senior Architect), and Scott Hurd (Manager, Web Projects & CMS Services).

MKSAP 17 Digital: Under the direction of Steven Spadt, Vice President, Digital Products & Services, the digital version of MKSAP 17 was developed within the ACP's Digital Product Development Department, led by Brian Sweigard (Director). Other members of the team included Dan Barron (Senior Web Application Developer/Architect), Chris Forrest (Senior Software Developer/Design Lead), Kara Kronenwetter (Senior Web Developer), Brad Lord (Senior Web Application Developer), John McKnight (Senior Web Developer), and Nate Pershall (Senior Web Developer).

The College also wishes to acknowledge that many other persons, too numerous to mention, have contributed to the production of this program. Without their dedicated efforts, this program would not have been possible.

MKSAP Resource Site (mksap.acponline.org)

The MKSAP Resource Site (mksap.acponline.org) is a continually updated site that provides links to MKSAP 17 online answer sheets for print subscribers; the latest details on Continuing Medical Education (CME) and Maintenance of Certification (MOC) in the United States, Canada, and Australia; errata; and other new information.

ABIM Maintenance of Certification

Check the MKSAP Resource Site (mksap.acponline.org) for the latest information on how MKSAP tests can be used to apply to the American Board of Internal Medicine for Maintenance of Certification (MOC) points.

Royal College Maintenance of Certification

In Canada, MKSAP 17 is an Accredited Self-Assessment Program (Section 3) as defined by the Maintenance of Certification (MOC) Program of The Royal College of Physicians and Surgeons of Canada and approved by the Canadian Society of Internal Medicine on December 9, 2014. Approval extends from July 31, 2015 until July 31, 2018 for the Part A sections. Approval extends from December 31, 2015 to December 31, 2018 for the Part B sections.

Fellows of the Royal College may earn three credits per hour for participating in MKSAP 17 under Section 3. MKSAP 17 also meets multiple CanMEDS Roles, including that of Medical Expert, Communicator, Collaborator, Manager, Health Advocate, Scholar, and Professional. For information on how to apply MKSAP 17 Continuing Medical Education (CME) credits to the Royal College MOC Program, visit the MKSAP Resource Site at mksap.acponline.org.

The Royal Australasian College of Physicians CPD Program

In Australia, MKSAP 17 is a Category 3 program that may be used by Fellows of The Royal Australasian College of Physicians (RACP) to meet mandatory Continuing Professional Development (CPD) points. Two CPD credits are awarded for each of the 200 *AMA PRA Category 1 Credits*™ available in MKSAP 17. More information about using MKSAP 17 for this purpose is available at the MKSAP Resource Site at mksap.acponline.org and at www.racp. edu.au. CPD credits earned through MKSAP 17 should be reported at the MyCPD site at www.racp.edu.au/mycpd.

Continuing Medical Education

The American College of Physicians (ACP) is accredited by the Accreditation Council for Continuing Medical Education (ACCME) to provide continuing medical education for physicians.

The ACP designates this enduring material, MKSAP 17, for a maximum of 200 *AMA PRA Category 1 Credits*™. Physicians should claim only the credit commensurate with the extent of their participation in the activity.

Up to 16 *AMA PRA Category 1 Credits*™ are available from July 31, 2015, to July 31, 2018, for the MKSAP 17 Gastroenterology and Hepatology section.

Learning Objectives

The learning objectives of MKSAP 17 are to:
- Close gaps between actual care in your practice and preferred standards of care, based on best evidence
- Diagnose disease states that are less common and sometimes overlooked or confusing
- Improve management of comorbid conditions that can complicate patient care
- Determine when to refer patients for surgery or care by subspecialists
- Pass the ABIM Certification Examination
- Pass the ABIM Maintenance of Certification Examination

Target Audience

- General internists and primary care physicians
- Subspecialists who need to remain up-to-date in internal medicine and in areas outside of their own subspecialty area
- Residents preparing for the certification examination in internal medicine
- Physicians preparing for maintenance of certification in internal medicine (recertification)

Earn "Instantaneous" CME Credits Online

Print subscribers can enter their answers online to earn instantaneous Continuing Medical Education (CME) credits. You can submit your answers using online answer sheets that are provided at mksap.acponline.org, where a record of your MKSAP 17 credits will be available. To earn CME credits, you need to answer all of the questions in a test and earn a score of at least 50% correct (number of correct answers divided by the total number of questions). Take any of the following approaches:

1. Use the printed answer sheet at the back of this book to record your answers. Go to mksap.acponline.org, access the appropriate online answer sheet, transcribe your answers, and submit your test for instantaneous CME credits. There is no additional fee for this service.

2. Go to mksap.acponline.org, access the appropriate online answer sheet, directly enter your answers, and submit your test for instantaneous CME credits. There is no additional fee for this service.

3. Pay a $15 processing fee per answer sheet and submit the printed answer sheet at the back of this book by mail or fax, as instructed on the answer sheet. Make sure you calculate your score and fax the answer sheet

to 215-351-2799 or mail the answer sheet to Member and Customer Service, American College of Physicians, 190 N. Independence Mall West, Philadelphia, PA 19106-1572, using the courtesy envelope provided in your MKSAP 17 slipcase. You will need your 10-digit order number and 8-digit ACP ID number, which are printed on your packing slip. Please allow 4 to 6 weeks for your score report to be emailed back to you. Be sure to include your email address for a response.

If you do not have a 10-digit order number and 8-digit ACP ID number or if you need help creating a user name and password to access the MKSAP 17 online answer sheets, go to mksap.acponline.org or email custserv@ acponline.org.

Permission/Consent for Use of Figures Shown in MKSAP 17 Gastroenterology and Hepatology Multiple-Choice Questions

Figures shown in Self-Assessment Test Item 39 and Item 69 appear courtesy of Dr. Amindra Arora, Mayo Clinic.

Disclosure Policy

It is the policy of the American College of Physicians (ACP) to ensure balance, independence, objectivity, and scientific rigor in all of its educational activities. To this end, and consistent with the policies of the ACP and the Accreditation Council for Continuing Medical Education (ACCME), contributors to all ACP continuing medical education activities are required to disclose all relevant financial relationships with any entity producing, marketing, re-selling, or distributing health care goods or services consumed by, or used on, patients. Contributors are required to use generic names in the discussion of therapeutic options and are required to identify any unapproved, off-label, or investigative use of commercial products or devices. Where a trade name is used, all available trade names for the same product type are also included. If trade-name products manufactured by companies with whom contributors have relationships are discussed, contributors are asked to provide evidence-based citations in support of the discussion. The information is reviewed by the committee responsible for producing this text. If necessary, adjustments to topics or contributors' roles in content development are made to balance the discussion. Further, all readers of this text are asked to evaluate the content for evidence of commercial bias and send any relevant comments to mksap_editors@acponline.org so that future decisions about content and contributors can be made in light of this information.

Resolution of Conflicts

To resolve all conflicts of interest and influences of vested interests, the American College of Physicians (ACP) precluded members of the content-creation committee from deciding on any content issues that involved generic or trade-name products associated with proprietary entities with which these committee members had relationships. In addition, content was based on best evidence and updated clinical care guidelines, when such evidence and guidelines were available. Contributors' disclosure information can be found with the list of contributors' names and those of ACP principal staff listed in the beginning of this book.

Hospital-Based Medicine

For the convenience of subscribers who provide care in hospital settings, content that is specific to the hospital setting has been highlighted in blue. Hospital icons (🏥) highlight where the hospital-based content begins, continues over more than one page, and ends.

High Value Care Key Points

Key Points in the text that relate to High Value Care concepts (that is, concepts that discuss balancing clinical benefit with costs and harms) are designated by the HVC icon (**HVC**).

Educational Disclaimer

The editors and publisher of MKSAP 17 recognize that the development of new material offers many opportunities for error. Despite our best efforts, some errors may persist in print. Drug dosage schedules are, we believe, accurate and in accordance with current standards. Readers are advised, however, to ensure that the recommended dosages in MKSAP 17 concur with the information provided in the product information material. This is especially important in cases of new, infrequently used, or highly toxic drugs. Application of the information in MKSAP 17 remains the professional responsibility of the practitioner.

The primary purpose of MKSAP 17 is educational. Information presented, as well as publications, technologies, products, and/or services discussed, is intended to inform subscribers about the knowledge, techniques, and experiences of the contributors. A diversity of professional opinion exists, and the views of the contributors are their own and not those of the American College of Physicians (ACP). Inclusion of any material in the program does not constitute endorsement or recommendation by the ACP. The ACP does not warrant the safety, reliability, accuracy, completeness, or usefulness of and disclaims any and all liability for damages and claims that may result from the use of information, publications, technologies, products, and/or services discussed in this program.

Errata

Errata for MKSAP 17 will be available through the MKSAP Resource Site at mksap.acponline.org as new information becomes known to the editors.

Table of Contents

Gastroenterology and Hepatology High Value Care Recommendations

The American College of Physicians, in collaboration with multiple other organizations, is engaged in a worldwide initiative to promote the practice of High Value Care (HVC). The goals of the HVC initiative are to improve health care outcomes by providing care of proven benefit and reducing costs by avoiding unnecessary and even harmful interventions. The initiative comprises several programs that integrate the important concept of health care value (balancing clinical benefit with costs and harms) for a given intervention into a broad range of educational materials to address the needs of trainees, practicing physicians, and patients.

HVC content has been integrated into MKSAP 17 in several important ways. MKSAP 17 now includes HVC-identified key points in the text, HVC-focused multiple choice questions, and, for subscribers to MKSAP Digital, an HVC custom quiz. From the text and questions, we have generated the following list of HVC recommendations that meet the definition below of high value care and bring us closer to our goal of improving patient outcomes while conserving finite resources.

High Value Care Recommendation: A recommendation to choose diagnostic and management strategies for patients in specific clinical situations that balance clinical benefit with cost and harms with the goal of improving patient outcomes.

Below are the High Value Care Recommendations for the Gastroenterology and Hepatology section of MKSAP 17.

- In a patient without alarm features (dysphagia, unintentional weight loss, hematemesis, or melena), symptom relief with an empiric trial of a proton pump inhibitor (PPI) confirms the diagnosis of gastroesophageal reflux disease (see Item 81); upper endoscopy should be reserved for patients whose symptoms are unresponsive to PPIs or have alarm features.
- Patients with gastroesophageal reflux disease with no alarm symptoms who have a partial response to once-daily proton pump inhibitor therapy should have their dose increased to twice daily (see Item 73).
- Gastroesophageal reflux disease is not a clinical indication for *Helicobacter pylori* testing.
- Endoscopic therapies for gastroesophageal reflux disease have not been shown to be effective in the long term.
- Current evidence does not support routine screening for Barrett esophagus based on gastroesophageal reflux disease symptoms.

- In patients with Barrett esophagus and no dysplasia, surveillance with upper endoscopy is recommended in 3 to 5 years (see Item 33).
- For patients younger than age 50 to 55 years who present with dyspepsia without alarm features, testing and treating for *Helicobacter pylori* infection or a trial of proton pump inhibitor therapy should be pursued before any further testing is done.
- Duodenal ulcers and low-risk gastric ulcers (for example, a young patient on NSAIDs) do not typically require endoscopic follow-up.
- Low-risk gastric ulcers are clean-based or have a nonprotuberant pigmented spot; they should be treated with oral proton pump inhibitor therapy, initiation of refeeding within 24 hours, and early hospital discharge (see Item 60).
- Peptic ulcers at low risk for bleeding (clean-based or with a nonprotuberant pigmented spot) can be managed with oral proton pump inhibitor therapy and early hospital discharge (see Item 93).
- Routine second-look endoscopy is not required after upper gastrointestinal bleeding unless rebleeding occurs or the initial examination was incomplete.
- Sporadic fundic gland polyps have been associated with proton pump inhibitor use and do not require excision or surveillance (see Item 41).
- Solitary juvenile polyps are one of the most commonly found polyps; they confer no future health risk once the polyp is removed and do not require surveillance endoscopy (see Item 89).
- Noninvasive testing to confirm eradication of *Helicobacter pylori* (with the urea breath test or fecal antigen test) should be performed given the high rate of treatment failure (roughly 25% in the United States); antibody testing is not appropriate for confirming eradication because antibodies can remain in the serum long after H. pylori has been eradicated.
- Endoscopic removal of type I gastric neuroendocrine tumors is curative when tumors are small (<1 cm) and few lesions are present (<5); further treatment or staging is not necessary (see Item 85).
- Contrast-enhanced CT is not usually required to diagnose acute pancreatitis; it is less sensitive than ultrasound for gallstones, exposes patients to the risk of contrast-medium–induced nephropathy (particularly in underresuscitated patients), and is expensive.
- Poor prognostic indicators for acute pancreatitis are elevated serum blood urea nitrogen level greater than

20 mg/dL (7.1 mmol/L), a hematocrit greater than 44%, or an elevated serum creatinine level.

- Enteral feeding has been shown to reduce infectious complications, multiple organ failure, operative interventions, and mortality compared with feeding by total parenteral nutrition in patients with severe acute pancreatitis (see Item 36).
- In patients with uncomplicated gallstone pancreatitis, a cholecystectomy should be performed prior to discharge.
- Because most cases of community-acquired diarrhea are self-limited, stool cultures or evaluation for ova and parasites are not required in most patients; studies may be indicated for symptoms lasting longer than 72 hours, particularly in patients with associated fever, tenesmus, or bloody stools (see Item 88).
- Artificial sweeteners have little or no absorption in the small intestine and, when taken in excess, can cause symptoms of carbohydrate malabsorption; patients with malabsorption should be screened for artificial sweetener use and, if positive, a trial of elimination should be done prior to proceeding with a malabsorption evaluation (see Item 2).
- Assessment for intentional or unintentional gluten ingestion is the first step in evaluating recurrent symptoms in a patient with celiac disease (see Item 77).
- Routine complete blood count, serum chemistry studies, thyroid function studies, stool studies for ova and parasites, and abdominal imaging are unnecessary in establishing the diagnosis of irritable bowel syndrome (see Item 14).
- Irritable bowel syndrome was previously considered a diagnosis of exclusion after eliminating organic causes; however, an accurate diagnosis can now be made with fulfillment of the diagnostic criteria without further testing in the absence of alarm features (anemia; weight loss; and family history of colorectal cancer, inflammatory bowel disease, or celiac disease).
- In a healthy, immunocompetent patient with diverticulitis and mild symptoms, outpatient therapy is appropriate and should consist of a liquid diet, oral antimicrobial agents that cover colonic organisms and include anaerobic coverage (such as ciprofloxacin and metronidazole), and as-needed analgesia (see Item 23).
- If clinical features are highly suggestive of diverticulitis, imaging studies are unnecessary.
- Despite a decrease in colorectal cancer mortality that is largely attributable to the use of screening, 35% of eligible Americans have not been screened for colorectal cancer with fecal occult blood testing, flexible sigmoidoscopy, or colonoscopy.
- Patients who are postpolypectomy with large (>2 cm) adenomas or adenomas with invasive cancer and favorable prognostic features may be managed with surveillance colonoscopy every 3 to 6 months and do not need surgical resection or radiation therapy (see Item 57).

- Because *MYH*-associated polyposis is an autosomal recessive disorder, a cost-effective approach to testing includes testing both parents for the *MYH* mutation before testing their children (see Item 63).
- Management of esophageal variceal bleeding includes placement of two large-bore intravenous lines, fluid resuscitation, and erythrocyte transfusion to a goal hemoglobin level of 7 g/dL (70 g/L); more liberal blood transfusion thresholds lead to increased portal pressures and risk of further bleeding.
- A presumptive diagnosis of nonalcoholic steatohepatitis can be made without liver biopsy in a patient with mild abnormalities of aminotransferase levels, risk factors for nonalcoholic fatty liver disease (such as diabetes mellitus, obesity, and hyperlipidemia), and imaging features consistent with hepatic steatosis (see Item 21).
- The finding of predominantly unconjugated hyperbilirubinemia indicates non–liver-disease states such as hemolysis or Gilbert syndrome, which is characterized by benign defects in bilirubin conjugation (see Item 79).
- Patients in the inactive carrier phase of hepatitis B virus (HBV) infection, characterized by a normal serum alanine aminotransferase level and a low HBV DNA level, do not require treatment (see Item 46).
- Acute hepatitis B infection will resolve in 90% of adult patients; thus, serial monitoring of liver enzymes is recommended in place of antiviral therapy for patients without evidence of marked liver dysfunction (see Item 71).
- The preferred method for screening patients with chronic hepatitis B infection for hepatocellular carcinoma is ultrasonography every 6 months, as this is the most widely available, safest, and least expensive imaging modality (see Item 92).
- Patients with a positive antibody to hepatitis C virus (HCV) but negative HCV RNA do not have HCV infection, and no further testing is required (see Item 62).
- There is no utility in monitoring serial ammonia values in patients with hepatic encephalopathy; head CT is warranted only in patients with unwitnessed falls or head trauma, or in cases of diagnostic uncertainty.
- Ultrasound is the most cost-effective diagnostic test for ascites.
- The vast majority of hepatocellular carcinoma can be diagnosed by radiology and does not require a biopsy.
- Observation (not cholecystectomy) is recommended for adult patients with asymptomatic gallstones (see Item 25).
- Patients with lower gastrointestinal bleeding do not require hospitalization when they meet four criteria (based on the 2008 Scottish Intercollegiate Guidelines Network): age less than 60 years, no hemodynamic instability, no evidence of gross rectal bleeding, and identification of an obvious anorectal source of bleeding on rectal examination or sigmoidoscopy (see Item 37).

Gastroenterology and Hepatology

Disorders of the Esophagus
Symptoms of Esophageal Disorders
Dysphagia

Dysphagia is the awareness of food not passing during the swallowing process. The swallowing mechanism is made up of two distinct components:

1. The oropharyngeal process is the passage of the food bolus from the mouth into the hypopharynx and upper esophagus.
2. The esophageal process is the passage of the food bolus through the upper esophagus into the stomach.

Patients typically describe a feeling of food "getting stuck" or being blocked while eating. Identifying which component of the swallowing process (oropharyngeal or esophageal) is abnormal is key for formulating the differential diagnosis and devising a diagnostic and management plan. There are many causes of dysphagia, which are described in **Table 1**.

Oropharyngeal Dysphagia

Patients with oropharyngeal dysphagia (also known as transfer dysphagia) are unable to initiate the swallowing process despite several attempts to swallow. Patients typically describe coughing, choking, and nasal regurgitation. Choking occurs owing to failure to clear food from the epiglottis and may lead to aspiration. Oropharyngeal dysphagia often occurs within 1 second of starting the swallowing process. Recurrent episodes of pulmonary infections (including pneumonia) can be a result of chronic aspiration. Symptoms of underlying systemic neurologic disease include hoarseness (laryngeal nerve dysfunction) and dysarthria (weakness of the soft palate or pharyngeal constrictors). Regurgitation of undigested food hours after eating or reports of a gurgling noise in the neck are symptoms of Zenker diverticulum. The initial test of choice for evaluation of oropharyngeal dysphagia is a modified barium swallow, also known as videofluoroscopy. The test begins with a liquid phase, which is followed by a solid phase if the liquid phase is not diagnostic. If results of the modified barium swallow are normal, oropharyngeal dysphagia is excluded and further evaluation should focus on the possibility of esophageal dysphagia. Oropharyngeal forms of dysphagia are often managed with dietary adjustment and incorporation of swallowing exercises with the assistance of a speech pathologist.

Esophageal Dysphagia

Patients with esophageal dysphagia often localize discomfort to the lower sternum and do not report problems initiating the swallowing process. Dysphagia to solid foods suggests mechanical obstruction; dysphagia to liquids or both solids and liquids suggests a motility disorder. Patients with achalasia describe regurgitation of nonacidic undigested food in combination with dysphagia to solids and liquids. Esophageal spasm is associated with chest pain that may be triggered by consuming liquids of extreme hot or cold temperatures. Systemic symptoms such as Raynaud phenomenon in the setting of heartburn suggest systemic sclerosis, a cause of both mechanical obstruction and motility disorders. Luminal causes of obstruction may include benign strictures, malignancy, esophageal webs, or a Schatzki ring (**Figure 1**). Upper endoscopy is the most appropriate test for esophageal dysphagia; it allows for both diagnostic intervention (biopsies and inspection) and therapeutic intervention (dilation). Treatment is guided by the underlying pathology causing the dysphagia, as discussed in later sections.

Reflux and Chest Pain

Reflux is the regurgitation of acidic contents from the stomach into the esophagus or back of the throat. Untreated reflux can lead to development of a peptic stricture, causing solid-food dysphagia. Pyrosis, also known as heartburn, is the most common digestive complaint in Western populations. Heartburn often occurs approximately 1 hour after eating and is temporarily relieved with antacids. Factors that can trigger or exacerbate reflux symptoms are listed in **Table 2**.

Patients may have esophageal chest pain symptoms that are identical to those of cardiac chest pain. Esophageal chest

TABLE 1. Causes of Dysphagia

Condition	Diagnostic Clues
Oropharyngeal Dysphagia	
Structural disorders	
Cervical osteophytes	High dysphagia, degenerative joint disease
Cricoid webs	High dysphagia, iron deficiency
Pharyngoesophageal (Zenker) diverticulum	Aspiration, neck mass, and regurgitation of foul-smelling food
Thyromegaly	Neck mass
Neurologic/myogenic disorders	
Amyotrophic lateral sclerosis	Upper and lower motoneuron signs, fasciculations
Central nervous system tumor	Headache, vision changes, nausea, seizures, balance problem
Stroke	Focal neurologic deficits
Muscular dystrophy	Slow progression of muscular weakness over years
Myasthenia gravis	Weakness with repetitive activity
Multiple sclerosis	Optic neuritis
Parkinson disease	Bradykinesia, rigidity, tremor
Dementia	Altered cognition
Sjögren syndrome	Dry mouth, dry eyes
Esophageal Dysphagia	
Structural disorders	
Dysphagia lusoria (vascular dysphagia)	Vascular extrinsic compression on the esophagus on imaging
Epiphrenic/traction diverticulum	Outpouching of the esophagus at any level on imaging
Esophageal strictures	Intermittent dysphagia, especially for solid food; history of reflux
Eosinophilic esophagitis	Food impactions, atopic history, rings or strictures on endoscopy
Esophageal webs or rings	Usually incidental finding, may be associated with iron deficiency anemia
Neoplasms	Rapidly progressive dysphagia for solids, then liquids; anorexia; weight loss
Motility disorders	
Achalasia	Concomitant liquid and solid dysphagia
Diffuse esophageal spasm	Chest pain
Systemic sclerosis	Tight skin, telangiectasias, sclerodactyly, GERD, Raynaud phenomenon

GERD = gastroesophageal reflux disease.

pain may be induced by physical activity, similarly to cardiac chest pain. The most common cause of noncardiac chest pain is untreated gastroesophageal reflux disease (GERD), followed by motility disorders. Cardiac causes must be ruled out before chest pain is attributed to an esophageal cause.

A trial of an acid-reducing agent such as a proton pump inhibitor (PPI) may alleviate symptoms, confirming the diagnosis of GERD. If symptoms are unresponsive to a PPI trial, additional evaluation with upper endoscopy, ambulatory pH testing, and/or esophageal manometry may be warranted. For diagnosis and management of reflux, see Gastroesophageal Reflux Disease. H

KEY POINT

- Cardiac causes must be ruled out before chest pain is attributed to an esophageal cause.

Odynophagia

Odynophagia is defined as pain with swallowing and is an indication of inflammation in the esophagus. Odynophagia is a sign of mucosal injury of the esophagus leading to ulceration. The most common causes of odynophagia are caustic ingestion, pill-induced damage, and infection with *Candida*, herpesvirus, or cytomegalovirus. Rarely, it has been associated with severe GERD or esophageal cancer. Upper endoscopy is the diagnostic test of choice for visual inspection and obtaining tissue biopsies.

Globus Sensation

Globus is the sensation of tightness or a lump in the throat. Globus occurs between swallows and is not related to meals. Stress, psychiatric disorders (anxiety, panic disorders,

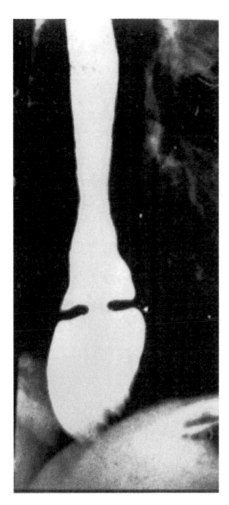

FIGURE 1. Barium esophagography showing a Schatzki ring.

TABLE 2.	Factors Associated with Reflux
Category	**Factor**
Lifestyle	Cigarette smoking
	Obesity
Eating habits	Eating large meals
	Eating late at night
	Lying supine shortly after eating
Foods and beverages	Alcohol
	Chocolate
	Citrus fruits and juices
	Coffee
	Fatty and fried foods
	Onions
	Peppermint
Medications	Anticholinergic agents
	Aspirin and NSAIDs
	Calcium channel blockers
	Nitrates
	Progesterone
	Opioids (due to delayed gastric emptying)
Body position	Bending over, exercising (both result in increased intra-abdominal pressure)
Other	Pregnancy
	Tight-fitting clothing
	Hiatal hernia

somatization), and frequent dry swallowing have been associated with globus. Globus should not be diagnosed in the setting of dysphagia or odynophagia. The management of globus should include ruling out an underlying pharyngeal lesion by nasal endoscopy or barium swallow. If these studies are negative, treatment with acid suppression (PPI) or cognitive behavioral therapy should be considered. Globus has been associated with GERD.

Nonmalignant Disorders of the Esophagus

Esophageal Motility Disorders

The esophagus is the conduit between the hypopharynx and stomach. The tubular esophagus is composed of both skeletal muscle (upper third) and smooth muscle (lower two thirds). Nerve innervations for the striated component are axons of lower motoneurons. The smooth muscle portion of the esophagus is innervated by the vagus nerve. Primary peristalsis begins with swallowing and runs the entire length of the tubular esophagus. The upper and lower esophageal sphincters relax during swallowing (**Figure 2**). Secondary peristaltic activity occurs when the esophagus is distended with air or fluid; peristalsis begins at the point of distention. High-resolution esophageal manometry is a valuable tool in evaluating esophageal physiology.

Hypertonic Motility Disorders
Achalasia and Pseudoachalasia
Achalasia is a motility disorder of the esophagus that results in aperistalsis and inadequate relaxation of the lower esophageal sphincter (LES). The cause of achalasia is unknown, but the pathophysiologic process involves ganglion cell and myenteric plexus degeneration in the esophageal body and LES. This nerve imbalance leads to uncontested action by cholinergic nerves and incomplete LES relaxation. It affects men and women equally, with an annual incidence of 1 in 100,000 individuals. It tends to occur between the ages of 30 and 60 years.

The clinical presentation of achalasia consists of dysphagia to both solids and liquids along with regurgitation of undigested bland food and saliva. Patients may also experience weight loss, chest pain, and even heartburn, resulting in a misdiagnosis of GERD. Symptoms of true achalasia do not respond to an empiric trial of acid reducers such as PPIs.

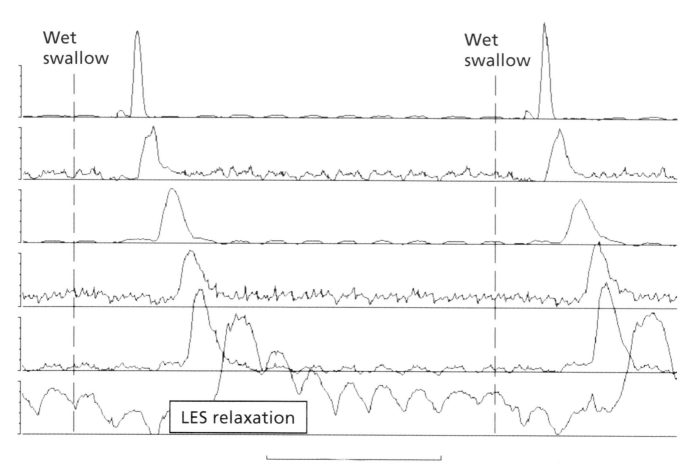

FIGURE 2. Normal esophageal manometric tracing, in which the lower esophageal sphincter (LES) pressure relaxes to baseline during the wet swallow, and peristaltic waves are seen (the scale for the esophageal leads is 100 mm Hg).

The initial test for achalasia is a barium esophagogram, which demonstrates dilation of the esophagus and narrowing at the gastroesophageal junction, described as a "bird's beak" (**Figure 3**). Manometry should be performed to confirm the diagnosis; it is the most sensitive test to demonstrate incomplete LES relaxation and aperistalsis (**Figure 4**). Upper endoscopy shows retained food and saliva, as well as no signs of mechanical obstruction or mass. Upper endoscopy is often performed to exclude mechanical obstruction, particularly if symptoms are concerning for underlying malignancy (shorter duration of symptoms, rapid weight loss).

Other conditions can mimic achalasia; for example, tumors at the gastroesophageal junction may lead to myenteric plexus infiltration, causing esophageal motor abnormalities that are known as pseudoachalasia. Patients with pseudoachalasia often have sudden weight loss and are in their sixth decade of life or older. Secondary achalasia is caused by extrinsic compression after fundoplication or gastric band weight loss surgery.

Achalasia is a chronic disease, and treatment is directed at lowering LES pressure and alleviating symptoms. Endoscopic

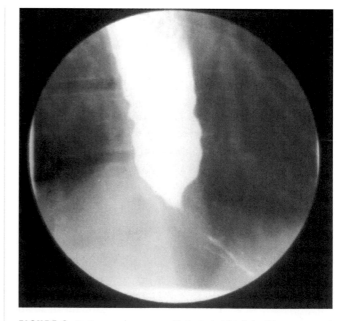

FIGURE 3. Barium esophagogram with the typical "bird's beak" appearance of the distal esophagus in a patient with achalasia.

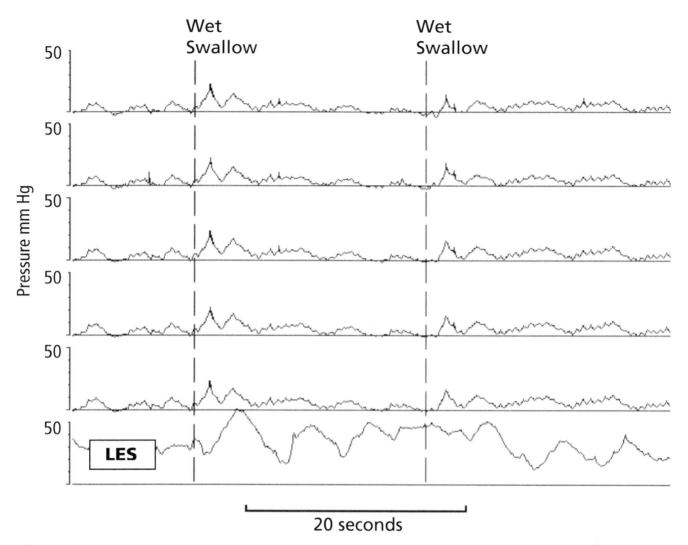

FIGURE 4. Esophageal manometric tracing in a patient with achalasia, in which the elevated lower esophageal sphincter (LES) pressure does not relax during the wet swallow. In addition, there is no esophageal body peristalsis (the waves seen are superimposable). The vertical scale is set in increments of 10 mm Hg (to a maximum of 50 mm Hg).

pneumatic dilation is an effective nonsurgical treatment for achalasia; the main complication is perforation, which occurs in 1.9% of patients. Laparoscopic surgical myotomy leading to disruption of circular muscle fibers is the surgical treatment of choice. Fundoplication is recommended after myotomy to prevent reflux, but PPI therapy may still be needed if heartburn symptoms are present. The choice between pneumatic dilation and surgical myotomy depends on local expertise, as both have comparable success rates. However, pneumatic dilation has been shown to be more cost-effective compared with surgical myotomy. If surgery and pneumatic dilation are not acceptable owing to surgical risk or patient preference, endoscopic injection of botulinum toxin may help relieve symptoms. Endoscopic injection of botulinum toxin inhibits acetylcholine release, resulting in LES relaxation. This treatment has a 50% relapse rate, requiring retreatment in about 6 months. Pharmacologic therapy is third-line therapy reserved for patients who are not candidates for endoscopic

intervention or surgery. These therapies include calcium channel blockers (nifedipine) or long-acting nitrates, which cause an inconsistent reduction in LES pressure.

There is an associated risk of squamous cell esophageal cancer in patients who have had achalasia for more than 10 years. Given the very low incidence of malignancy, endoscopic surveillance has not been widely recommended in these patients.

KEY POINTS

- The clinical presentation of achalasia consists of dysphagia to both solids and liquids along with regurgitation of undigested bland food and saliva; weight loss, chest pain, and heartburn may be present.

- The initial test for achalasia is a barium esophagogram, which demonstrates dilation of the esophagus and narrowing at the gastroesophageal junction, described as a "bird's beak."

(Continued)

- Endoscopic pneumatic dilation and laparoscopic surgical myotomy are the primary treatments for achalasia; the choice of therapy depends on local expertise, as both have comparable success rates.

Diffuse Esophageal Spasm and Nutcracker Esophagus
Hypertonic motility disorders of the esophagus often present with dysphagia and/or chest pain. These disorders are differentiated based on manometry findings.

Diffuse esophageal spasm is a rare motility disorder that presents with chest pain or dysphagia. Clinical manifestations are similar to those of angina pectoris. Although the cause of diffuse esophageal spasm is unknown, it may be associated with reflux. On esophageal manometry, simultaneous high-amplitude (>30 mm Hg) esophageal contractions are seen with intermittent aperistaltic contractions. The barium esophagogram finding of a "corkscrew" esophagus (**Figure 5**) is typical of diffuse esophageal spasm. It may progress to achalasia in some patients.

Nutcracker esophagus is characterized by high-amplitude peristaltic contractions of greater than 220 mm Hg.

Management of hypertonic disorders of the esophagus is aimed at symptom relief. The ideal therapy is not clear, but pharmacologic therapy has included calcium channel blockers, hydralazine, botulinum toxin injections, and anxiolytics.

Hypotonic Motility Disorders

Hypotensive disorders of the esophagus can involve a hypotense LES, aperistaltic contractions, or both. A weakened LES can lead to GERD, and poor peristaltic activity can result in dysphagia. In most cases, the cause of the hypotensive esophageal disorder is unknown. However, secondary causes include smooth-muscle relaxants, anticholinergic agents, estrogen, progesterone, connective tissue disorders (such as systemic sclerosis), and pregnancy. Manometry demonstrates hypotensive or nonperistaltic contractions in the distal esophagus. Management consists of therapy for GERD to prevent complications such as erosive esophagitis and stricture formation.

Infectious, Pill-Induced, and Eosinophilic Esophagitis

Infectious Esophagitis

Infectious esophagitis can be caused by bacterial (uncommon), fungal, viral, and parasitic pathogens. Patients may be asymptomatic, but common symptoms are odynophagia or dysphagia. *Candida* infection can occur in both immunocompetent and immunocompromised patients. Upper endoscopy reveals small, white, raised plaques (**Figure 6**), and esophageal brushings confirm the diagnosis. The most common species is *Candida albicans*, which is treated with oral fluconazole. Cytomegalovirus (CMV) is seen in immunocompromised patients and rarely occurs in patients with an intact immune system. Although herpes simplex virus (HSV) can be seen in both immunocompetent and immunocompromised patients, it is much more likely to be found in an immunocompromised individual. Upper endoscopy is needed to confirm the diagnosis, and biopsies of the ulcer base (to detect CMV) and ulcer edge (to detect HSV) should be performed. HSV is treated with acyclovir, and CMV responds to ganciclovir and valganciclovir. **H**

- The most common cause of infectious esophagitis is *Candida albicans*, which is treated with oral fluconazole.

Pill-Induced Esophagitis

Many medications have been associated with esophageal mucosal injury. Risk factors associated with pill-induced

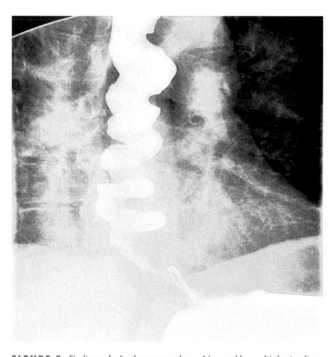

FIGURE 5. Findings of a "corkscrew esophagus" (caused by multiple simultaneous contractions) on esophagogram are typical of diffuse esophageal spasm.

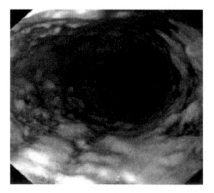

FIGURE 6. Upper endoscopy showing white adherent plaques suggestive of *Candida* esophagitis.

esophagitis include decreased salivary output, esophageal dysmotility, ingestion of large pills, medications that alter LES tone (such as opioid analgesics), and ingestion of medications in the supine position. Pill-induced esophagitis is characterized by chest pain, dysphagia, and odynophagia. Symptoms occur several hours to days after taking the medication. Pill-induced esophagitis has been observed with alendronate, quinidine, tetracycline, doxycycline, potassium chloride, ferrous sulfate, and mexiletine. Medications associated with stricture formation include alendronate, ferrous sulfate, NSAIDs, and potassium chloride. Preventive strategies to decrease pill-induced esophagitis are to drink plenty of water with the medication and avoid lying down for 30 minutes after ingestion.

KEY POINT

- Preventive strategies to decrease pill-induced esophagitis are to drink plenty of water with the medication and avoid lying down for 30 minutes after ingestion.

Eosinophilic Esophagitis

Eosinophilic esophagitis (EoE) is defined as esophageal squamous mucosal inflammation caused by eosinophilic infiltration. The classic presentation of EoE is an atopic man in the third decade of life with solid-food dysphagia and food impactions requiring removal by endoscopy. EoE has been associated with food allergies, asthma, and eczema. Children may have a nonspecific presentation characterized by feeding issues, vomiting, and pain. The reported prevalence is as high as 54 per 100,000 persons in the United States. Upper endoscopy findings include rings, longitudinal furrows, luminal narrowing, and white exudates and plaques (**Figure 7**). Esophageal biopsies show greater than 15 eosinophils per high-power field. GERD has been associated with esophageal eosinophilia and can mimic EoE.

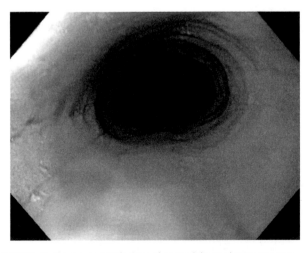

FIGURE 7. The macroscopic findings of eosinophilic esophagitis on upper endoscopy are nonspecific, but mucosal furrowing (appearing as stacked esophageal rings), white specks, and mucosal friability have been consistently described.

Patients with esophageal eosinophilia should undergo an 8-week trial of a PPI; clinical response to the PPI trial indicates GERD-associated eosinophilia rather than EoE. Repeat upper endoscopy with biopsies should be considered; if esophageal eosinophilia is still present, this confirms a diagnosis of EoE. Treatment endpoints include resolution of clinical symptoms and reduction of eosinophil infiltration in esophageal mucosa. Dietary treatments (elemental diet or targeted elimination diet) can be tried in adults and children. Medical therapy for EoE consists of swallowed aerosolized topical glucocorticoids (fluticasone or budesonide); if symptoms are not responsive, oral prednisone should be used. Esophageal dilation should be considered in patients with a persistent esophageal stricture despite medical therapy. Patients should be advised that EoE is a chronic disease that often recurs after treatment is stopped; therefore, repeat or maintenance therapy may be needed.

KEY POINT

- The classic presentation of eosinophilic esophagitis is an atopic man in the third decade of life with symptoms of solid-food dysphagia and food impactions requiring removal by endoscopy.

Gastroesophageal Reflux Disease

GERD is a common clinical problem that occurs when acid and food from the stomach reflux into the esophagus and throat. GERD-related symptoms occur in 10% to 20% of individuals in the Western world, but prevalence is lower in Asia. In the United States, about 40% of adults have monthly and 20% have weekly GERD symptoms. GERD affects patients' quality of life, causing poor sleep, low productivity, and missed days at work. Symptoms include heartburn, regurgitation, and chest pain. GERD-related chest pain must be differentiated from cardiac chest pain before treatment can begin. Dysphagia can occur with GERD, but additional evaluation is required to rule out an underlying ring, web, malignancy, or motility disorder. Nonacid reflux may occur in patients who are already on maximal acid suppression or in those with achlorhydria; patients note symptoms of regurgitation of liquids similar to those with acid-related reflux.

The major physiologic mechanisms to protect against esophageal acid injury include clearing mechanisms (peristalsis), a competent LES, and intact gastric emptying. A breakdown in these protective mechanisms can lead to symptomatic GERD.

GERD is common in pregnancy and can happen during any trimester, but severity can increase throughout the pregnancy. GERD related to pregnancy is a clinical diagnosis and testing is not required; heartburn symptoms typically resolve after delivery. There is a strong relationship between GERD and obesity. Complications of GERD include erosive esophagitis, stricture, Barrett esophagus, and esophageal cancer.

Diagnosis

The diagnosis of GERD can be established by clinical history, response to medical therapy, and testing. Symptoms of heartburn and regurgitation are strong predictors for the clinical diagnosis of GERD. In a patient without alarm features (dysphagia, unintentional weight loss, hematemesis, or melena), symptom relief with an empiric trial of a PPI confirms the diagnosis of GERD.

Upper endoscopy is the primary tool to evaluate the esophagus and identify damage in the form of erosive esophagitis, stricture, or Barrett esophagus. Upper endoscopy should be performed in patients whose symptoms are not responsive to an empiric PPI trial, and it should be the first step in evaluation of patients with alarm symptoms. Most patients with symptoms of heartburn and regurgitation have normal upper endoscopy findings.

Ambulatory pH testing or impedance-pH testing is valuable to identify acid exposure within the esophagus. Impedance-pH testing can identify both acid and nonacid reflux. Testing can be done with a 48-hour wireless capsule or 24-hour transnasal catheter to detect active acid reflux. The wireless capsule has been shown to have better patient tolerability.

Esophageal manometry has limited value as a tool to identify GERD; however, manometry should be done before antireflux surgery to rule out a motility disorder such as achalasia or a hypomotility disorder (systemic sclerosis).

Barium radiographs for the diagnosis of GERD have low sensitivity and should not be performed.

HVC

Treatment

An algorithm describing the management of GERD is shown in **Figure 8**.

Lifestyle Changes

Diet and lifestyle changes are often recommended as part of GERD therapy. Weight reduction is suggested for patients with recent weight gain or for those who are overweight. Interventions such as raising the head of the bed and eliminating meals within 2 to 3 hours of bedtime are helpful for nocturnal GERD. Global elimination of proposed trigger foods (caffeine, chocolate, spicy foods, acidic foods such as oranges, and fatty foods) is not recommended; however, targeted elimination of foods associated with symptoms is a reasonable approach. Cessation of alcohol and tobacco use is universally supported.

Medical Therapy

Pharmacologic therapy for GERD consists of antacids, H₂ blockers, or PPI therapy. PPI therapy once daily for 8 weeks is the therapy of choice for symptom relief. PPI therapy is superior to

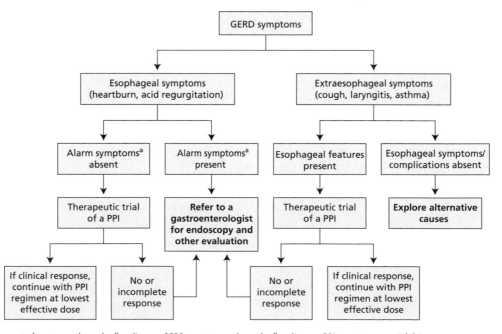

FIGURE 8. Management of gastroesophageal reflux disease. GERD = gastroesophageal reflux disease; PPI = proton pump inhibitor.

ᵃAlarm symptoms = dysphagia, unintentional weight loss, hematemesis, or melena.

H_2 blockers for treatment of GERD. It has been shown to offer faster healing rates for erosive esophagitis and decreased relapse compared with other agents, and it also has been shown to offer faster and more complete relief of symptoms. A PPI should be taken once daily 30 to 60 minutes before the first meal of the day. Patients with a partial response to PPI therapy should have their dose increased to twice daily. Patients who require long-term maintenance therapy should receive the lowest effective PPI dose, including on-demand or intermittent usage.

Common adverse reactions to PPIs are headache and diarrhea; dyspepsia may occur with sudden discontinuation of PPI therapy. Switching to a different PPI may be helpful if the patient has an adverse reaction or if there is no clinical response; however, outcomes may remain the same with a different PPI. Other possible adverse reactions include vitamin (B_{12}) and mineral (calcium and magnesium) malabsorption as well as increased risk of community-acquired pneumonia, *Clostridium difficile* infection, hip fractures, osteoporosis, and cardiovascular events. Hip fracture risk may not be increased unless other risk factors are present. Short-term PPI use has been linked to community-acquired pneumonia, but long-term use has not been similarly associated. Despite earlier concerns that concurrent PPI therapy decreased the activation of clopidogrel, two randomized clinical studies have since failed to show an increased risk of adverse outcomes in patients treated with clopidogrel and PPIs. PPIs are safe in pregnant patients.

Sucralfate has no role in the treatment of GERD. Prokinetic agents (metoclopramide) should not be used in the treatment of GERD unless gastroparesis is present.

Antireflux Surgery
Surgical treatments for GERD consist of laparoscopic fundoplication or bariatric surgery (the latter for obese patients). Indications for surgery include patient preference to stop taking medication, medication side effects, large hiatal hernia, and refractory symptoms despite maximal medical therapy (although patients with medically refractory symptoms may be less likely to benefit from surgery). Patients should undergo objective testing (such as pH-impedance monitoring to demonstrate true reflux with symptom correlation and manometry to rule out a motility disorder) prior to surgery. Surgery is most effective in patients with typical symptoms of heartburn and regurgitation that are responsive to therapy. However, approximately one third of patients will require resumption of PPI therapy 5 to 10 years after surgery. Postoperative complications include dysphagia, diarrhea, and inability to belch because of a tight fundoplication. Carbonated beverages should be avoided.

Endoscopic Therapy
Endoscopic therapies for GERD have not been shown to be effective in the long term. Therapies have included thermal radiofrequency to augment the LES, silicone injection to the LES, and suturing of the LES. Early improvement of reflux

symptoms has been seen, but long-term benefits have not been shown. Normalized esophageal pH levels have not been demonstrated after endoscopic therapies. Transoral incisionless fundoplication is a newer therapy that uses a full-thickness suture to create an endoscopic fundoplication; however, there are no long-term data that demonstrate efficacy.

KEY POINTS

- Proton pump inhibitor therapy is superior to H_2 blockers for treatment of gastroesophageal reflux disease.
- In patients with gastroesophageal reflux disease, indications for antireflux surgery include patient preference to stop taking medication, medication side effects, large hiatal hernia, and refractory symptoms despite maximal medical therapy.
- Endoscopic therapies for gastroesophageal reflux disease have not been shown to be effective in the long term.   **HVC**

Extraesophageal Manifestations
GERD has been associated with asthma, chronic cough, and laryngitis (**Figure 9**). It is important to eliminate other non-GERD causes when these symptoms are present. Laryngoscopy often demonstrates edema and erythema as signs of reflux-induced laryngitis; however, over 80% of healthy persons also have these findings. Laryngoscopy should not be used to diagnose GERD-related laryngitis. A PPI trial is recommended in patients who have typical GERD symptoms and extraesophageal symptoms.

Refractory Gastroesophageal Reflux Disease
The first step in treating refractory GERD is to optimize PPI therapy by verifying correct administration (30-60 minutes before meals), increasing to twice-daily dosing, or switching to another PPI. If symptoms remain unresponsive, alternative causes should be considered. In patients with typical symptoms, upper endoscopy should be performed to rule out eosinophilic esophagitis or erosive esophagitis. If the endoscopy does not reveal eosinophilic esophagitis or reflux-related changes, pH-impedance testing should be performed. A negative pH-impedance test likely indicates that PPI therapy should be discontinued and that the patient does not have GERD. For those with prominent extraesophageal manifestations, referral to an otolaryngologist, pulmonologist, or allergist should be considered.

Metaplastic and Neoplastic Disorders of the Esophagus

Barrett Esophagus

Epidemiology and Screening
Barrett esophagus (BE) is present when columnar epithelium replaces the normal squamous epithelium in the distal esophagus. Risk factors associated with BE are older age, male

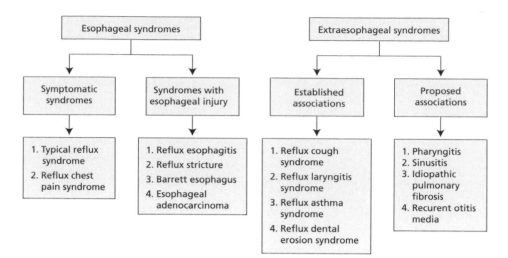

FIGURE 9. Classification of gastroesophageal reflux disease and its subsets.

Reprinted by permission from Macmillan Publishers Ltd: American Journal of Gastroenterology (Vakil N, van Zanten SV, Kahrilas P, Dent J, Jones R; Global Consensus Group. The Montreal definition and classification of gastroesophageal reflux disease: a global evidence-based consensus. 101(8):1900-20. [PMID: 16928254]), copyright 2006.

gender, white ethnicity, GERD, hiatal hernia, high BMI, smoking, and an abdominal distribution of fat. Protective factors are moderate wine consumption and a diet rich in fruits and vegetables. BE is a consequence of GERD whether or not patients experience clinical symptoms.

BE is classified as a premalignant condition that could progress to esophageal cancer. The annual incidence of progression to high-grade dysplasia and adenocarcinoma is variable. The cancer risk associated with BE is believed to be 0.5% per year, but a recent study from Denmark reports an estimate of 0.12% per year. Approximately 10% of patients with GERD are found to have BE on upper endoscopy, although 40% of patients diagnosed with adenocarcinoma of the esophagus report no symptoms of GERD. Current evidence does not support routine screening for BE based on GERD symptoms. However, the American College of Physicians suggests that screening for BE may be appropriate in men older than 50 years with chronic GERD (symptoms for more than 5 years) and additional risk factors, including nocturnal reflux symptoms, hiatal hernia, elevated BMI, tobacco use, and intra-abdominal fat distribution. If screening is performed and is negative for BE, no additional endoscopic screening is indicated, even for patients continuing treatment for GERD, unless other symptoms or clinical findings develop.

KEY POINTS

- Barrett esophagus is classified as a premalignant condition that could progress to esophageal cancer.

HVC

- Current evidence does not support routine screening for Barrett esophagus based on gastroesophageal reflux disease symptoms.

Diagnosis and Management

The diagnosis of BE is based on the endoscopic finding of columnar epithelium above the normally located gastroesophageal junction (**Figure 10**), followed by histologic confirmation

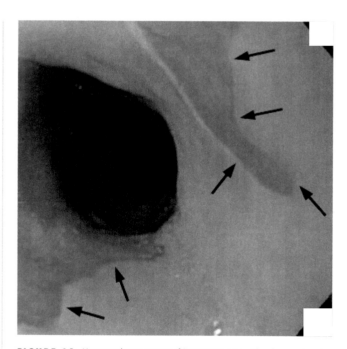

FIGURE 10. Upper endoscopic view of Barrett mucosa, with salmon-colored mucosa (*arrows*) representing Barrett mucosa compared with the normal pearl-colored squamous mucosa.

demonstrating specialized intestinal metaplasia with acid-mucin–containing goblet cells. Upper endoscopy measurements have categorized BE into short segment (less than 3 cm) or long segment (greater than 3 cm) (**Figure 11**). The pathway of progression of BE is from intestinal metaplasia to low-grade dysplasia to high-grade dysplasia to invasive adenocarcinoma.

Recommended surveillance intervals are based on the grade of BE and the presence of dysplasia (**Table 3**); however, the potential risks and benefits of surveillance should be weighed in patients with significant comorbidities or limited life expectancy. Although most patients with BE are treated

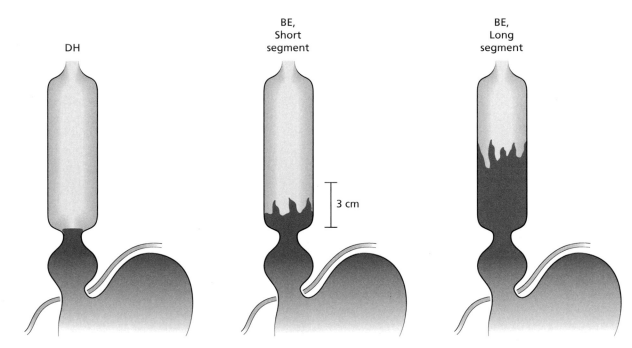

DH

BE, Short segment

BE, Long segment

3 cm

FIGURE 11. Diagram of the esophageal and gastric junction showing replacement of normal esophageal squamous epithelium by specialized intestinal epithelium (shown in red) in Barrett esophagus. BE = Barrett esophagus; DH = diaphragmatic (hiatal) hernia.

Courtesy of Dr. Alan Cameron.

TABLE 3. Practice Guidelines for Endoscopic Surveillance of Barrett Esophagus	
Dysplasia Grade	**Recommendation**
None	If no dysplasia is present, repeat upper endoscopy every 3 to 5 years
Low-grade	Confirmation by expert pathologist
	Repeat upper endoscopy 6 to 12 months after diagnosis to detect prevalent dysplasia
High-grade	Confirmation by expert pathologist
	Endoscopic evaluation for any focal lesion (may indicate more advanced neoplasia); if present, focal lesion(s) should be removed by endoscopic mucosal resection for diagnosis and staging
	Options for further management: esophagectomy, endoscopic ablation, surveillance every 3 months

Data from: American Gastroenterological Association, Spechler SJ, Sharma P, Souza RF, Inadomi JM, Shaheen NJ. American Gastroenterological Association medical position statement on the management of Barrett's esophagus. Gastroenterology. 2011 Mar;140(3):1084-91. [PMID: 21376940]

with PPI therapy for GERD symptom control or to heal erosive esophagitis (if present), the use of acid suppression primarily to prevent progression of BE to dysplasia or adenocarcinoma has not been established. Therefore, long-term PPI use in patients with BE should be individualized. There are some data from case-control studies suggesting that aspirin and other NSAIDs may reduce the risk for esophageal adenocarcinoma in patients

with BE, but guidelines do not recommend treatment as chemoprevention. Additionally, there is no strong evidence that antireflux surgery can prevent the progression of BE to adenocarcinoma. Treatment to remove BE is recommended for patients with confirmed high-grade dysplasia and can be done with endoscopic therapies that include radiofrequency ablation, photodynamic therapy, or endoscopic mucosal resection. Endoscopic therapies have had similar outcomes to surgery (esophagectomy), but local expertise and patient preference should determine the best course of therapy.

KEY POINTS

- Chemoprevention with a proton pump inhibitor, aspirin or NSAID therapy, or antireflux surgery has not been definitively shown to decrease the risk of progression of dysplasia or development of adenocarcinoma in patients with Barrett esophagus.
- Treatment to remove Barrett esophagus is recommended for patients with confirmed high-grade dysplasia and can be done with endoscopic therapies that include radiofrequency ablation, photodynamic therapy, or endoscopic mucosal resection.

Esophageal Carcinoma
Epidemiology
Esophageal cancer is the sixth leading cause of cancer-related mortality worldwide. The most common types are squamous cell carcinoma (SCC) and adenocarcinoma; the latter is more common in the United States. Esophageal cancer has a male

CONT.

predominance and often occurs in the fifth to sixth decades of life. SCC is more common in black men. In the United States, about 16,000 new cases of esophageal cancer are reported annually, with 14,000 deaths occurring within the same year. The overall 5-year survival rate is between 15% and 25% depending on the stage at time of initial diagnosis. **H**

KEY POINT

- The overall 5-year survival rate of patients with esophageal carcinoma is between 15% and 25% depending on the stage at time of initial diagnosis.

Risk Factors

The risk factors associated with SCC are tobacco and alcohol use, caustic injury, achalasia, past thoracic radiation, nutritional deficiencies (zinc, selenium), poor socioeconomic status, poor oral hygiene, nonepidermolytic palmoplantar keratoderma (tylosis), human papillomavirus infection, and nitrosamine exposure. Adenocarcinoma risk factors include GERD, BE, obesity, tobacco use, past thoracic radiation, diet low in fruits and vegetables, increased age, male sex, and possibly medications that relax the LES.

Diagnosis and Staging

The most common clinical manifestation of esophageal cancer is solid-food dysphagia; however, esophageal cancer has been diagnosed in asymptomatic individuals during surveillance upper endoscopy. Other symptoms include weight loss, anorexia, and anemia (secondary to gastrointestinal bleeding). Upper endoscopy with biopsy is the preferred initial diagnostic test. SCC is located in the proximal esophagus, whereas adenocarcinoma is usually found in the distal esophagus.

TNM staging is often done with CT scan (to evaluate for metastatic disease), endoscopic ultrasound (to assess locoregional disease), and PET imaging (to follow up on indeterminate lesions). For treatment of esophageal carcinoma, see MKSAP 17 Hematology and Oncology. **H**

KEY POINTS

- The most common clinical manifestation of esophageal cancer is solid-food dysphagia.
- Upper endoscopy with biopsy is the preferred initial diagnostic test for esophageal carcinoma.

Disorders of the Stomach and Duodenum

Peptic Ulcer Disease

Clinical Features, Diagnosis, and Complications

Peptic ulcer disease (PUD) can present as an uncomplicated gastric and/or duodenal ulcer or as a complicated ulcer. Although the widespread use of potent acid suppressants and the dramatic reduction in *Helicobacter pylori* prevalence have

lowered the overall incidence of PUD, the incidence of complicated PUD remains largely unchanged. This phenomenon is largely due to the increased use of aspirin and NSAIDs (see Gastrointestinal Complications of NSAIDs, Aspirin, and Anticoagulants), as well as to the aging population.

The cardinal symptom in uncomplicated PUD is epigastric pain or discomfort. Accompanying symptoms may include nocturnal pain, relief of pain with eating, early satiety, nausea, bloating, or abdominal fullness.

Peptic ulcers are diagnosed not by symptoms but instead by the presence of a mucosal break 5 mm or larger in the stomach or duodenum. Upper endoscopy is considered the gold standard in the diagnosis of PUD.

Complicated PUD can present in a variety of ways depending on the specific complication that has developed. The four major complications of PUD are bleeding, perforation, penetration, and obstruction. The most common presentation of complicated PUD is acute or chronic upper gastrointestinal bleeding (see Gastrointestinal Bleeding). Symptoms of acute gastrointestinal bleeding can include epigastric pain, hematemesis, melena, and/or orthostatic symptoms. Chronic PUD bleeding commonly presents as an iron deficiency anemia. Perforation is likely to present with severe, sudden abdominal pain with peritoneal signs on abdominal examination (tenderness, guarding, rigidity), or possibly with septic shock. Penetration occurs when an ulcer crater erodes through and into adjacent organs including the small bowel, pancreas, liver, and/or biliary tree. It typically presents with a gradual increase in the severity and frequency of abdominal pain, with pancreatitis as a common presentation. Obstruction can be acute or insidious in onset, with symptoms of nausea, vomiting, anorexia, and weight loss accompanying abdominal pain. PUD in the elderly may present atypically, with complications in the absence of abdominal pain. **H**

When uncomplicated PUD is suspected, definitive diagnosis is made by upper endoscopy (or upper gastrointestinal barium radiography when endoscopy is contraindicated or unavailable). The differential diagnosis for the symptoms of uncomplicated PUD is broad; for further discussion, see Dyspepsia. For patients with complicated PUD or other alarm features (age >55 years with unexplained new-onset epigastric pain, or patients with abdominal pain and unexplained weight loss, gastrointestinal bleeding, microcytic anemia, or recurrent vomiting), a prompt structural evaluation with upper endoscopy, abdominal cross-sectional imaging, or upper gastrointestinal imaging using water-soluble contrast is essential, depending on the complication suspected.

KEY POINTS

- Peptic ulcers are diagnosed not by symptoms but instead by the presence of a mucosal break 5 mm or larger in the stomach or duodenum.
- Upper endoscopy is the gold standard for diagnosis of peptic ulcer disease.

(Continued)

- The four major complications of peptic ulcer disease are bleeding, perforation, penetration, and obstruction.

Management

The primary goals of uncomplicated PUD management are to identify the cause and correct modifiable risk factors for ulcer complications and ulcer recurrence (**Table 4**). There are no guideline recommendations that support follow-up endoscopy in all patients with gastric ulcers given the decreasing incidence of gastric cancer in the United States. If a gastric ulcer is found in a patient who is at low risk for gastric cancer (for example, a young patient on NSAIDs), follow-up endoscopy to assess healing may not be required. However, when a gastric ulcer has an endoscopic appearance that is concerning for malignancy despite initial biopsies being negative, then endoscopy should be repeated after 8 to 12 weeks of antisecretory therapy to assess for healing. Additional biopsies should be obtained if healing has not occurred. Duodenal ulcers do not typically require endoscopic follow-up. An assessment for *H. pylori* infection should be performed in all patients with PUD (see *Helicobacter pylori* Infection).

- The primary goals of uncomplicated peptic ulcer disease management are to identify the cause and correct modifiable risk factors for ulcer complications and ulcer recurrence.

(Continued)

- Duodenal ulcers and low-risk gastric ulcers (for example, a young patient on NSAIDs) do not typically require endoscopic follow-up.

Dyspepsia
Clinical Features

Dyspepsia encompasses a heterogeneous symptom complex that may include epigastric pain or burning, abdominal fullness, nausea, vomiting, bloating, belching, and/or weight loss. After identifiable causes (**Table 5**) have been evaluated and excluded, the term functional dyspepsia (FD) can be used. Approximately two thirds of dyspepsia cases are attributed to FD. Although the cause of FD remains unknown, proposed pathophysiologic mechanisms include abnormal upper gastrointestinal motor and reflex functions, visceral hypersensitivity, altered brain-gut interactions, disrupted gut-immune interactions, psychological factors, and genetic factors. Lacking a definable biomarker, FD is defined by fulfillment of diagnostic criteria developed by the Rome III consensus group, an international panel of experts in the field of functional bowel disorders. FD diagnostic criteria consist of one or more of the following: (1) bothersome postprandial fullness, (2) early satiety, (3) epigastric pain, and/or (4) epigastric burning. These criteria should be met for the past 3 months, with symptom onset at least 6 months prior to diagnosis and with no evidence of structural disease to explain the symptoms.

TABLE 4. Risk Factors for and Interventions to Prevent Peptic Ulcer Disease Recurrence and Complications

Risk Factor	Intervention to Prevent PUD Recurrence
Advanced age (>65 years)	Indefinite use of antisecretory therapy[a]
Aspirin use (high or low dose)	Co-therapy with antisecretory therapy if chronic aspirin use is indicated
Helicobacter pylori infection	Treat and confirm eradication
	If other risk factors for PUD recurrence are present, continue antisecretory therapy indefinitely
NSAID use	Co-therapy with antisecretory therapy if no alternative therapy is available
Tobacco use	Smoking cessation
	Indefinite use of antisecretory therapy
Alcohol use	Reduce or eliminate alcohol use
	Indefinite use of antisecretory therapy
Comorbidities (COPD; chronic kidney disease; coronary artery disease; diabetes mellitus; obesity; chronic anticoagulation, immunosuppression, or glucocorticoid use)	Indefinite use of antisecretory therapy
	Optimization of chronic disease
Other nonmodifiable risk factors (male gender, black ethnicity, complicated PUD)	Indefinite use of antisecretory therapy

PUD = peptic ulcer disease.

[a]Antisecretory therapy: proton pump inhibitor, H_2 blocker.

TABLE 5.	Identifiable Causes of Dyspepsia
Erosive gastroesophageal reflux disease	
Nonerosive gastroesophageal reflux disease	
Esophageal malignancy	
Peptic ulcer disease	
Helicobacter pylori infection	
Gastric malignancy	
Gastroparesis	
Celiac disease	
Carbohydrate maldigestion (lactose, fructose, small intestinal bacterial overgrowth)	
Biliary tract disease	
Pancreatitis or pancreatic malignancy	
Infiltrative and inflammatory diseases involving the upper gastrointestinal tract	
Ischemic bowel disease	
Abdominal wall pain (muscle strain, nerve entrapment, myositis)	
Medications (most commonly aspirin and NSAIDs)	
Alcohol	
Systemic and metabolic disorders (diabetes mellitus, thyroid dysfunction, ischemic heart disease)	
Pregnancy	

KEY POINT

- Diagnostic criteria for functional dyspepsia consist of one or more of the following: (1) bothersome postprandial fullness, (2) early satiety, (3) epigastric pain, and/or (4) epigastric burning; these criteria should be met for the past 3 months, with symptom onset at least 6 months prior to diagnosis and with no evidence of structural disease to explain the symptoms.

Management

Management of dyspepsia is described in **Figure 12**. For patients younger than 50 to 55 years who present with dyspepsia without alarm features (melena, rectal bleeding, unintentional weight loss, anorexia, early satiety, persistent or recurrent vomiting, dysphagia, odynophagia, family history of upper gastrointestinal malignancy, personal history of PUD or malignancy, prior gastric surgery, abdominal mass, or anemia), testing and treating for *H. pylori* infection or a trial of proton pump inhibitor (PPI) therapy should be pursued before any further testing is done. Further structural testing should be performed in patients older than 50 to 55 years, those with alarm features at any age, or those with persistent dyspeptic symptoms despite eradication of *H. pylori* and/or a trial of PPI therapy. Upper endoscopy is considered the gold standard for the exclusion of upper gastrointestinal structural causes of dyspepsia. No other biochemical, structural, or physiologic studies should be performed routinely for evaluation of dyspepsia. Such additional testing may be considered on a case-by-case basis given the patient's age, presence of alarm features, accompanying symptoms, comorbid illnesses, and results of prior testing.

The treatment of FD is largely empiric and consists of dietary and lifestyle modification, over-the-counter and prescription medications, psychological treatments, and complementary and alternative medicine therapies. Dietary and lifestyle strategies may include a food diary to identify behaviors or specific foods that trigger symptoms. Other suggestions include the ingestion of low-fat, smaller, more frequent meals and the avoidance of late-evening meals. Both PPIs and H₂ blockers have demonstrated efficacy in a select subgroup of patients with FD, typically those with a predominant symptom of epigastric pain. There does not appear to be a dose effect with either agent alone. There is no clear synergistic effect when both agents are used concomitantly. Antidepressants, such as tricyclics and selective serotonin reuptake inhibitors, should be reserved for more severe or refractory FD. Psychological therapies such as psychodrama, cognitive-behavioral therapy, relaxation therapy, guided imagery, and hypnotherapy may be beneficial in patients with symptoms related to anxiety or stress, a history of abuse, or comorbid psychological conditions. The best-studied herbal remedies in FD include STW 5 (a liquid formulation of nine herbal extracts), peppermint, and caraway, and limited data exist on artichoke leaf extract and capsaicin. Referral to a gastroenterologist should be considered for patients whose symptoms do not respond to a test-and-treat approach for *H. pylori*, a trial of antisecretory therapy, and dietary modifications.

KEY POINTS

- For patients younger than age 50 to 55 years who present with dyspepsia without alarm features, testing and treating for *Helicobacter pylori* infection or a trial of proton pump inhibitor therapy should be pursued before any further testing is done. **HVC**

- The treatment of functional dyspepsia is largely empiric and consists of dietary and lifestyle modification, over-the-counter and prescription medications, psychological treatments, and complementary and alternative medicine therapies.

Helicobacter pylori Infection
Indications for *Helicobacter pylori* Testing

Despite the decreasing prevalence of *H. pylori* infection in developed countries such as the United States, it remains linked to a number of important clinical conditions and is deemed a human carcinogen by the World Health

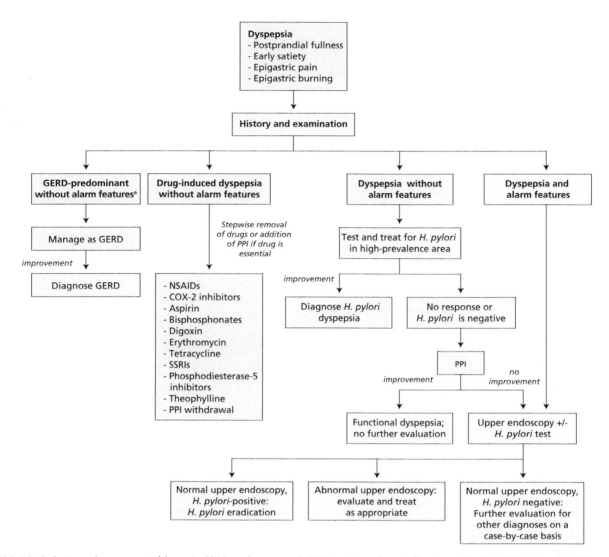

FIGURE 12. Evaluation and management of dyspepsia. COX-2 = cyclooxygenase-2; GERD = gastroesophageal reflux disease; *H. pylori* = *Helicobacter pylori*; PPI = proton pump inhibitor; SSRI = selective serotonin reuptake inhibitor.

[a]Alarm features = melena, rectal bleeding, unintentional weight loss, anorexia, early satiety, persistent or recurrent vomiting, dysphagia, odynophagia, family history of upper gastrointestinal malignancy, personal history of peptic ulcer disease or malignancy, prior gastric surgery, abdominal mass, or anemia.

Organization. Clearly established indications for *H. pylori* testing are active PUD (gastric and/or duodenal ulcer), a confirmed history of PUD, gastric mucosa–associated lymphoid tissue (MALT) lymphoma, uninvestigated dyspepsia, and following endoscopic resection of early gastric cancer. Less-established indications for *H. pylori* testing include unexplained iron deficiency anemia and primary immune thrombocytopenia (previously termed idiopathic thrombocytopenic purpura). Controversial indications for *H. pylori* testing include chronic NSAID and/or aspirin use and a first-degree family member with gastric cancer. Gastroesophageal reflux disease is not a clinical indication for *H. pylori* testing; however, the coexistence of gastroesophageal reflux disease with one of the above-stated indications should not preclude testing for *H. pylori*.

KEY POINTS

- Clearly established indications for *Helicobacter pylori* testing are active peptic ulcer disease (gastric and/or duodenal ulcer), a confirmed history of peptic ulcer disease, gastric mucosa–associated lymphoid tissue lymphoma, uninvestigated dyspepsia, and following endoscopic resection of early gastric cancer.

- Gastroesophageal reflux disease is not a clinical indication for *Helicobacter pylori* testing.

HVC

Diagnosis

Noninvasive tests that identify active infection include the urea breath test and fecal antigen test. To improve the diagnostic accuracy of the urea breath test and fecal antigen test, antimicrobial agents and bismuth should be avoided for 28 days prior to testing. PPIs should be avoided for 7 to 14 days prior to testing, and H_2 blockers should be avoided for 1 to 2 days prior to testing.

Serum testing for IgG antibodies to *H. pylori* does not identify active infection in populations with low prevalence of disease; however, it remains popular given its ease of administration, rapidity of results, and low cost. Given its marginal sensitivity (85%) and specificity (79%), antibody testing should not be used when there is a low background prevalence of *H. pylori* (prevalence <20%).

Invasive (endoscopic) tests for *H. pylori* include the rapid urease test, histology, and culture; all invasive testing modalities identify active infection.

Owing to the increased risk of false-negative endoscopic and fecal antigen test results in patients with bleeding PUD, serologic antibody testing should also be performed as a second test in this clinical setting, and treatment should be pursued if either test modality is positive.

Table 6 provides a summary of *H. pylori* testing in clinical practice.

Treatment

Treatment regimens should consist of a minimum of three agents, including two antimicrobial agents and one antisecretory agent. Treatment duration should be 10 to 14 days. Second-line therapy following treatment failure should consist of an alternative drug regimen. Recommended treatment regimens are shown in **Table 7**. Reasons for treatment failure include antimicrobial resistance (clarithromycin, metronidazole), patient noncompliance, and tobacco smoking and alcohol ingestion during treatment. Patients in whom two courses of eradication therapy are unsuccessful should be referred to a gastroenterologist for endoscopy. During upper endoscopy, tissue should be obtained for culture of *H. pylori* and determination of antibiotic sensitivities.

TABLE 6. Diagnostic Testing for *Helicobacter pylori* Infection

Test Modality	Advantages	Disadvantages	Use in Clinical Practice
Serum IgG antibody test	Low cost Widely available Allows for office-based testing Rapid results Good negative predictive value (a negative result is helpful)	Does not identify active infection Poor positive predictive value (a positive test is not helpful when pretest probability is low)	Most useful when there is high pretest probability (in individuals from urban areas or communities with large immigrant populations, and in patients with a peptic ulcer) Do not use to confirm *H. pylori* eradication following therapy or to assess for reinfection
Urea breath test	Identifies active *H. pylori* infection (through urease activity) Accurate (sensitivity and specificity >95%)	Limited by need for specialized equipment and personnel Radiation risk if radioactive ^{14}C isotope used (nonradioactive ^{13}C is available) Accuracy decreased by bismuth, antibiotic, and PPI use Costly	Use to confirm a positive antibody test when pretest probability is low (population with low background prevalence of *H. pylori*) Use to confirm eradication after therapy (at least 4 weeks after therapy) Use to assess for reinfection
Fecal antigen test	Identifies active *H. pylori* infection (identifies bacterial antigen by EIA) Costs less than urea breath testing	Requires collection of stool specimen Polyclonal test not as accurate as monoclonal after eradication therapy Accuracy decreased by bismuth, antibiotic, and PPI use	Use to confirm a positive antibody test when pretest probability is low (population with low background prevalence of *H. pylori*) Can use to confirm eradication after therapy (at least 4 weeks after therapy; monoclonal test preferred) Use to assess for reinfection
Endoscopic-based testing (rapid urease test, histology, and culture)	Allows for visualization of stomach Excellent sensitivity and specificity of histology Allows for determination of antibiotic sensitivities	Requires endoscopy Expensive Accuracy decreased by bismuth, antibiotic, and PPI use Limited availability for culture	Use if endoscopy is indicated for other reasons Use to obtain tissue for culture of *H. pylori* and determination of antibiotic sensitivities (after failure of two or more courses of eradication therapy)

EIA = enzyme immunoassay; PPI = proton pump inhibitor.

TABLE 7. First- and Second-Line Treatment Regimens for *Helicobacter pylori* Infection

First-Line Treatment Options	Caveats
Standard-dose PPI[a] twice daily or esomeprazole daily; clarithromycin, 500 mg twice daily; amoxicillin, 1000 mg twice daily	Avoid where clarithromycin resistance rates are >15%-20%
Standard-dose PPI[a] twice daily or esomeprazole daily; clarithromycin, 500 mg twice daily; metronidazole, 500 mg twice daily	Use metronidazole only when penicillin allergy exists
Ranitidine, 150 mg twice daily, or standard-dose PPI[a] twice daily; bismuth subsalicylate, 525 mg four times daily; metronidazole, 250 mg four times daily; tetracycline, 500 mg four times daily	Doxycycline, 100 mg twice daily, can be used in place of tetracycline if unavailable
Second-Line Treatment Options	
Consider first-line options listed above not used as initial therapy	
Standard-dose PPI[a] twice daily; levofloxacin, 500 mg/d; amoxicillin, 1000 mg twice daily	

PPI = proton pump inhibitor.

[a]Standard-dose PPI: omeprazole, 20 mg; lansoprazole, 30 mg; pantoprazole, 40 mg; rabeprazole, 20 mg

Data from: Chey WD, Wong BC; Practice Parameters Committee of the American College of Gastroenterology. American College of Gastroenterology guideline on the management of *Helicobacter pylori* infection. Am J Gastroenterol. 2007 Aug;102(8):1808-25. [PMID: 17608775]

KEY POINT

- Treatment regimens for *Helicobacter pylori* should consist of a minimum of three agents, including two antimicrobial agents and one antisecretory agent; treatment duration should be 10 to 14 days.

Eradication Testing

Testing to confirm eradication of *H. pylori* should ideally be pursued in all cases given the high rate of treatment failure (roughly 25% in the United States). Eradication testing should definitively be pursued in patients with an *H. pylori*–associated peptic ulcer, *H. pylori*–associated MALT lymphoma, gastric cancer resection, or persistent dyspepsia. Eradication testing should be performed no sooner than 4 weeks after completing antimicrobial therapy. PPI therapy should be stopped at least 2 weeks prior to testing. Antibody testing is not appropriate for confirming eradication because antibodies can remain in the serum long after *H. pylori* has been eradicated. Unless upper endoscopy is indicated for other reasons, noninvasive testing modalities appropriate for confirmation of eradication or assessment for reinfection include the urea breath test or the fecal antigen test. Both testing modalities are equivalent with regard to accuracy; therefore, the specific test chosen should be based on patient preference and/or test availability.

KEY POINT

HVC
- Noninvasive testing to confirm eradication of *Helicobacter pylori* (with the urea breath test or fecal antigen test) should be performed given the high rate of treatment failure (roughly 25% in the United States); antibody testing is not appropriate for confirming eradication because antibodies can remain in the serum long after *H. pylori* has been eradicated.

Miscellaneous Gastropathy

Mucosal gastropathic conditions such as intestinal metaplasia, autoimmune atrophic gastritis, lymphocytic gastritis, and eosinophilic gastritis may be identified at the time of upper endoscopy based on the histopathologic findings of gastric biopsies. Although these relatively uncommon conditions are largely managed by the gastroenterologist, important clinical aspects are relevant to the internist, who often has requested the upper endoscopy.

Atrophic Gastritis

The two forms of atrophic gastritis are *H. pylori*–associated and autoimmune. *H. pylori*–associated atrophic gastritis typically resolves with *H. pylori* eradication. Autoimmune atrophic gastritis, however, has no cure. Important clinical manifestations include pernicious anemia, iron deficiency anemia, and hypergastrinemia, which result from the long-term effects of the associated parietal cell loss and subsequent development of achlorhydria. Pernicious anemia and iron deficiency anemia are likely to require lifelong vitamin B_{12} and/or iron replacement, respectively. Hypergastrinemia is associated with an increased risk for the development of gastric carcinoid and adenocarcinoma; however, the risk is low enough that no endoscopic surveillance program is endorsed in the United States. There is a surveillance program in Europe.

Intestinal Metaplasia

Intestinal metaplasia is a relatively common precancerous lesion of the gastric mucosa. There can be an association with *H. pylori*; however, the infection may be patchy and may be missed on biopsies. Therefore, a second testing modality such as the urea breath test or fecal antigen test should be considered to further evaluate for active *H. pylori* infection. Although there is an increased risk for gastric adenocarcinoma, the risk is low enough that endoscopic surveillance is not performed unless the patient has additional risk factors, such as emigration from a geographic location with a high gastric cancer risk (Eastern Asia, Eastern Europe, and South America) or a family history of gastric cancer. However, given the association of gastric adenocarcinoma with *H. pylori*, this infection should be treated if identified.

Eosinophilic Gastritis

Eosinophilic gastritis is a rare, heterogeneous inflammatory condition that can involve the mucosal, muscular, or serosal layers of the stomach and/or duodenum. Eosinophilic gastritis is not considered a premalignant condition, and there are no specific nutritional deficiencies that are known to develop. Symptoms associated with eosinophilic gastritis can be quite variable and may include epigastric pain, nausea, vomiting, other dyspeptic symptoms, gastric outlet obstruction, and in rare cases ascites. Dietary treatment or glucocorticoid therapy may have a role in severe cases.

Lymphocytic Gastritis

Lymphocytic gastritis is a rare, benign chronic inflammatory condition of the gastric mucosa. Clinical manifestations may include dyspepsia, iron deficiency anemia, and diarrhea. Protein-losing gastroenteropathy has also been reported. Lymphocytic gastritis has been associated with celiac disease and *H. pylori* gastritis. Other less common associations include varioliform gastritis (a rare form of chronic gastritis characterized by endoscopic findings of nodules, thickened rugal folds, and erosions), Crohn disease, HIV infection, lymphocytic gastroenterocolitis (when the lymphocytic inflammation involves more than the stomach and is found on small-bowel and colon biopsies), and gastric lymphomas. Treatment is directed at the underlying condition, which in most cases is celiac disease or *H. pylori* infection. Lymphocytic gastritis is not considered a premalignant condition. Endoscopic surveillance is not required; however, small-bowel and colon biopsies should be obtained to determine the extent of the inflammation and to identify underlying conditions.

Gastrointestinal Complications of NSAIDs, Aspirin, and Anticoagulants

Epidemiology and Risk Factors

Low-dose aspirin used for cardioprophylaxis is associated with a two- to fourfold increase in upper gastrointestinal complications. Nearly 25% of chronic NSAID users will develop PUD, and 2% to 4% will develop complications of bleeding or perforation. Risk factors for NSAID-related gastrointestinal complications include a history of PUD or other gastrointestinal bleeding event; *H. pylori* infection; age 65 years or older; concomitant use of aspirin (of any dose), anticoagulants, other

NSAIDs, or glucocorticoids; high-dose NSAID use; and chronic comorbid illness.

> **KEY POINT**
>
> - Risk factors for NSAID-related gastrointestinal complications include a history of peptic ulcer disease or other gastrointestinal bleeding event; *Helicobacter pylori* infection; age 65 years or older; concomitant use of aspirin (of any dose), anticoagulants, other NSAIDs, or glucocorticoids; high-dose NSAID use; and chronic comorbid illness.

Prevention of NSAID-Induced Injury

PPIs are the preferred agent for treatment and prophylaxis of NSAID- and aspirin-related gastrointestinal injury. Misoprostol at full dose (800 µg/d) is effective in preventing PUD and ulcer complications with NSAID use; however, its use is limited by side effects (diarrhea, abortifacient). In patients with a history of PUD, testing and treating for *H. pylori* infection should be performed before starting chronic antiplatelet therapy. Prevention recommendations based on risk stratification of NSAID-induced gastrointestinal injury are summarized in **Figure 13**.

Selective cyclooxygenase-2 (COX-2) inhibitors preferentially inhibit the COX-2 isoenzyme, which primarily modulates pain and inflammation, and minimally inhibit the COX-1 isoenzyme, which promotes generation of the gastric mucosal protective barrier, decreases gastric acid secretion, and helps to maintain good mucosal blood flow. The risk of gastroduodenal ulcers and ulcer complications is significantly lower in patients taking COX-2 inhibitors compared with nonselective NSAIDs. However, in high-risk individuals, such as those with previous PUD, a COX-2 inhibitor alone is no better than a nonselective NSAID coadministered with a PPI in preventing ulcer complications. Moreover, the beneficial effect of COX-2 inhibitors is lost when taken concomitantly with low-dose aspirin. There is also evidence that COX-2 inhibitors and nonselective NSAIDs, with the possible exception of naproxen, increase the risk of cardiovascular complications. Therefore, the decision to use a COX-2 inhibitor requires a risk-benefit analysis that weighs the gastrointestinal risks of an NSAID with the potential cardiovascular risks of a COX-2 inhibitor.

> **KEY POINT**
>
> - Proton pump inhibitors are the preferred agent for treatment and prophylaxis of NSAID- and aspirin-related gastrointestinal injury.

Gastroparesis

Diagnosis

Gastroparesis is a heterogeneous clinical syndrome that is diagnosed based on the presence of specific symptoms and objective documentation of delayed delivery of the stomach contents into the proximal small bowel in the absence of a

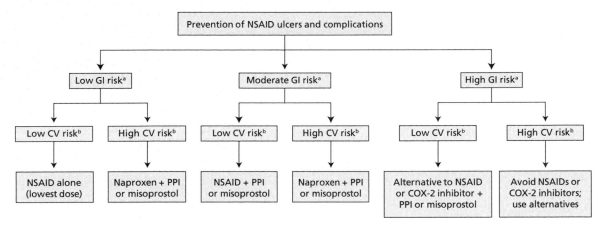

FIGURE 13. Prevention of NSAID-induced ulcers and complications. CV = cardiovascular; COX-2 = cyclooxygenase-2; GI = gastrointestinal; PPI = proton pump inhibitor.

[a]Gastrointestinal risk is stratified into low (no risk factors), moderate (presence of one or two risk factors), and high (multiple risk factors or previous ulcer complications or concomitant use of glucocorticoids or anticoagulants).

[b]High CV risk = need for aspirin to prevent cardiovascular events. Low-dose aspirin is indicated in patients with high CV risk.

Adapted by permission from Macmillan Publishers Ltd: American Journal of Gastroenterology (Lanza FL, Chan FK, Quigley EM; Practice Parameters Committee of the American College of Gastroenterology. Guidelines for prevention of NSAID-related ulcer complications. 104(3):728-38. [PMID: 19240698]), copyright 2009.

mechanical obstruction. Commonly reported symptoms include early satiety, postprandial fullness, nausea, vomiting, upper abdominal pain, bloating, and weight loss. These symptoms correlate poorly with the findings on objective gastric emptying tests. For example, patients with accelerated gastric emptying may report similar symptoms to those with delayed gastric emptying. A variety of other upper gastrointestinal disorders, including PUD, partial gastric or small-bowel obstruction, functional dyspepsia, gastric cancer, *H. pylori* infection, and pancreaticobiliary disorders, can present with similar symptoms. Exclusion of other upper gastrointestinal disorders, objective documentation of delayed gastric emptying, and an attempt to identify the cause of the gastroparesis are essential prior to treatment.

KEY POINT

- Commonly reported symptoms of gastroparesis include early satiety, postprandial fullness, nausea, vomiting, upper abdominal pain, bloating, and weight loss.

Testing

A structural assessment of the upper gastrointestinal tract must be performed before pursuing a gastric emptying study. Upper endoscopy is the most accurate test for this initial assessment; however, upper gastrointestinal barium radiography is a reasonable alternative when upper endoscopy is not available or noninvasive testing is desired. The standard test for assessment of gastric emptying is the scintigraphic gastric emptying of solids. A 4-hour emptying study is more accurate than a 2-hour study. A wireless motility capsule is also available to assess gastric emptying and offers the advantage of also providing small-bowel and colon transit information. Drugs that affect gastric emptying (**Table 8**) should be stopped a

TABLE 8.	Medications that Impair Gastric Emptying
Opioid analgesics	
Anticholinergic agents	
Tricyclic antidepressants	
Calcium channel blockers	
Progesterone	
Octreotide	
Proton pump inhibitors	
H_2 blockers	
Sucralfate	
Aluminum hydroxide	
Interferon alfa	
L-dopa	
Fiber	
β-Agonists	
Glucagon	
Calcitonin	
Dexfenfluramine	
Diphenhydramine	
Nicotine	
Tetrahydrocannabinol	

minimum of 48 hours before testing. Patients with diabetes mellitus should have a plasma glucose level less than 275 mg/dL (15.3 mmol/L) during testing because marked hyperglycemia can acutely impair gastric emptying.

Patients diagnosed with gastroparesis should be assessed for diabetes, thyroid dysfunction, neurologic disease, previous gastric or bariatric surgery, and autoimmune disorders.

Patients should be asked about viral illness prior to symptom onset to identify a postviral gastroparesis.

- Diagnostic testing for gastroparesis consists of an initial assessment with upper endoscopy to exclude mechanical obstruction, followed by a gastric emptying study.

Management

Initial management consists of the prompt identification and treatment of dehydration, electrolyte disturbances, and micronutrient deficiencies, as these can worsen symptoms associated with gastroparesis. Dietary modification and optimization of glycemic control in patients with diabetes should be the first treatment intervention. Specific diet recommendations include small, low-fat meals consumed four to five times per day. Insoluble fiber (found in fresh fruits, fresh vegetables, and bran) should be avoided. High-calorie liquids can be used to increase the liquid nutrient component of meals. Carbonated beverages, alcohol, and tobacco smoking should be minimized or ideally avoided.

On-demand use of antiemetic agents is effective in addressing nausea and vomiting associated with gastroparesis; however, these agents have no effect on gastric emptying. Prokinetic agents can be used in conjunction with dietary management and aggressive glycemic control to improve gastric emptying. Metoclopramide is the only prokinetic agent approved by the FDA for the treatment of gastroparesis. Given the risk of side effects, including dystonia, parkinsonism-type movements, and tardive dyskinesia, the lowest dose should be used (starting at 5 mg three times daily), should be taken with meals, and should be advanced slowly to a maximum total dose of 40 mg a day (10 mg four times daily). Patients should be informed of the potential for neurologic side effects and should be instructed to stop therapy if they occur. Erythromycin also improves gastric emptying; however, it is generally reserved for short-term intravenous use in patients hospitalized for gastroparesis exacerbations. Low-dose tricyclic antidepressants can also be considered to address refractory nausea and vomiting, but these agents may further slow gastric emptying. If symptoms persist despite these interventions, patients should be referred to a gastroenterologist.

Gastric Polyps and Subepithelial Lesions

Gastric Polyps

Gastric polyps are found on up to 5% of upper endoscopies; 90% are either hyperplastic or fundic gland polyps (FGPs). Sporadic FGPs have been associated with PPI use and do not require excision or surveillance. They are usually 1 to 5 mm in size and fewer than 10 in number. FGPs related to familial adenomatous polyposis (FAP) or *MYH*-associated polyposis are usually numerous (>30 polyps), frequently harbor dyspla-

sia, and warrant excision if they are 10 mm or larger. Colonoscopy to rule out FAP and *MYH*-associated polyposis is recommended in patients younger than 40 years with dysplastic or numerous FGPs. Adenomatous and hyperplastic polyps are associated with atrophic gastritis, intestinal metaplasia, and *H. pylori* infection. Adenomas are dysplastic and warrant excision, whereas only 20% of hyperplastic polyps harbor dysplasia. Polypectomy of lesions larger than 5 mm is recommended. Less common gastric polyps include inflammatory fibroid polyps, hamartomas, pancreatic rests, and carcinoids.

- Colonoscopy to rule out familial adenomatous polyposis or *MYH*-associated polyposis is recommended in patients younger than 40 years with dysplastic or numerous fundic gland polyps.

Gastric Subepithelial Lesions

Lesions arising beneath the gastric epithelium are frequently asymptomatic and are often found incidentally during upper endoscopy or radiologic imaging of the gastrointestinal tract. The differential diagnosis of gastric subepithelial lesions (SELs) is broad and includes a variety of intramural lesions as well as compression from extraluminal organs or lesions. Benign SELs include lipoma, leiomyoma, pancreatic rests, inflammatory fibroid polyps, and duplication cysts. The malignant and potentially malignant SELs include gastrointestinal stromal tumors (GISTs), lymphoma, carcinoid, glomus tumors, and rarely metastases. Because endoscopic biopsy is often unable to provide a diagnosis, endoscopic ultrasound (EUS) is the imaging modality of choice for the evaluation of SELs. EUS ascertains characteristic features suggestive of the diagnosis by identification of the layer of origin of the lesion. Because benign and malignant lesions may not always be differentiated by sonographic features, EUS-guided fine-needle aspiration may be performed for cytopathologic specimen analysis.

Gastrointestinal Stromal Tumors

GISTs represent less than 1% of tumors of the gastrointestinal tract and are most commonly found in the stomach. Most are discovered incidentally, but large tumors may cause pain, obstruction, or hemorrhage. GISTs are mesenchymal tumors believed to arise from the interstitial cells of Cajal (ICC). Approximately 95% of GISTs have evidence of a *KIT* oncogene mutation, which stains positive for the CD117 antigen, a marker expressed by ICC. GISTs may range from indolent to aggressive. The prognosis is based upon mitotic index (mitoses per 50 high-power fields), tumor size, and location.

See MKSAP 17 Hematology and Oncology for staging and treatment of GISTs.

Gastric Carcinoid Tumors

Carcinoid tumors, known as neuroendocrine tumors (NETs), represent 1% of gastric neoplasms. They are derived from enterochromaffin cells of the gastric mucosa. Three subtypes of gastric NETs exist. Type I accounts for 80% and is associated with autoimmune atrophic gastritis and hypergastrinemia. Type II is associated with multiple endocrine neoplasia type 1 and Zollinger-Ellison syndrome. Endoscopic polypectomy is curative for type I and II NETs that are smaller than 1 cm. Type III lesions account for 15% of gastric NETs; they are gastrin independent and have the poorest prognosis. Gastric NETs secrete 5-hydroxytryptophan rather than serotonin; therefore, classic carcinoid syndrome is rare, while wheezing, lacrimation, swelling, flushing, and carcinoid heart and valvular disease may be seen owing to high systemic amine concentrations.

See MKSAP 17 Hematology and Oncology for treatment of gastric NETs.

KEY POINT

- Endoscopic ultrasound is the imaging modality of choice for evaluation of gastric subepithelial lesions.

Gastric Adenocarcinoma

Epidemiology and Risk Factors

Gastric cancer is the fourth most common cancer worldwide. The highest rates are seen in developing countries, including those in Asia (particularly China), South America, and Eastern Europe. Gastric cancer rates have decreased in most parts of the world owing to a reduction in risk factors (**Table 9**). The rate of stomach cancer in white women in the United States is 4 per 100,000, which is lower than the rate in white men (8.4 per 100,000). The

TABLE 9. Risk Factors Associated with Gastric Adenocarcinoma

Type	Risk Factor
Environmental factors	*Helicobacter pylori* infection
	Diet low in fresh fruits and vegetables
	Diet high in salted and preserved foods
	Smoking
Underlying conditions	Chronic atrophic gastritis and intestinal metaplasia
	Previous gastric surgery
	Gastric adenomas
Genetic factors	Familial adenomatous polyposis
	MYH-associated polyposis
	Lynch syndrome
	Li-Fraumeni syndrome
	Juvenile polyposis syndrome
	Peutz-Jeghers syndrome
	Gastric hyperplastic polyposis
	Hereditary diffuse gastric cancer

incidence is higher in nonwhites, with the highest rates in black patients. Overall 5-year survival is approximately 28%. Gastric adenocarcinoma accounts for more than 90% of gastric cancers and is subdivided into intestinal and diffuse histology. Intestinal type predominates and is often related to environmental factors. Diffuse gastric cancer is more often seen in women and young patients. Germline mutations in the gene *E-cadherin* cause hereditary diffuse gastric cancer, which is associated with an 80% lifetime risk of gastric cancer. Prophylactic gastrectomy is recommended in gene carriers who are 20 years of age or older. Other genetic syndromes associated with an increased risk for gastric cancer include Lynch syndrome, FAP, *MYH*-associated polyposis, Li-Fraumeni syndrome, hyperplastic gastric polyposis, juvenile polyposis syndrome, and Peutz-Jeghers syndrome.

Screening and Surveillance

Gastric cancer screening for average-risk patients is not recommended in the United States. Patients with a genetic gastric cancer predisposition should undergo syndrome-specific surveillance. Surveillance upper endoscopy is recommended 1 year after adenomatous gastric polyp removal and, if negative, every 3 to 5 years. There is insufficient evidence to support surveillance for individuals with gastric intestinal metaplasia; however, surveillance can be considered in patients who have intestinal metaplasia as well as an increased risk owing to ethnicity or family history. Surveillance in intestinal metaplasia should incorporate a biopsy protocol that maps the entire stomach. Patients with low-grade dysplasia should undergo biopsy every 3 months for the first year, and surveillance should cease when two consecutive endoscopies are negative. The presence of high-grade dysplasia warrants surgical resection. Surveillance after early gastric cancer treatment should be individualized.

KEY POINT

- Gastric cancer screening for average-risk patients is not recommended in the United States; patients with a genetic gastric cancer predisposition should undergo syndrome-specific surveillance.

Clinical Manifestations and Diagnosis

Gastric cancer symptoms are nonspecific and may include anorexia, weight loss, abdominal discomfort, early satiety, gastrointestinal bleeding, or nausea and vomiting. Upper endoscopy with biopsy is the diagnostic test of choice.

For staging and treatment of gastric cancer, see MKSAP 17 Hematology and Oncology.

KEY POINT

- Upper endoscopy with biopsy is the diagnostic test of choice for gastric cancer.

Complications of Gastric Surgical Procedures

Bariatric Surgery Complications

For a general discussion of bariatric surgery, see MKSAP 17 General Internal Medicine.

Postoperative Mortality

In general, mortality rates are low for bariatric surgery and are reported to be 0.3% to 0.4% at 30 days and 0.8% at 2 years. Laparoscopic and restrictive procedures (gastric banding, sleeve gastrectomy) are associated with lower mortality than open and malabsorptive/restrictive procedures (Roux-en-Y gastric bypass, biliopancreatic diversion with duodenal switch). Several clinical factors that increase mortality are a history of deep venous thrombosis or pulmonary embolism, obstructive sleep apnea, impaired functional status, advanced age, and a surgeon and/or hospital with lower volumes of bariatric surgery. The major causes of perioperative mortality are anastomotic leaks, pulmonary embolism, bleeding, and cardiovascular complications.

Restrictive Procedure Complications

Complications unique to gastric banding include slippage of the gastric band resulting in pouch dilatation, intragastric band erosion with the potential for gastric perforation and/or abscess formation, and esophageal dilatation. Less frequent complications include tube migration, tube disconnection, and port-site infection. Tubing-related small-bowel obstruction is a relatively rare yet serious complication that carries the risk of closed-loop bowel obstruction.

Complications unique to sleeve gastrectomy include staple-line bleeding, stenosis, and staple-line leakage; leaks are the most concerning complication. Stenosis is typically due to angulation or kinking of the stomach resulting in functional obstruction; it presents as dysphagia to solids and liquids with nausea and vomiting.

The most common complication associated with vertical banding gastroplasty is stenosis at the site of the band placement. Other less common complications include esophagitis, band migration, and staple-line disruption.

Malabsorptive Procedure Complications

Complications following Roux-en-Y gastric bypass include cholelithiasis, nephrolithiasis (due to increased urine oxalate excretion), dumping syndrome, anastomotic stricture, anastomotic ulceration, small-bowel obstruction from internal hernias, and gastrogastric fistula. Although small intestinal bacterial overgrowth can occur following any bariatric procedure, it occurs most often with Roux-en-Y gastric bypass. Similar complications are seen following biliopancreatic diversion with duodenal switch, although most concerning are the nutritional deficiencies.

Nutritional and Endocrine-Related Complications

Protein-calorie malnutrition can occur 1 to 2 years after malabsorptive procedures (Roux-en-Y gastric bypass or biliopancreatic diversion), typically presenting as rapid weight loss, generalized edema, muscle wasting, and hypoalbuminemia. Micronutrient deficiencies can also develop following bariatric surgery and are more common with malabsorptive procedures (**Table 10**). Deficiencies may include thiamine (vitamin B_1); pyridoxine (vitamin B_6); folate; cobalamin (vitamin B_{12}); vitamins C, A, D, E, and K; iron; zinc; selenium; magnesium; and copper. Acceleration in loss of bone mineral density also

TABLE 10.	Possible Micronutrient Deficiency Following Bariatric Surgery
Nutrient	**Features of Deficiency**
Calcium	Short term: muscle contractions, pain, spasms, paresthesia
	Long term: decrease in bone density, osteopenia/osteoporosis
Cobalamin (vitamin B_{12})	Macrocytic anemia, neurocognitive impairment, peripheral neuropathy, proprioceptive loss, spasticity, weakness, glossitis, cheilosis, angular stomatitis
Copper	Microcytic anemia, leukopenia, myelopathy (weakness, numbness, spasticity, hyperreflexia, painful paresthesia), poor wound healing
Folate	Macrocytic anemia, glossitis, cheilosis, palpitations, fatigue
Iron	Microcytic anemia, fatigue, white fingernail beds
Magnesium	Muscle spasm and pain
Selenium	Dilated cardiomyopathy, myopathy, myositis, connective tissue abnormalities (hair, nails, skin)
Thiamine (vitamin B_1)	Cerebellar ataxia, nystagmus, ophthalmoplegia, confusion, confabulation (Wernicke-Korsakoff syndrome), heart failure, edema, ascites, peripheral neuropathy, weakness
Vitamin A	Night vision impairment, Bitot spots, corneal ulceration, blindness, itching, dry hair, loss of immunity
Vitamin D	Osteomalacia, osteoporosis, myalgia, arthralgia, depression, fasciculations
Zinc	Dermatitis, poor wound healing, blunting of taste sense, hair loss, glossitis

Data from: Stein J, Stier C, Raab H, Weiner R. Review article: The nutritional and pharmacological consequences of obesity surgery. Aliment Pharmacol Ther. 2014 Sep;40(6): 582-609. [PMID: 25078533]

occurs, primarily with malabsorptive procedures, due to calcium and vitamin D deficiency leading to secondary hyperparathyroidism.

In patients undergoing malabsorptive procedures, Endocrine Society guidelines recommend testing for albumin/prealbumin, iron/ferritin, vitamin B_{12}, folate, serum calcium, parathyroid hormone, and 25-hydroxyvitamin D every 6 months postoperatively for the first 2 years and then annually thereafter; measurement of vitamins A, vitamin B_1, and zinc is considered optional. Bone mineral density measurement is also recommended annually after the procedure until stable.

Postprandial hypoglycemia can occur in some patients following Roux-en-Y gastric bypass secondary to maladaptive secretion of insulin, dumping syndrome, or nesidioblastosis, which is characterized by hyperplasia of pancreatic islet cells. Ingestion of small, frequent meals along with avoidance of simple carbohydrates can decrease the frequency and improve the symptoms of postprandial hypoglycemia. In severe cases, partial pancreatectomy can be utilized for hypoglycemic symptoms associated with nesidioblastosis.

Other Gastric Resection Complications

Total and partial gastrectomy for the treatment of PUD, gastric malignancy, and pancreatic tumors can result in a variety of short- and long-term complications. Complications following gastrectomy include intraluminal bleeding, anastomotic leaks, and anastomotic strictures. Delayed gastric emptying, dumping syndrome, and/or fat malabsorption may also develop following partial gastrectomy with or without vagotomy, resulting in symptoms of nausea and vomiting, loss of appetite, bloating and fullness, or early satiety. Pancreaticoduodenectomy (Whipple resection) entails removal of the pancreatic head, duodenum, common bile duct, gallbladder, and distal stomach. Common complications are weight loss, reflux, dumping syndrome, and bacterial overgrowth. **H**

Disorders of the Pancreas
Acute Pancreatitis

Acute pancreatitis is the leading gastrointestinal cause of hospitalization in the United States. Acute pancreatitis is an acute inflammatory process involving the pancreas and is typically associated with severe upper abdominal pain. Inflammation may be localized to the pancreas or, through a number of pathophysiologic mechanisms, may also be systemic. Systemic inflammation is characterized by involvement of distant organs as part of a capillary leak syndrome known as the systemic inflammatory response. Multiple factors contribute to the disease pathogenesis, one of which is premature intracellular activation of digestive enzymes that cause pancreatic "autodigestion."

Eighty percent of patients with acute pancreatitis experience mild disease, characterized by an uncomplicated, reversible course of interstitial pancreatitis leading to recovery within several days. Twenty percent develop moderate or severe disease and may have a protracted hospital course. Moderate severity is characterized by development of local pancreatic complications (pancreatic necrosis, acute fluid collections) or transient organ system failure (circulatory, renal, respiratory). Severe pancreatitis is defined by persistent organ system failure for 3 consecutive days; persistent failure is the strongest predictor of death. Median overall mortality rate from acute pancreatitis is 5% (range 2%-9%).

Gallstones and alcohol use are the most common causes of acute pancreatitis, accounting for 80% of cases in the United States (**Table 11**).

TABLE 11.	Causes of Acute Pancreatitis
Common	
Biliary disease	
Gallstones	
Microlithiasis (1- to 2-mm stones that are not detected by imaging studies)	
Alcohol use	
Occasional	
Medications	
Furosemide	
Didanosine	
Asparaginase	
Mesalamine	
Hydrochlorothiazide	
6-Mercaptopurine/azathioprine	
Simvastatin	
Hypertriglyceridemia	
Hypercalcemia	
Pancreas divisum (controversial)	
Choledochocele	
Post-ERCP	
Rare	
Autoimmune	
Infectious	
Viral (mumps, coxsackie B virus, cytomegalovirus)	
Parasitic (*Toxoplasma* species, *Ascaris lumbricoides*)	
Ischemia	
Trauma	
Neoplasia	
Celiac disease	
Genetic (only if attacks are recurrent)	
ERCP = endoscopic retrograde cholangiopancreatography.	

Clinical Presentation and Diagnosis

Diagnosis of acute pancreatitis requires two of three criteria: (1) acute onset of upper abdominal pain, (2) serum amylase or lipase level increased by at least three times the upper limit of normal, and (3) characteristic findings on cross-sectional imaging (contrast CT, MRI, or ultrasound).

Sudden onset of severe epigastric abdominal pain is a hallmark feature of acute pancreatitis. Pain often radiates to the back, diminishes by sitting or leaning forward, and is associated with nausea, vomiting, and fever. Dyspnea is typically a manifestation of the systemic inflammatory response, and associated ventilation-perfusion mismatch may develop from a symptomatic pleural effusion, which is thought to impair diaphragmatic and chest-wall motion during respiration. Acute liver enzyme elevation at the time of presentation with acute pancreatitis is strongly suggestive of obstruction of the common bile duct by gallstones.

Both amylase and lipase levels increase within hours of disease onset. Lipase is the preferred test owing to its longer half-life than amylase and greater sensitivity and specificity. Amylase can be elevated in other settings, such as parotitis, peptic ulcer disease, acute cholecystitis, and diabetic ketoacidosis. Benign pancreatic hyperenzymemia is a rare cause of asymptomatic amylase and lipase elevations without significant imaging abnormalities. Macroamylasemia, a cause of isolated hyperamylasemia, is due to poor excretion of large amylase multimers from the blood and is diagnosed by serum protein electrophoresis.

In most patients, the diagnosis of acute pancreatitis may be made based on a consistent clinical picture with an elevation of the serum lipase (or amylase) level. Because gallstones are the most common cause of pancreatitis, all patients should be evaluated with a transabdominal ultrasound unless another obvious cause of pancreatitis is present; transabdominal ultrasound has excellent sensitivity for detecting cholelithiasis and evidence of biliary obstruction. It is also cost effective. Contrast-enhanced CT is not usually required to diagnose acute pancreatitis; it tends to be less sensitive than ultrasound for gallstones, exposes patients to the risk of contrast-medium–induced nephropathy (particularly in underresuscitated patients), and is expensive. CT imaging is indicated, however, when the diagnosis is uncertain (abdominal pain but minimal pancreatic enzyme elevations), the patient's presentation is severe and concerning for an undiagnosed intraabdominal complication, or the patient does not improve within 48 to 72 hours of hospital admission. Imaging features and complications of acute pancreatitis seen on CT scanning include pancreatic or peripancreatic edema, inflammatory stranding, fluid collections, pancreatic necrosis, or splenic vein thrombosis (**Figure 14**).

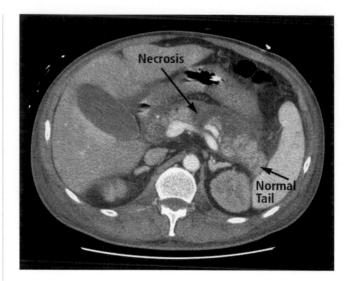

FIGURE 14. CT scan demonstrating acute pancreatitis, with hypoperfusion of the pancreatic body indicating necrosis. Note that the distal tail is perfusing normally.

HVC

Prognostic Criteria

Acute pancreatitis guidelines recommend assessment of all patients into high- and low-risk categories. Implementation of this recommendation is sometimes lacking, owing perhaps in part to poor familiarity with both the recommendations and available risk stratification tools. Multiple clinical scoring systems are available to stratify risk of developing severe disease; this can help determine the appropriate level of care and enable key early management decisions. All scoring systems have modest accuracy, but some of the more recent systems (Glasgow, Japanese scoring system, Systemic Inflammatory Response Syndrome [SIRS] score) are simpler to use compared with older criteria, such as the Ranson criteria and the Acute Physiology and Chronic Health Evaluation (APACHE) II score. Laboratory findings that are associated with a severe course are an elevated serum blood urea nitrogen level greater than

CONT. 20 mg/dL (7.1 mmol/L), a hematocrit greater than 44%, or an elevated serum creatinine level. Similarly, a rising blood urea nitrogen level or hematocrit early in the course of acute pancreatitis portends a severe course. Patient characteristics that predispose to more severe disease or longer hospital stay include the presence of multiple comorbid illnesses, age greater than 70 years, and BMI greater than 30.

KEY POINT

HVC
- Poor prognostic indicators for acute pancreatitis are elevated serum blood urea nitrogen level greater than 20 mg/dL (7.1 mmol/L), a hematocrit greater than 44%, or an elevated serum creatinine level.

Management

Most patients with acute pancreatitis require hospitalization for hydration, brief bowel rest, pain control, and antiemetics. Intravascular fluid volume falls in response to inflammation and capillary leak syndrome. Therefore, aggressive fluid resuscitation (250-500 mL/h) with isotonic crystalloid should be administered on presentation. Similar to the sepsis paradigm of an early therapeutic window, this intervention appears to be most beneficial within the first 12 to 24 hours and may have a limited impact thereafter. In patients with evidence of developing organ system failure, careful monitoring and treatment at higher levels of care are appropriate.

In patients with severe acute pancreatitis, enteral feeding should begin approximately 72 hours after presentation. This evidence-based intervention reduces infectious complications, organ failure, and mortality compared with total parenteral nutrition. Enteral feeding prevents infections by promoting gut mucosal health and barrier function necessary for preventing leakage or translocation of bacteria that can infect other tissues. Both nasogastric and nasojejunal enteral feeding are safe and have comparable effectiveness. Total parenteral nutrition should be avoided when possible. In mild acute pancreatitis, oral feeding may start when nausea, vomiting, and abdominal pain resolve (or are absent) but should not be withheld on the basis of persistent elevations in pancreatic enzyme levels.

Pain control is not standardized but typically requires opiates, which may be administered by a nurse or a patient-controlled analgesia pump.

In patients with uncomplicated gallstone pancreatitis, a cholecystectomy should be performed prior to discharge. In those with gallstone pancreatitis who have ascending cholangitis, endoscopic retrograde cholangiopancreatography (ERCP) should be performed within 24 hours of presentation. ERCP is probably beneficial for patients with biliary pancreatitis and nonresolving bile duct obstruction (without cholangitis), but the timing of ERCP (24-72 hours) is less certain. In the absence of gallstone pancreatitis and/or a significant history of alcohol abuse, investigation is necessary to identify a cause of pancreatitis to reduce the risk of a recurrent, more

devastating attack. Typical hospital evaluation includes testing for hypertriglyceridemia, hypercalcemia, drug-induced pancreatitis, infectious exposures and triggers, and abdominal trauma. In patients who are aged 40 years or older with unexplained pancreatitis, assessment for a benign or malignant pancreatic tumor may also be part of the evaluation. Consultation with a specialist is appropriate, particularly for idiopathic pancreatitis. Because of autodigestion, areas of pancreatic necrosis are frequently identified on imaging. Patients with uninfected pancreatic necrosis do not benefit from antibiotic use, which can unnecessarily increase the risk of intra-abdominal fungal infections. Therefore, patients with pancreatic necrosis should not routinely receive antibiotic agents; antibiotics should be reserved for those with proven infection. Patients whose condition does not improve or deteriorates 7 to 10 days after presentation may have infected necrosis. CT-guided fine-needle aspiration helps guide treatment decisions regarding antibiotic use, drainage, and continued supportive care. In stable patients with infected necrosis, the preferred approach is to initiate antibiotics and to ideally delay drainage procedures for at least 4 weeks to allow the collection to become encapsulated, which facilitates drainage.

KEY POINT

HVC
- In patients with uncomplicated gallstone pancreatitis, a cholecystectomy should be performed prior to discharge.

Complications

In interstitial pancreatitis, fluid collections arise from disruption of the pancreatic ductal system. They are known as acute peripancreatic fluid collections for the first 4 weeks after presentation and are subsequently called pancreatic pseudocysts when the collection becomes encapsulated. Most resolve and do not require treatment; however, in patients who are symptomatic from the effects of these fluid collections, transgastric or transduodenal drainage can be performed. Persistent leaks manifest as enlarging fluid collections and are often accompanied by ongoing symptoms; they warrant treatment with bowel rest or mid-distal jejunal feeding, pancreatic enzymes, octreotide, and pancreatic duct stenting.

In patients with pancreatic necrosis, fluid collections are known as acute necrotic collections for the first 4 weeks after presentation and involve pancreatic and/or peripancreatic tissues. They are subsequently known as walled-off necrosis, when the collection becomes encapsulated (**Figure 15**). Many resolve spontaneously, but some persist, enlarge, have a mass effect, and/or cause symptoms. They may require decompression or debridement if symptomatic. Diabetes mellitus may develop from extensive pancreatic necrosis.

Nonpancreatic local complications include gastric outlet dysfunction, splenic vein thrombosis, gastric variceal bleeding, and colonic necrosis.

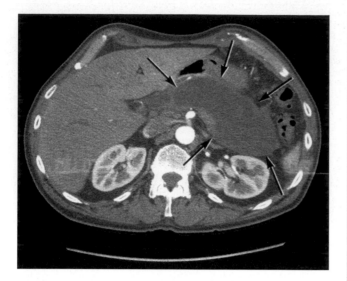

FIGURE 15. CT scan demonstrating walled-off pancreatic necrosis (*arrows*) virtually replacing the entire pancreatic body and tail.

Chronic Pancreatitis

Chronic pancreatitis affects approximately 5 in 100,000 persons in the United States. It is an inflammatory disease that results in irreversible pancreatic injury, which leads to varying degrees of abdominal pain, reduced pancreatic exocrine function, diabetes mellitus, and pancreatic calcifications.

Alcohol is the most common historical cause of chronic pancreatitis (**Table 12**), but it should be considered a disease cofactor because only 3% of patients with alcoholism develop chronic pancreatitis. Most patients with alcohol-related chronic pancreatitis are heavy users (>50-80 g/d) for more than 5 to 10 years. A standard "drink" contains approximately 14 g of alcohol. Tobacco is an independent risk factor for chronic pancreatitis.

KEY POINT

- Alcohol is the most common historical cause of chronic pancreatitis.

Clinical Presentation and Diagnosis

The hallmark symptom of chronic pancreatitis is abdominal pain that often radiates to the back; however, pain can be absent. Pain is typically intermittent, with attacks interrupted by varying pain-free intervals. Constant pain may occur from local anatomic causes (compressing pseudocyst, biliary or pancreatic duct stricture) or from visceral hyperalgesia (increased sensation in response to stimuli) from chronic narcotic use and centralization of pain. Other hallmark clinical features, particularly in severe disease, are (1) exocrine pancreatic insufficiency with bulky and greasy stools, fat-soluble vitamin deficiencies, and weight loss; (2) diabetes; and (3) pancreatic calcifications.

Chronic pancreatitis is classified anatomically as either large- or small-duct (also known as minimal change) disease.

TABLE 12.	Causes of Chronic Pancreatitis
Toxic	
Alcohol	
Tobacco	
Hypercalcemia (controversial)	
Idiopathic	
Early onset (commonly associated with genetic mutations)	
Late onset	
Genetic Mutations	
Cationic trypsinogen gene	
Cystic fibrosis transmembrane conductance regulator gene	
Serine protease inhibitor, Kazal type I gene	
Chymotrypsinogen C gene	
Calcium-sensing receptor gene	
Claudin-2 gene	
Obstructive	
Pancreatic solid tumor	
Intraductal papillary mucinous neoplasm	
Trauma (with pancreatic duct stricture)	
Recurrent or Severe Acute Pancreatitis	
Postnecrotic	
Recurrent acute pancreatitis from any cause	
Vascular diseases/ischemia	
Postirradiation	
Other	
Celiac disease	
Autoimmune pancreatitis	

Small-duct disease is characterized by attacks of pain with normal or minimally abnormal pancreatic imaging.

The diagnosis of chronic pancreatitis remains challenging. Serum amylase and lipase levels are often not elevated and are unreliable for diagnosing chronic pancreatitis or an exacerbation of the disease. Common criteria employ a combination of clinical features (pain, recurrent attacks of pancreatitis, weight loss) with objective findings of calcifications, imaging features of ductal dilatation or inflammatory masses (**Figure 16**), exocrine pancreatic insufficiency, diabetes, and rarely histologic findings. Disease onset in older patients requires exclusion of autoimmune pancreatitis and pancreatic cancer.

An abdominal radiograph should be performed to detect pancreatic calcifications. If calcifications are absent, a dedicated pancreas-protocol CT or magnetic resonance cholangiopancreatography should be done to detect abnormalities of the main and side-branch pancreatic ducts. A gastroenterologist

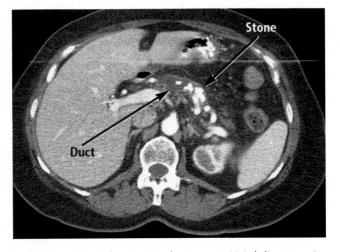

FIGURE 16. CT scan demonstrating chronic pancreatitis including pancreatic ductal dilatation and parenchymal stones.

may perform endoscopic ultrasound (EUS), which can allow application of EUS-based criteria to aid in making the diagnosis in cases where cross-sectional imaging is unremarkable. Endoscopic retrograde cholangiopancreatography should be reserved for patients requiring therapeutic interventions.

Pancreatic malabsorption, measured by quantitative 72-hour fecal fat testing, occurs when residual pancreatic enzyme secretion is only 5% to 10% of normal.

Diagnosis of chronic pancreatitis is difficult and may lack firm data, such as when imaging abnormalities are absent or minor. In this situation, clinicians may follow patients prospectively to detect more obvious manifestations of the disease or consider referring patients to specialized centers that perform direct cholecystokinin or secretin stimulation tests, the most sensitive and specific tests for detecting mild to moderate reductions in pancreatic function and aiding diagnosis of early or small-duct chronic pancreatitis.

KEY POINTS

- The hallmark symptom of chronic pancreatitis is abdominal pain, often radiating to the back.
- The common diagnostic criteria for chronic pancreatitis include clinical features (pain, recurrent attacks of pancreatitis, weight loss) with objective findings of calcifications, imaging features of ductal dilatation or inflammatory masses, exocrine pancreatic insufficiency, diabetes mellitus, and histologic findings.

Management

Patients with chronic pancreatitis should be counseled to stop smoking and drinking alcohol.

Management focuses on reducing pain and detecting and treating complications. Recognizing the pain pattern is central to pain management for patients with chronic pancreatitis.

Acute intermittent attacks of pain are treated with supportive care, acetaminophen, and ibuprofen in combination

with tramadol, a nonopioid with opiate action. Tramadol has been shown to provide analgesia comparable to other opioid analgesics in patients with chronic pancreatitis and causes fewer gastrointestinal side effects. If the pain pattern changes or becomes constant, further evaluation is necessary to exclude other causes (for example, pseudocyst, mass, ductal obstruction or stones, and peptic ulcers).

Persistent pain is treated in a stepwise approach beginning with simple analgesics, tramadol, low-dose tricyclic antidepressants, and gabapentinoids (gabapentin and pregabalin). Initiating opioids other than tramadol is reasonable while developing a pain management program, but an important goal is to control pain with opioid-sparing adjunctive agents to minimize chronic narcotic use, owing to concerns of opioid dependence and gastrointestinal side effects. Pancreatic enzymes help relieve symptoms of steatorrhea, and immediate-release (non–enteric-coated) enzymes may help reduce pain in patients with nonalcoholic chronic pancreatitis by decreasing pancreatic stimulation. The use of antioxidants for pain relief is controversial. Percutaneous or EUS-guided celiac plexus blockade using glucocorticoids provides only short-term pain relief in 50% of patients, but it helps guide therapy by classifying pain as visceral or nonvisceral (central).

In persistent or refractory pain, several treatment options are available based on anatomic location. In patients with a dilated pancreatic duct and intraductal calcifications, options include endoscopic stenting, lithotripsy, and surgical drainage (pancreaticojejunostomy). Pancreaticojejunostomy provides superior short- and long-term pain relief. Disease limited to a specific segment of the pancreas may warrant localized resection, such as a pancreaticoduodenectomy for symptomatic obstruction or concern for cancer within the pancreatic head, versus a distal pancreatectomy for disease limited to the pancreatic tail. In patients with a nondilated pancreatic duct ("small-duct" disease), there is no established medical or surgical treatment for pain, but some patients are offered partial or total pancreatectomy.

Exocrine pancreatic insufficiency is treated with enzymes containing 90,000 United States Pharmacopeia (USP) units of lipase (equivalent to 30,000 international units [IU]) with meals, and a half dose with snacks. Patients should be screened and treated for fat-soluble vitamin deficiencies. Diabetes associated with chronic pancreatitis is typically labile and may be difficult to manage.

KEY POINT

- Patients with chronic pancreatitis should be counseled to stop smoking and drinking alcohol.

Pancreatic Adenocarcinoma

The 5-year survival rate for pancreatic adenocarcinoma remains low at 5%. Diagnoses exceed 45,000 annually, and more than 80% of patients die owing to unresectable disease at presentation and ineffective treatments except curative surgical resection.

Strong risk factors for pancreatic cancer are age greater than 50 years, family history of pancreatic cancer (present in 16%), cigarette smoking, chronic pancreatitis, obesity, diabetes, and intraductal papillary mucinous neoplasms. Hereditary pancreatitis is a rare condition associated with a 40% to 55% lifetime risk of pancreatic cancer; the diagnosis is usually made by recognizing an autosomal dominant pattern of inheritance and by commercially available genetic screening to detect cationic trypsinogen (*PRSS1*) gene mutations.

KEY POINTS

- The 5-year survival rate for pancreatic adenocarcinoma remains low at 5%.
- Strong risk factors for pancreatic cancer are age greater than 50 years, family history of pancreatic cancer, cigarette smoking, chronic pancreatitis, obesity, diabetes mellitus, and intraductal papillary mucinous neoplasms.

Clinical Presentation

The most common presenting symptoms of pancreatic cancer are weight loss, abdominal pain, and jaundice. Jaundice is characteristic of tumors located in the pancreatic head (the most common location). Back pain is characteristic of tumors that are located in the body or tail of the pancreas and affect the celiac ganglia. Patients rarely present with acute pancreatitis. Most patients have abnormal glucose tolerance, and approximately 50% have diabetes. Two thirds of patients have new-onset diabetes within the 36 months prior to the cancer diagnosis.

Patients with pancreatic cancer and jaundice occasionally have Courvoisier sign (palpable gallbladder due to distal bile duct compression) and rarely paraneoplastic manifestations, such as pancreatic panniculitis (tender red-purple ulcerated subcutaneous nodules) or Trousseau syndrome (migratory thrombophlebitis). Signs of advanced disease include an abdominal mass, ascites, and supraclavicular lymphadenopathy (Virchow node).

KEY POINT

- The most common presenting symptoms of pancreatic cancer are weight loss, abdominal pain, and jaundice.

Diagnosis and Staging

Screening tests for pancreatic cancer do not improve survival but are recommended for (1) patients aged 50 years or older with idiopathic pancreatitis or with abdominal symptoms and new-onset diabetes; (2) patients older than 40 to 50 years with a family history or hereditary syndrome conferring more than 5% lifetime risk (such as selected patients with Peutz-Jeghers syndrome, familial atypical multiple mole melanoma syndrome, Lynch syndrome, hereditary pancreatitis, or germline mutations in the *BRCA2* gene); and (3) patients with pancreatic cancer precursors, intraductal papillary mucinous neoplasm, and high-grade pancreatic intraepithelial neoplasia. Recommended screening and surveillance tests are EUS or

MRI/magnetic resonance cholangiopancreatography, but there is a lack of consensus of how often to screen patients and when to refer to surgery for many high-risk groups.

In patients in whom pancreatic cancer is suspected, contrast-enhanced multidetector CT has 90% sensitivity for detecting malignancy (**Figure 17**). CT also provides staging information. EUS does not significantly affect staging but has greater sensitivity in detecting tumors smaller than 2 cm and allows tissue diagnosis by fine-needle aspiration (FNA) when required.

The need for EUS-FNA is variable. It may be indicated to establish a diagnosis prior to neoadjuvant or palliative radiochemotherapy and to exclude unusual tumors or pseudotumors that would not benefit from surgery. FNA is usually unnecessary in surgical candidates with potentially resectable tumors because negative results (with a relatively low negative predictive value) do not affect management.

For staging and treatment of pancreatic adenocarcinoma, see MKSAP 17 Hematology and Oncology.

KEY POINT

- Contrast-enhanced multidetector CT has 90% sensitivity for detecting pancreatic malignancy.

Ampullary Adenocarcinoma

Ampullary adenocarcinoma is rare and develops from premalignant adenomas. Compared with pancreatic adenocarcinoma, the 5-year survival rate is much higher, ranging from 37% to 68%. Tumors causing obstructive jaundice lead to diagnosis at an earlier stage. Up to 50% of adenomas contain a focus of adenocarcinoma. Reliable differentiation between adenoma and adenocarcinoma often requires EUS. Whereas endoscopic mucosal biopsies have a high false-negative rate (25%-50%), EUS-directed biopsy has 90% diagnostic accuracy. EUS is superior to MRI and CT for staging.

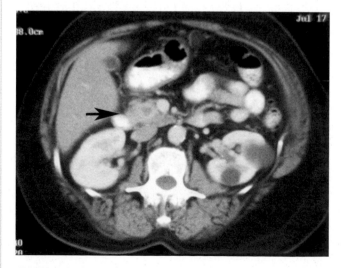

FIGURE 17. CT scan of pancreatic adenocarcinoma, with a large mass in the head of the pancreas (*arrow*).

Only 10% of tumors are limited to the ampulla of Vater at the time of diagnosis (stage T1); these tumors are amenable to endoscopic ampullectomy. Careful staging is essential because 8% to 45% of T1 lesions have lymph node metastases that confer a 70% reduction in median survival compared with lymph node–negative T1N0 tumors. Greater T-stage tumors and/or lymph node metastases require pancreaticoduodenectomy. However, only 40% of patients undergo surgery, primarily because many patients with ampullary adenocarcinoma are older (median 65 years) and/or have a poor operative status.

Autoimmune Pancreatitis and IgG4 Disease

Autoimmune pancreatitis (AIP) is rare and has an unclear pathogenesis. Type I AIP is a systemic fibroinflammatory disease, defined as an inflammatory condition causing tissue damage and scarring. Pancreatic involvement is only one manifestation of a systemic IgG4 disease that encompasses multiple autoimmune conditions, including Sjögren syndrome, primary sclerosing cholangitis, and inflammatory bowel disease. Type II AIP is characterized by an idiopathic duct-centric chronic pancreatitis without elevated levels of IgG4 or systemic disease. Type II is frequently associated with inflammatory bowel disease (30%).

For more information on IgG4-related disease, see MKSAP 17 Rheumatology.

Clinical Presentation and Diagnosis

Patients with AIP typically have painless obstructive jaundice and cross-sectional imaging evidence of focal or diffuse "sausage-shaped" pancreatic enlargement with a featureless border (**Figure 18**). Pancreatic adenocarcinoma must be excluded. AIP presents rarely with acute pancreatitis.

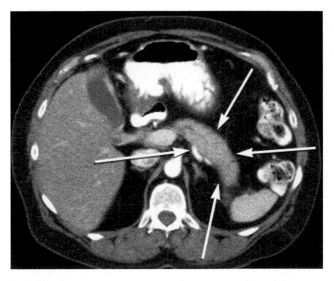

FIGURE 18. CT scan demonstrating autoimmune pancreatitis with the classic "sausage-shaped" pancreas (*arrows*).

Type I AIP typically presents in older men (mean age of onset in the fifth decade of life). Biliary involvement is common and is known as IgG4-associated cholangitis. Diagnosis is fulfilled by a combination of five criteria: (1) cross-sectional imaging abnormalities as described in the previous paragraph and pancreatography showing duct narrowing without upstream dilation, (2) increased serum IgG4 level, (3) extrapancreatic organ involvement, (4) compatible histopathology, and (5) response to glucocorticoid therapy.

Type II AIP has an equal gender distribution and an age of onset in the fourth decade of life. Definitive diagnosis requires histology because imaging findings and response to glucocorticoids are similar to type I, but serologic abnormalities and extrapancreatic organ involvement are absent.

KEY POINT

- Autoimmune pancreatitis is typically characterized by painless obstructive jaundice and cross-sectional imaging evidence of focal or diffuse "sausage-shaped" pancreatic enlargement with a featureless border.

Treatment

Almost all patients (>90%) enter clinical remission in response to glucocorticoids. Those with jaundice typically require biliary stenting. Relapse is more common in type I AIP versus type II (30% versus 10%). Patients with relapse typically respond to glucocorticoid retreatment. To avoid glucocorticoid-induced complications, glucocorticoid-sparing immunomodulators (azathioprine, 6-mercaptopurine, and mycophenolate mofetil) may be offered to patients who have single or multiple relapses and cannot be weaned from glucocorticoids. Rituximab, a monoclonal antibody, has also been found to be successful in those with recurrent disease or glucocorticoid dependency.

KEY POINT

- Almost all patients with autoimmune pancreatitis enter clinical remission in response to glucocorticoids; however, relapse is common.

Cystic Neoplasms of the Pancreas

Pancreatic cysts are common, affecting 2.5% of asymptomatic individuals; prevalence is 10% in persons aged 70 years or older.

Pancreatic cysts are classified as pancreatic cystic neoplasms (the most common), nonneoplastic pancreatic cysts, and pseudocysts. The two most common pancreatic cystic neoplasms are mucinous cystic neoplasms (MCNs) and intraductal papillary mucinous neoplasms (IPMNs) (**Figure 19**), which involve the main duct, branch ducts, or both. Most pancreatic cysts are branch-duct IPMNs.

Figure 20 summarizes the general clinical approach to pancreatic cystic lesions and a specific approach to suspected IPMNs and MCNs.

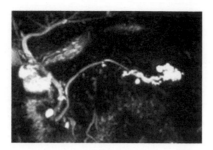

FIGURE 19. Magnetic resonance cholangiopancreatography demonstrating main-duct intraductal papillary mucinous neoplasm in the pancreatic tail.

Recent American Gastroenterological Association (AGA) guidelines recommend surveillance based on cyst characteristics (size < or ≥3 cm, presence of a solid component, pancreatic duct dilation); recommend MRI for surveillance; and provide parameters for stopping surveillance for stable cysts.

Main-duct and mixed-type IPMNs appear radiologically as a main-duct dilation often extending into branch ducts; 80% of patients have symptoms and 65% develop malignancy. Resection is recommended for surgical candidates. Branch-duct IPMNs are typically asymptomatic and have a lower incidence of malignancy (20%). Surveillance is usually indicated rather than resection.

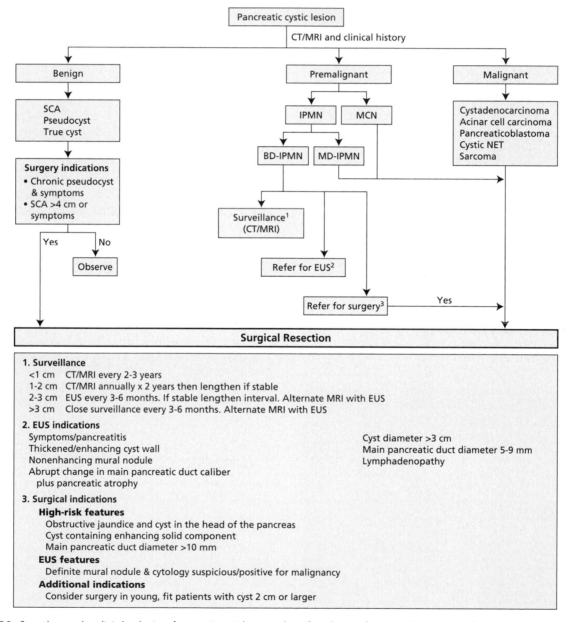

FIGURE 20. General approach to clinical evaluation of pancreatic cystic lesions and specific evaluation of suspected intraductal papillary mucinous neoplasms and mucinous cystic neoplasms. BD-IPMN = branch-duct intraductal papillary mucinous neoplasm; EUS = endoscopic ultrasound; IPMN = intraductal papillary mucinous neoplasm; MCN = mucinous cystic neoplasm; MD-IPMN = main-duct intraductal papillary mucinous neoplasm; NET = neuroendocrine tumor; SCA = serous cyst adenoma.

Adapted with permission of Current Science, Inc., from Turner BG, Brugge WR. Pancreatic cystic lesions: when to watch, when to operate, and when to ignore. Curr Gastroenterol Rep. 2010 Apr;12(2):98-105. [PMID: 20424981]; permission conveyed through Copyright Clearance Center, Inc.

MCNs most frequently occur in the body and tail of the pancreas, have ovarian stroma present on histology, and have an 18% incidence of malignancy. Resection is recommended.

Diagnosis of solitary cysts is challenging. It may require EUS-FNA to distinguish between cystic neoplasms (branch-duct IPMNs, MCNs, and serous tumors) and pseudocysts based on cytology (see Figure 20). Diagnosis may also require cyst fluid measurement; IMPNs and MCNs are high in carcinoembryonic antigen, and pseudocysts are high in amylase.

KEY POINT

- The two most common pancreatic cystic neoplasms are mucinous cystic neoplasms and intraductal papillary mucinous neoplasms, which involve the main duct, branch ducts, or both.

Pancreatic Neuroendocrine Tumors

Pancreatic neuroendocrine (islet cell) tumors arise from pluripotent cells in the pancreatic ductal/acinar system and represent 3% of primary pancreatic neoplasms. Of all pancreatic neuroendocrine tumors, 75% to 90% are nonfunctional and are typically large (mean, 4 cm) and symptomatic (pancreatitis, abdominal pain, jaundice, weight loss) related to local mass effect or metastatic disease. Frequent use of abdominal imag-ing occasionally identifies patients with incidental, asymptomatic, and earlier-stage neoplasms. Ten percent to 25% of neuroendocrine tumors are functional and hypersecrete hormones, most commonly gastrin and insulin (**Table 13**). Most patients are older and have sporadic tumors. Younger patients may have heritable conditions. Those with von Hippel-Lindau disease typically have nonfunctional tumors, and those with multiple endocrine neoplasia type 1 typically have nonfunctional tumors or gastrinomas.

Testing focuses on determining the functional status of the tumor (see Table 13) and localizing it by cross-sectional CT or MRI imaging. Occult lesions require EUS (90% sensitivity) and pentetreotide scintigraphy (octreotide scanning). Insulinomas and gastrinomas are typically small. Insulinomas are differentiated from gastrinomas by having a typical solitary appearance and inadequate expression of somatostatin receptors to be detected by octreotide scanning. Insulinomas cause hypoglycemia, and gastrinomas produce symptoms related to oversecretion of gastric acid (diarrhea, esophagitis, peptic ulcer disease). Less common pancreatic neuroendocrine tumors are typically larger (>5 cm) and have other clinical profiles (see Table 13).

Localized tumors should be resected owing to the risk of metastases. Metastatic disease has limited treatment options. Hormone-derived symptoms are typically treated

TABLE 13. Clinical Characteristics of Pancreatic Neuroendocrine Tumors

Tumor Type	Hormone	Symptoms	Diagnostic Criteria
Nonfunctional (75%-90%)			
Nonfunctional	None	None or symptoms related to local mass effect or metastatic disease May metastasize Associated with MEN1 and VHL	Mass on imaging, typically large (mean, 4 cm) and symptomatic from mass effect (pancreatitis, abdominal pain, jaundice, weight loss) No elevated hormones
Functional (10%-25%)			
Most common			
Gastrinoma	Gastrin	Peptic ulcer disease, diarrhea, esophagitis (Zollinger-Ellison syndrome) Associated with MEN1	Elevated serum gastrin >1000 pg/mL (1000 ng/L), secretin stimulation test
Insulinoma	Insulin	Hypoglycemia Associated with MEN1	Inappropriately high insulin and C-peptide levels during hypoglycemia
Uncommon and rarely associated with MEN1			
VIPoma	Vasoactive intestinal peptide	Watery diarrhea, hypokalemia, hypochlorhydria	Elevated serum VIP level >75 pg/mL (75 ng/L)
Glucagonoma	Glucagon	Dermatitis (necrolytic migratory erythema), diabetes mellitus	Elevated serum glucagon >1000 pg/mL (1000 ng/L)
Somatostatinoma	Somatostatin	Triad of gallstones, diabetes, and diarrhea	Elevated somatostatin
GHRHoma	Growth hormone-releasing hormone	Acromegaly	Elevated GHRH

GHRH = growth hormone-releasing hormone; MEN1 = multiple endocrine neoplasia type 1; VHL = von Hippel-Lindau disease; VIP = vasoactive intestinal peptide.

with somatostatin analogues or therapy to control symptoms of hormone secretion (for example, proton pump inhibitors for gastrinoma). Other treatments include molecularly targeted agents (everolimus or sunitinib), chemotherapy, hepatic artery embolization, and possibly radiolabeled somatostatin analogues.

KEY POINTS

- Of all pancreatic neuroendocrine tumors, 75% to 90% are nonfunctional; 10% to 25% are functional and hypersecrete hormones, most commonly gastrin and insulin.

- Localized pancreatic neuroendocrine tumors should be resected owing to the risk of metastases.

Disorders of the Small and Large Bowel

Diarrhea

Characterization

Diarrhea can be defined by high stool frequency (>3 per day) or abnormally loose stools; however, some patients use the term to describe urgency or fecal incontinence. In addition, some patients refer to an increase in stool frequency without an increase in stool liquidity as diarrhea. This phenomenon is referred to as hyperdefecation and often is seen in irritable bowel syndrome (IBS) and hyperthyroidism. However, hyperdefecation also can be seen in conditions that decrease rectal compliance, such as rectal cancer, and therefore deserves evaluation even if it is not true diarrhea. Normal stool weight should be 200 g/d or less. Stool weights above 200 g/d are sometimes used to define diarrhea, but stool weight is influenced by factors such as fiber intake. In the absence of abnormal consistency, weight alone is not an ideal indicator.

Most cases of diarrhea in developed countries are acute (<4 weeks' duration). Chronic diarrhea (>4 weeks' duration) occurs in 1% to 5% of adults in developed countries.

Chronic diarrhea is classified into five broad categories based on history, physical examination, and diagnostic tests (**Table 14**). Approaching chronic diarrhea using these subclassifications helps focus the differential diagnosis, direct the evaluation, and decrease costs of testing. However, some causes of chronic diarrhea do not fit into only one category.

Evaluation and Management

The majority of acute diarrhea in developed countries is due to viral gastroenteritis or foodborne illness and is self-limited. In these cases, the yield of testing (such as stool cultures) is low,

TABLE 14.	Classification of Chronic Diarrhea	
Category	**Clinical Features**	**Examples**
Secretory	Large-volume, watery stools	Medications (e.g., colchicine, NSAIDs)
	Does not stop with fasting	SIBO
		Hormone-producing tumors (e.g., gastrinoma, VIPoma, carcinoid, somatostatinoma)
		Bile acid malabsorption
		Noninvasive infections (e.g., cholera)
Osmotic	Diarrhea stops with fasting	Medications (e.g., magnesium sulfate laxative)
	Bloating, gas	Carbohydrate malabsorption
Steatorrhea	Bulky, greasy, oily, malodorous stools	Pancreatic insufficiency
	Weight loss	Small-bowel mucosal disease (e.g., celiac disease)
		SIBO
		Bile acid deficiency
		Lymphatic obstruction
Impaired motility	Bloating, nausea	Diabetes mellitus
	Features of underlying disorder	Postsurgery
		Hyperthyroidism
		Scleroderma
Inflammatory	Abdominal pain +/− fever, bleeding, weight loss	Inflammatory bowel disease
		Invasive/inflammatory infections (e.g., *Clostridium difficile*)
		Ischemia

SIBO = small intestinal bacterial overgrowth; VIP = vasoactive intestinal peptide.

and the monetary cost per positive test is unacceptably high. In the absence of alarm features (**Table 15**), supportive care with attention to fluid balance is often sufficient. In immunocompetent patients, acute infectious diarrhea usually resolves within 1 week. Elderly patients and those with multiple or severe comorbidities require close follow-up. A careful review of medication history (including nonprescription medications and supplements) is indicated to look for drugs that cause diarrhea. If diarrhea does not resolve in 1 week, evaluation is recommended. Stool testing for common bacterial pathogens, including *Clostridium difficile*, should be performed. See MKSAP 17 Infectious Disease for further discussion of infectious diarrhea.

In patients with chronic diarrhea, clinical features help direct the evaluation (**Table 16**). A basic laboratory evaluation (complete blood count, electrolytes, creatinine) is recommended to assess for anemia (suggesting blood loss or malabsorption as part of the diarrheal process), leukocytosis

TABLE 15. Alarm Features Requiring Evaluation in Patients with Acute Diarrhea

Severe abdominal pain

Bloody stools

Fever

Recent hospitalization or antimicrobial use

Special populations

    Elderly patients

    Immunocompromised patients

    Patients with inflammatory bowel disease

    Pregnant patients

TABLE 16. Key Clinical Features of Chronic Diarrhea

Symptoms

    Diarrhea pattern and duration

    Rome criteria for irritable bowel syndrome

Associated symptoms

    Extraintestinal manifestations of inflammatory bowel disease

Medical history

Family history

Exposures

    Changes in diet

    Ingestion of nonabsorbable carbohydrates (lactose, fructose, dietary sweeteners)

    Recent travel

    Sick contacts

    Medications

Physical examination

    Rash

(suggesting an inflammatory cause of diarrhea), electrolyte disturbances, and dehydration. Additional testing is dictated by the prioritized differential diagnosis, as discussed below.

Infectious causes of chronic diarrhea are uncommon in immunocompetent adults in developed countries, except for infection with *Giardia lamblia* (see MKSAP 17 Infectious Disease). Giardia infection should be considered in patients with exposure to young children or potentially contaminated water such as lakes and streams.

As in acute diarrhea, a careful review of medications (including nonprescription medications and supplements) is indicated to assess for drugs that cause diarrhea.

Patients older than 50 years should undergo colonoscopy to screen for colorectal cancer. Patients younger than 50 years should also have colonoscopy if features of inflammatory bowel disease are present. Any patient undergoing colonoscopy to evaluate diarrhea should have inspection of the terminal ileum (to assess for Crohn disease) and random biopsies of the colonic mucosa (to assess for microscopic colitis). Sigmoidoscopy is not recommended in most patients because it does not evaluate the proximal colon or terminal ileum.

If this initial evaluation does not disclose an underlying diagnosis, a combination of stool tests should be performed to subclassify the type of diarrhea. A 48- to 72-hour stool collection with analysis of fat content measures the amount of diarrhea and steatorrhea. Normal fat excretion is less than 7 g/d (in patients consuming 100 g/d of fat); however, this may be increased nonspecifically by any diarrheal disorder to 12 to 14 g/d. Fat excretion above 14 g/d is diagnostic of steatorrhea. Patients with steatorrhea should undergo evaluation for small-bowel mucosal disorders (celiac disease, Whipple disease), small intestinal bacterial overgrowth (SIBO), and pancreatic insufficiency. See Malabsorption for further discussion of malabsorption syndromes, including celiac disease and SIBO. Pancreatic insufficiency may be difficult to diagnose, particularly in early disease. Abdominal imaging may show calcification, but this finding may also be absent. CT scan is more sensitive than plain radiographs in detecting pancreatic calcifications. Endoscopic ultrasound is more sensitive than CT scan or endoscopic retrograde cholangiopancreatography in diagnosing chronic pancreatitis, but it does not assess pancreatic function. Tests of pancreatic function are not widely available and have several limitations. Therefore, an empiric trial of pancreatic enzymes is often used as a diagnostic test when chronic pancreatitis is suspected.

In patients with true diarrhea but without steatorrhea, measurement of stool electrolytes can be helpful to categorize the diarrhea so that more targeted testing can later be performed. Measurement of fecal sodium and potassium allows calculation of the osmotic gap, as follows:

$$290 - 2 \times [\text{stool sodium} + \text{stool potassium}]$$

A gap greater than 100 mOsm/kg (100 mmol/kg) indicates an osmotic diarrhea, signifying that some ingested osmotic agent is promoting the diarrheal process. If the gap is less than 50 mOsm/kg (50 mmol/kg), the diarrhea is secretory rather than osmotic. A gap between 50 and 100 mOsm/kg (50 and 100 mmol/kg) is equivocal. Although the measured osmolality is typically not used to calculate the gap (as the stool osmolality should always be 290 mOsm/kg [290 mmol/kg]), it can be helpful if there is concern about the adequacy of the stool collection, given that the osmolality is less than 290 mOsm/kg (290 mmol/kg) when water or dilute urine has been added. Alternatively, bacterial fermentation in the stool sample can lead to falsely elevated results of the measured osmolality.

Finally, a stool test for inflammation (such as fecal leukocytes, calprotectin, or lactoferrin) should be completed if colonoscopy has not already been performed.

Based on clinical features and the results of the fecal fat study, stool electrolyte measurements, and testing for inflammation, diarrhea can often be categorized into one of the five subtypes (see Table 14), which directs further evaluation.

The evaluation of acute and chronic diarrhea is described in **Figure 21**.

KEY POINTS

HVC
- The majority of acute diarrhea in developed countries is due to viral gastroenteritis or foodborne illness and is self-limited; the yield of diagnostic testing (such as stool cultures) is low, and the monetary cost per positive test is unacceptably high.

- Patients with chronic diarrhea who are older than 50 years should undergo colonoscopy to screen for colorectal cancer.

Malabsorption

Malabsorption can be a generalized process or can involve each specific nutrient class (carbohydrate, lipid, protein) individually. For a discussion of the diagnosis and approach to fat malabsorption, see Diarrhea.

Celiac Disease

Celiac disease is a chronic inflammatory enteropathy caused by an immune-mediated reaction to gluten and gliadins, proteins that are present in wheat and other grains. Celiac disease is present in 0.5% to 1% of the population; however, many patients are undiagnosed owing to the nonspecific and variable manifestations of this disorder. The classic presentation of malabsorption (weight loss, steatorrhea, nutritional deficiencies) now occurs in a small proportion of patients owing to better recognition of earlier presentations. Chronic diarrhea and abdominal pain are common features; however, diarrhea may be absent. Other signs and symptoms include a unique, characteristic skin rash (dermatitis herpetiformis), osteopenia, iron deficiency anemia, abnormal liver chemistry studies, infertility, and a variety of neurologic symptoms. Long-standing celiac disease is associated with intestinal lymphoma and adenocarcinoma. Although these associations are strong, the absolute risk of a malignant complication is low, especially in patients who respond to a gluten-free diet.

The diagnosis of celiac disease requires positive serologic markers and a compatible small-bowel biopsy.

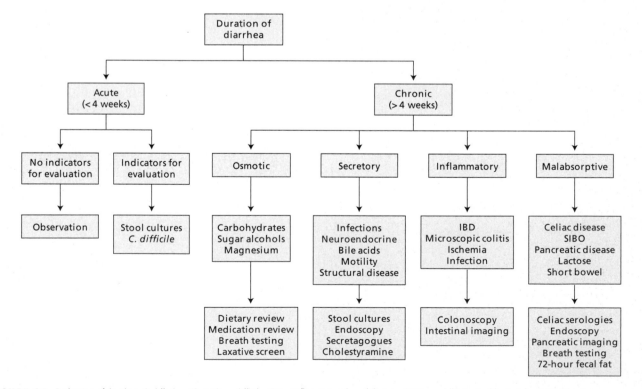

FIGURE 21. Evaluation of diarrhea. *C. difficile* = *Clostridium difficile*; IBD = inflammatory bowel disease; SIBO = small intestinal bacterial overgrowth.

IgA tissue transglutaminase (tTG) antibodies and endomysial antibodies (EMA) are sensitive and specific serologic markers; testing for these should be done while the patient is consuming gluten. Celiac serologic studies may be negative in patients with IgA deficiency, in those with mild disease and limited small-bowel damage, and in those who have restricted dietary gluten. Other serologic studies, such as gliadin antibodies, have poor sensitivity and specificity and should not be used. Newer serologic studies for deaminated gliadin peptides (DGPs) have superior test characteristics compared with traditional gliadin antibodies, which are no longer recommended in clinical practice. Although serologic testing for anti-DGPs has not proved to be superior to tTG antibody testing (IgA tTG remains the serologic screening test of choice), studies for anti-DGPs could be performed in patients with borderline tTG results or discordant serologic and histologic findings to help ascertain the diagnosis.

The classic findings on small-bowel histology are intraepithelial lymphocytosis, crypt elongation, and villous blunting (**Figure 22**). Mild cases may show only lymphocytosis (stage 1) or hyperplasia (stage 2). Villous blunting can be partial (stage 3) or complete (stage 4). However, these changes are not specific for celiac disease (**Table 17**); therefore, the diagnosis also relies on positive serologic tests.

If the diagnosis is unclear (such as in patients with equivocal or conflicting biopsies or serologies) or if a patient is following a gluten-free diet when serologic studies are performed, *HLA* haplotyping may be helpful.

The treatment of celiac disease is with a strict gluten-free diet. Symptom improvement often occurs within a few weeks, but histologic remission may take several months or years. Patients whose symptoms do not respond to the diet or who relapse while on it should be assessed for gluten exposure, microscopic colitis, collagenous or refractory sprue,

TABLE 17. Differential Diagnosis of Small-Bowel Villous Blunting
Celiac disease
Tropical sprue
Radiation enteropathy
Severe giardiasis
SIBO
Chronic ischemia
Chemotherapy
Graft-versus-host disease
Crohn disease
Autoimmune enteropathy
Enteropathy-associated T-cell lymphoma
Common variable immunodeficiency
Cow's milk or other dietary protein allergy
Medications (olmesartan)

SIBO = small intestinal bacterial overgrowth.

small-bowel lymphoma or adenocarcinoma, and other causes of diarrhea as discussed previously. Risk factors for a malignant complication include advanced age and long-standing, poorly controlled disease.

Repeat small-bowel biopsies are no longer required to show healing if there is a clear response to a gluten-free diet; however, patients with atypical features at disease onset may benefit from follow-up histology to ensure mucosal healing. Mucosal healing may take years in adults despite strict adherence to a gluten-free diet and may never be complete.

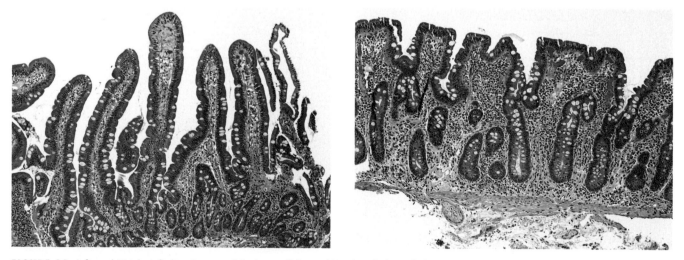

FIGURE 22. *Left panel:* Histologic findings in a normal duodenum. *Right panel:* Histologic findings of celiac disease, with villous atrophy, crypt hyperplasia, and increased inflammatory infiltration of the lamina propria.

Courtesy of Thomas C. Smyrk, MD, Division of Anatomic Pathology, Mayo Clinic.

- The diagnosis of celiac disease requires positive serologic markers (IgA tissue transglutaminase antibodies or endomysial antibodies) and a compatible small-bowel biopsy.
- The treatment of celiac disease is with a strict gluten-free diet.

Small Intestinal Bacterial Overgrowth

Small intestinal bacterial overgrowth (SIBO) causes diarrhea, often with bloating, flatulence, and weight loss. A clue to the diagnosis of SIBO is the combination of vitamin B_{12} deficiency (due to bacterial consumption) and an elevated serum folate level (due to bacterial production). Several conditions can predispose patients to SIBO, owing to effects on stomach acid, intestinal transit, or disruption of normal antibacterial defense mechanisms (**Table 18**). Gastric bypass surgery is an increasingly common cause of SIBO owing to the obesity epidemic and more frequent use of bariatric surgery as a treatment.

The small intestine normally has very few bacteria, with proximal jejunal bacterial counts less than 10^4/mL. SIBO is therefore typically defined as a bacterial count greater than 10^5/mL; however, in practice it is difficult to obtain cultures from the proximal jejunum. Furthermore, this practice is expensive because endoscopy is required to obtain the sample. Although not without shortcomings (low sensitivity and specificity), hydrogen breath testing provides the simplest and most widely available diagnostic modality for suspected SIBO. Alternatively, and in areas where hydrogen breath testing is not available, SIBO has been diagnosed based on a response to a trial of antimicrobial therapy. However, this practice may lead to inappropriate use of antibiotics in patients who do not have SIBO (for example, those with IBS). Therefore, empiric antibiotics should only be considered in patients with symptoms compatible with SIBO and one or more risk factors (see Table 18).

A variety of antimicrobial agents are effective for the treatment of SIBO. Because many conditions that predispose to SIBO are irreversible, patients often need repeat courses of antimicrobial agents. In these cases, many clinicians use rotating antimicrobial agents (cycling between three to four different classes) to avoid the development of bacterial resistance. Patients with SIBO may also have lactose intolerance, perhaps owing to the effect of small-bowel inflammation on brush border enzymes. Therefore, a lactose-free diet should be considered if the response to antimicrobial agents is incomplete.

- Small intestinal bacterial overgrowth may be characterized by diarrhea, bloating, flatulence, weight loss, vitamin B_{12} deficiency, and an elevated serum folate level.

Short-Bowel Syndrome

Short-bowel syndrome (SBS) arises when a large portion of the small intestine is resected or diseased. Causes of SBS are massive resection or bowel dysfunction related to ischemia, radiation enteropathy, Crohn disease, or trauma. SBS typically does not occur until less than 200 cm of healthy small intestine remains. However, the risk for SBS is lower if the colon is intact. The colon can adapt to increase fluid and electrolyte absorption, and colonic bacteria can salvage malabsorbed nutrients through fermentation to short-chain fatty acids. When SBS is present, the remaining bowel has insufficient absorptive area to meet minimal nutrient, fluid, and/or electrolyte needs. Patients with SBS present with voluminous diarrhea, weight loss, and evidence of malnutrition. Treatment focuses on ensuring adequate caloric, electrolyte, and fluid balance through the oral, enteral, and/or parenteral routes.

- Short-bowel syndrome arises when a large portion of the small intestine is resected or diseased; it typically does not occur until less than 200 cm of healthy small intestine remains.

Carbohydrate Malabsorption

Carbohydrate malabsorption is relatively common but is often overlooked. Malabsorbed carbohydrates are fermented by colonic bacteria and produce osmotically active substances that cause diarrhea and gas, which causes bloating, discomfort, and flatulence. A careful dietary history is essential in the evaluation of a patient with chronic diarrhea.

Lactose, the primary carbohydrate in cow's milk and other dairy products, is the most commonly malabsorbed carbohydrate. Lactose must be cleaved to glucose and galactose by the enzyme lactase in the brush border of the small intestine in order to be absorbed. In many adults, the amount of lactase present may be marginal or its expression is lost, leading to lactose intolerance. The prevalence of lactose intolerance shows geographic and racial

TABLE 18. Conditions Associated with Small Intestinal Bacterial Overgrowth
Disorders of Acid Secretion
Achlorhydria
Antrectomy/vagotomy
Prolonged used of high-dose acid suppressive medications
Disorders of Bowel Transit
Blind limbs
Small-bowel diverticula
Small-bowel strictures
Dysmotility (diabetic enteropathy, systemic sclerosis, pseudo-obstruction)
Disruption of Normal Antibacterial Mechanisms
Resection of ileocecal valve
Immunoglobulin deficiency (for example, CVID, IgA deficiency)
Loss of biliary or pancreatic secretions
CVID = common variable immunodeficiency.

variation. For example, it is lowest in northern Europeans (approximately 10%), more common in southern European and Middle Eastern populations (approximately 40%), and most common in Asian populations (up to 90%). Lactose intolerance is not absolute; patients are usually able to tolerate variable amounts of lactose.

Lactose malabsorption often is diagnosed by history (bloating, cramps, and/or diarrhea related to dairy intake) and confirmed by resolution of symptoms with lactose avoidance. In equivocal cases, the diagnosis can be made with hydrogen breath testing. Treatment includes avoidance of lactose-containing products or administration of lactase whenever dairy products are consumed.

Fructose malabsorption is also relatively common. It is often overlooked because clinicians and patients do not recognize the presence of fructose in many processed foods, typically in the form of high-fructose corn syrup. Fresh fruits and fruit juices can also cause diarrhea if ingested in excess because the absorption of fructose has a maximum threshold. Fructose intolerance also may be diagnosed by careful history, including resolution of symptoms with dietary avoidance. In equivocal cases, hydrogen breath testing can be helpful.

Sugar alcohols (sorbitol, xylitol, maltitol, and others) are used as artificial sweeteners in sugar-free diet foods, candies, gums, and drinks. These carbohydrates have little or no absorption in the small intestine and, when taken in excess, cause symptoms of carbohydrate malabsorption. Breath tests exist for some sugar alcohols, but the diagnosis is generally made by a careful history.

KEY POINTS

- Lactose, the primary carbohydrate in cow's milk and other dairy products, is the most commonly malabsorbed carbohydrate.
- Fructose malabsorption is often overlooked because clinicians and patients do not recognize the presence of fructose in many processed foods, typically in the form of high-fructose corn syrup.

Inflammatory Bowel Disease

Inflammatory bowel disease (IBD) is characterized by idiopathic gastrointestinal inflammation and is divided primarily into Crohn disease (CD) and ulcerative colitis (UC). A subset of patients has indeterminate colitis, which is characterized by clinical features and test results that do not allow a definitive classification.

Risk Factors

IBD is believed to be related to interplay between genetic and environmental factors. There is an increased risk of IBD in family members, which provides evidence for a genetic component. Monozygotic twins have a higher risk than dizygotic twins or siblings. The risk of IBD in an offspring is higher if both parents are affected. Certain ethnic groups (for example, Jewish patients) are at a higher risk than others (for example, black patients). Genes associated with IBD have been identified in recent years, but the contribution of each individual gene to the overall population with IBD is small.

Environmental risk factors have also been recognized. Cigarette smoking is a risk factor for the development of CD, whereas it is a protective factor for UC. A variety of dietary factors have been proposed, but the results of studies in this area have been inconsistent. IBD is more common in developed countries, which suggests that environmental factors in developed countries are causative or that factors in underdeveloped countries are protective. For example, the hygiene hypothesis suggests that exposure to infectious or other environmental factors in underdeveloped countries may promote immune tolerance and a lower risk of autoimmune diseases like IBD. A north-south gradient (with a higher risk of IBD in northern climates) has been identified, suggesting that a factor such as vitamin D may be involved.

Clinical Manifestations

Symptoms in an individual patient with IBD are related to the location and severity of inflammation and the presence of complications or extraintestinal manifestations. These factors are nonspecific and variable between patients, which may lead to diagnostic difficulty.

Ulcerative Colitis

UC typically presents with bloody diarrhea and abdominal discomfort, the severity of which is related to the extent and severity of inflammation. The distribution of UC is generally divided into proctitis (involving the rectum only), left-sided colitis (inflammation does not extend beyond the splenic flexure), and pancolitis (inflammation extends above the splenic flexure). Some patients with distal inflammation can present with constipation owing to rectal spasm and stasis of stool. Because UC typically involves the rectum, tenesmus, urgency, rectal pain, and fecal incontinence are common. Fever and weight loss are uncommon and suggest severe disease.

With mild disease, the physical examination may be normal. Severe disease may be characterized by fever, tachycardia, dehydration, abdominal tenderness, or pallor. Abdominal distention, hypoactive bowel sounds, and rebound tenderness suggest perforation or megacolon. Laboratory findings, such as significant anemia, leukocytosis, hypoalbuminemia, and electrolyte abnormalities, also reflect the severity of disease.

KEY POINT

- Ulcerative colitis typically presents with bloody diarrhea and abdominal discomfort; tenesmus, urgency, rectal pain, and fecal incontinence are common.

Crohn Disease

Common symptoms of CD are abdominal pain, diarrhea, and weight loss; fever and overt gastrointestinal bleeding are less common than is typically seen in UC. Additionally, unlike UC, the transmural inflammation seen in CD may predispose to fistula formation. Given the variable distribution of inflammation in CD, the symptoms can vary considerably between patients. Thirty percent of patients have isolated small-bowel disease, 40% have ileocolonic inflammation, and 25% have isolated colonic disease. The other 5% of patients have isolated upper gastrointestinal or perianal manifestations. Symptoms correlate with disease location. Disease involving primarily the small bowel usually presents with abdominal pain with or without diarrhea; overt gastrointestinal bleeding is uncommon. In ileocolonic disease, right lower quadrant pain is common, and diarrhea and bleeding are less common. Colonic disease is more likely to present with bloody diarrhea; it is also associated with perianal disease, which causes perineal pain and seepage of stool or mucus from fistulas. Small-volume diarrhea with urgency and tenesmus suggests proctitis. Upper gastrointestinal disease presents with epigastric pain, nausea, vomiting, and occasionally gastric outlet obstruction.

Physical examination findings can range from normal to significantly abnormal depending on disease location and severity. Patients may appear pale, malnourished, or chronically ill. Fever may be present; if high it suggests an abscess or peritonitis. Abdominal tenderness, sometimes with a mass or fullness, is often located in the right lower quadrant. Perianal examination may reveal skin tags, induration, or fistulas.

As in UC, laboratory findings correlate with disease severity. Leukocytosis, anemia, hypoalbuminemia, and vitamin deficiencies indicate more severe disease. The erythrocyte sedimentation rate and C-reactive protein levels are often elevated; if so, these levels can be monitored as signs of response to therapy and subsequent disease flare.

KEY POINT

- Common symptoms of Crohn disease are abdominal pain, diarrhea, and weight loss; however, given the variable distribution of inflammation in Crohn disease, the symptoms can vary considerably between patients.

Extraintestinal Manifestations

Extraintestinal manifestations (EIMs) are found in approximately 10% of patients with IBD. The most common EIMs are oral aphthous ulcers, arthralgia, and back pain (indicating ankylosing spondylitis or sacroiliitis). Eye symptoms (redness, pain, swelling) may be due to uveitis, scleritis, or other causes of ocular inflammation and warrant immediate examination by an ophthalmologist. Skin manifestations are common and include pyoderma gangrenosum and erythema nodosum (see MKSAP 17 Dermatology). Liver involvement can also be seen, most commonly in the form of primary sclerosing cholangitis.

In CD, EIMs are more common with colitis than small-bowel disease. In either CD or UC, EIMs may precede gastrointestinal symptoms. Some EIMs correlate with IBD activity, whereas others do not.

KEY POINT

- Common extraintestinal manifestations of inflammatory bowel disease are oral aphthous ulcers, arthralgia, back pain, eye symptoms, and skin manifestations.

Diagnosis

Because the symptoms of IBD are nonspecific, visualization of the gastrointestinal tract, often by colonoscopy and biopsy of

the colon and ileum, is required to make the diagnosis. All patients suspected of having IBD should undergo stool examination to exclude infectious colitis, including *C. difficile*.

In UC, inflammation typically begins in the rectum and extends proximally in a circumferential manner. At presentation, 25% of patients have only proctitis, 25% have disease up to the splenic flexure (left-sided colitis), and 50% have extensive colonic involvement. Some patients with pancolitis have inflammation extending into the ileum for a few centimeters, known as backwash ileitis. This finding alone is not indicative of CD. Mild UC is characterized by mucosal edema, erythema, and loss of the normal vascular pattern. More significant disease produces granularity, friability, ulceration, and bleeding (**Figure 23**). Histology shows altered crypt architecture with shortened, branched crypts, as well as acute and chronic inflammation of the lamina propria.

In CD, endoscopic findings vary from superficial aphthous ulcers to discrete, deep ulcers that can be linear, stellate, or serpiginous and that may coalesce into a "cobblestone" appearance (**Figure 24**). Rectal sparing is typical, as are areas of inflammation separated by normal mucosa (known as skip lesions). The ileum should be inspected during colonoscopy to detect ileal inflammation characteristic of CD. Histology may show patchy transmural inflammation, but more superficial inflammation does not rule out CD. Aphthous ulcers and granulomas are characteristic findings but are often not seen.

CD can affect any part of the gastrointestinal tract, and in some patients inflammation is beyond the reach of colonoscopy. In these patients, supportive evidence can be obtained with CT or magnetic resonance (MR) enterography, capsule endoscopy, or directly by deep enteroscopy. These tests may not only assist in confirming the diagnosis but may also determine the extent and severity of involvement. Enterography also rules out complications such as obstruction, perforation, fistulas, and

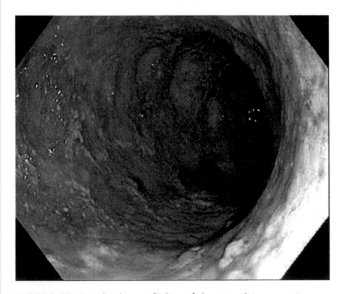

FIGURE 23. Typical endoscopic findings of ulcerative colitis are a continuous pattern of inflammation with varying severity of mucosal granularity, edema, loss of the normal vascular pattern, friability, and ulceration. A diffuse pattern of microulcerations is commonly seen, and frank ulcers are atypical.

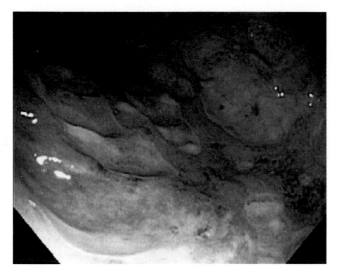

FIGURE 24. Endoscopic view of Crohn colitis demonstrating deep, geographic ulcerations on a background of diffuse mucosal inflammation.

abscesses. Radiographs are more often used in CD than UC owing to the frequent involvement of the small intestine. Plain films can evaluate bowel obstruction and dilatation. Small-bowel barium radiographs were often used in the past to evaluate the small bowel, but these examinations have largely been replaced by the more sensitive CT or MR enterography. Patients with CD often need repeat imaging, raising concern about cumulative doses of diagnostic ionizing radiation. Therefore, imaging should be used only when the results affect management, and modalities that do not use radiation (ultrasound, MRI) should be used in place of CT scanning whenever possible.

A subset of patients (10%-15%) has IBD that cannot be categorized; this is known as indeterminate colitis. In these patients, serologic tests have been proposed as a way to distin-guish UC from CD. However, these tests are expensive, are relatively insensitive or nonspecific, and often do not add useful information to standard diagnostic tests such as colonoscopy and enterography. Therefore, they should be used only sparingly when the diagnosis remains unclear. In particular, these tests should not be used as initial tests in patients with nonspecific symptoms such as diarrhea; their operating characteristics are particularly poor in these circumstances.

KEY POINTS

- Because the symptoms of inflammatory bowel disease are nonspecific, visualization of the gastrointestinal tract, often by colonoscopy and biopsy of the colon and ileum, is required to make the diagnosis.

- Patients with Crohn disease often need repeat imaging, raising concern about cumulative doses of diagnostic ionizing radiation; therefore, imaging should be used only when the results affect management, and modalities that do not use radiation (ultrasound, MRI) should be used in place of CT scanning whenever possible.

Treatment

Many therapies are available for patients with IBD, including 5-aminosalicylate (5-ASA) drugs, antimicrobial agents, gluco-corticoids, immunosuppressive medications (such as azathio-prine [AZA], 6-mercaptopurine [6-MP], methotrexate, and cyclosporine), and biologic drugs (such as anti–tumor necrosis factor [TNF] agents and leukocyte trafficking inhibitors). Some of these medications deliver the drug to specific areas of the bowel, whereas others act systemically. For the former, an understanding of the distribution of inflammation is required to choose the optimal drug formulation. Many of these treatments can be used for both UC and CD, with some exceptions. The side effects of these medications are listed in **Table 19**. The

TABLE 19.	Side Effects of Medications for Inflammatory Bowel Disease
Medication	**Side Effects**
Mesalamine, balsalazide	More common: dyspepsia, headache, nausea, alopecia
	Less common: interstitial nephritis, pericarditis, pancreatitis, hypersensitivity colitis
Sulfasalazine	In addition to side effects noted for mesalamine, autoimmune hemolytic anemia, bone marrow toxicity, reversible male infertility
Olsalazine	In addition to side effects noted for mesalamine, secretory diarrhea
Glucocorticoids	Hypertension, hyperglycemia, edema, redistribution of body fat, striae, cataracts, osteopenia
Azathioprine and 6-mercaptopurine	Fever, nausea, allergic reactions, pancreatitis, bone marrow suppression, hepatitis, infections, increased risk of lymphoma and skin cancer
Methotrexate	Liver toxicity, stomatitis, pneumonitis, bone marrow toxicity, infections, fetal toxicity; possibly lymphoma and skin cancers
Cyclosporine	Headache, paresthesias, seizures, kidney disease, hypertension, infections
Anti-TNF biologic agents	Infusion or injection site reactions, delayed hypersensitivity reaction, autoimmune disorders (such as drug-induced lupus), infections (including in particular tuberculosis and fungal infections), psoriasis; possibly lymphoma and skin cancers
Natalizumab	Headache, rash, nausea, infections (including PML), infusion reaction
PML = progressive multifocal leukoencephalopathy; TNF = tumor necrosis factor.	

treatment of IBD has become increasingly complex, and most of the medications are immune suppressing. Most patients with CD and patients with UC who require more than 5-ASA products should be referred to a gastroenterologist with expertise in managing these medications.

Ulcerative Colitis

Treatment of UC is based on disease severity (**Table 20**). For mild to moderate UC, the 5-ASA drugs are first-line therapy for inducing and maintaining remission. With these agents, 5-ASA is delivered topically to the bowel lumen, primarily to the colon, with the exception of the time-release formulation of mesalamine, which is able to deliver the drug throughout the small bowel as well as the colon (**Table 21**). Sulfasalazine may cause folate deficiency, and supplementation is recommended.

More severe UC is often treated with oral glucocorticoids such as prednisone, 40 to 60 mg/d. Doses above 60 mg provide little if any additional efficacy with more side effects. Budesonide is a glucocorticoid with high first-pass metabolism available in a controlled ileal-release formulation frequently used in CD. However, another formulation (multi-matrix [MMX] system) provides release of the drug throughout the colon and may be useful in treating UC. It has similar efficacy as prednisone but has fewer glucocorticoid-related side effects owing to its high first-pass metabolism. However, this benefit must be balanced against the high cost of this new medication. Patients whose disease does not respond to oral glucocorticoids should be hospitalized and given intravenous glucocorticoids or should be treated with a biologic agent. Glucocorticoids are not effective for maintaining remission in UC. Therefore, in patients whose disease responds to glucocorticoids, the dose should be tapered over 2 to 4 months while transitioning to a maintenance medication (AZA, 6-MP, or a biologic agent).

Patients with glucocorticoid-responsive disease are often treated with AZA or 6-MP for maintenance. AZA is converted in the body to 6-MP, which is then either inactivated (by xanthine oxidase or thiopurine methyltransferase [TPMT]) or activated to 6-thioguanine nucleotide. The level of TPMT should be checked before starting AZA or 6-MP; 1 in 300 patients (0.3%) lack enzyme activity and are at high risk of toxicity, and AZA and 6-MP should not be used in these patients. Intermediate TPMT activity is present in 10% of patients, whose increased risk of toxicity can be minimized by dose reduction and careful follow-up; 90% of patients have normal enzyme activity and can be treated with full-dose AZA or 6-MP.

AZA at daily doses between 1.5 and 2.5 mg/kg is effective for glucocorticoid sparing and maintaining remission in UC. However, the onset of action is slow, and consequently AZA is typically not used for induction.

Patients whose symptoms do not respond to glucocorticoids are treated with cyclosporine, a biologic agent, or colectomy. Cyclosporine is effective for avoiding colectomy in the short term in most patients. However, many patients eventually require colectomy, and many clinicians do not believe the risks (see Table 19) are worth the long-term benefit. The three anti-TNF antibodies approved for inducing and maintaining remission in UC are infliximab, adalimumab, and golimumab. The integrin-blocking antibody vedolizumab blocks leukocyte trafficking and is also approved for the treatment of UC.

TABLE 20.	Ulcerative Colitis Severity	
Variable	**Mild**	**Severe**
Stools (number per day)	<4	>6
Blood in stool	Intermittent	Frequent
Temperature	Normal	>37.5 °C (99.5 °F)
Pulse (beats per minute)	Normal	>90
Hemoglobin	Normal	<75% of normal
Erythrocyte sedimentation rate (mm/h)	<30	>30

Data from: Truelove SC, Witts LJ. Cortisone in ulcerative colitis; final report on a therapeutic trial. Br Med J. 1955 Oct 29;2(4947):1041-8. [PMID: 13260656]

TABLE 21.	5-Aminosalicylate Preparations for Treatment of Ulcerative Colitis		
Generic Name	**Proprietary Name**	**Formulation**	**Sites of Delivery**
Mesalamine	Canasa®	Suppository	Rectum
	Rowasa®	Enema	Left colon
	Pentasa®	Controlled-release granules	Small bowel and colon
	Asacol®, Delzicol®	Tablets with pH-dependent coating (pH ≥7)	Terminal ileum, colon
	Apriso®	Capsule with pH-dependent coating (pH ≥6) around polymer matrix	Terminal ileum, colon
	Lialda®	Tablet with pH-dependent coating (pH ≥7) around polymer matrix	Terminal ileum, colon
Olsalazine	Dipentum®	5-ASA dimer linked by azo bond	Colon
Sulfasalazine	Azulfidine®	5-ASA linked to sulfapyridine by azo bond	Colon
Balsalazide	Colazal®, Giazo®	5-ASA linked to inert carrier by azo bond	Colon

ASA = aminosalicylate.

Crohn Disease

In contrast to UC, the role of 5-ASA drugs in CD is less clear, with meta-analyses showing little or no benefit. Antimicrobial agents are important in patients with fistulas or abscesses, but they have no role in treating luminal disease. Therefore, patients with mild to moderate inflammatory CD are often treated initially with glucocorticoids. Prednisone is often used, with the same dosing comments as noted above for UC. For patients with ileocolonic CD, controlled-release budesonide is an alternative to prednisone, with fewer side effects but higher cost.

As in UC, glucocorticoids are not effective for maintaining remission in CD. Therefore, patients whose disease responds to glucocorticoids should be transitioned to an immunomodulator while the glucocorticoid is tapered. In addition to AZA and 6-MP, methotrexate is an option in CD. Trials have demonstrated that AZA, 2 to 3 mg/kg/d; 6-MP, 1.5 mg/kg/d; and methotrexate, 25 mg/week, are effective for inducing and maintaining remission in CD. In addition, AZA and 6-MP are effective for closing fistulas. Some adverse events from methotrexate can be minimized by the use of folic acid. Methotrexate should not be used in pregnant or lactating women.

Patients with more severe disease are treated with a biologic agent. The three anti-TNF agents that are FDA approved for CD are infliximab, adalimumab, and certolizumab. These medications are effective for inducing and maintaining remission and closing fistulas, and are generally considered to be safe in pregnancy (FDA pregnancy category B). Recent evidence indicates that efficacy is better when an anti-TNF agent is used together with an immunomodulator. In addition, the risk of developing antibodies against the anti-TNF agent is lower with combination therapy. Patients whose disease does not respond to one anti-TNF agent are often switched to a second or third anti-TNF agent. Those with no response to or intolerance of anti-TNF agents should be treated with either surgery or a leukocyte trafficking blocker (natalizumab or vedolizumab).

Natalizumab is a monoclonal antibody that interferes with leukocyte migration out of the bloodstream by blocking α4 integrin. It is effective for induction and maintenance of remission in CD that has failed to respond to other medications. Natalizumab increases the risk of infections, including progressive multifocal leukoencephalopathy (PML). Interest in natalizumab has been renewed owing to the availability of testing for exposure to the JC virus that causes PML; patients who are seronegative have very low risk of PML. In those who are seropositive, the risk is unacceptably high with natalizumab and it should not be used. Vedolizumab is another leukocyte trafficking blocker that is specific to the gastrointestinal tract owing to its inhibition of α4β7-integrin. It is approved for the treatment of CD. Because vedolizumab does not affect leukocyte trafficking in the brain, it should not be associated with PML.

Health Maintenance for the Patient with Inflammatory Bowel Disease

Patients with IBD have health risks related to their disease or its treatment. Patients with long-standing colitis are at increased risk for colon cancer and should undergo surveillance colonoscopy every 1 to 2 years beginning after 8 to 10 years of disease. This recommendation applies to patients with UC involving more than the rectum and those with Crohn colitis involving at least one third of the colon. Patients with severely active disease, particularly CD, are at risk for malnutrition and various vitamin deficiencies and should undergo screening for these conditions. In particular, distal ileal disease is associated with vitamin B_{12} malabsorption. Other health risks in IBD are related to immunosuppressive medications. Cumulative glucocorticoid use for longer than 3 months is a risk factor for osteoporosis and is an indication to assess bone density. Patients who will be treated with immunosuppressive medications are at risk for various infections, and vaccinations can decrease this risk. In addition to routine adult vaccines, these patients should receive annual vaccination against influenza with the killed vaccine and not the attenuated intranasal vaccine, hepatitis A and B virus (if not already immune), and pneumococcus. College students should receive meningococcal vaccine. Before starting an anti-TNF agent, patients should be assessed for exposure to tuberculosis (with a skin antigen test or interferon-γ release assay) and for immunity to hepatitis A and B viruses.

KEY POINT

- Patients with long-standing colitis associated with inflammatory bowel disease are at increased risk for colon cancer and should undergo surveillance colonoscopy every 1 to 2 years beginning after 8 to 10 years of disease.

Microscopic Colitis

Microscopic colitis (MC) accounts for 10% to 15% of patients with chronic, watery diarrhea. In contrast to IBD, MC is more common in older persons and does not cause endoscopically visible inflammation. The symptoms of MC are similar to other chronic causes of nonbloody diarrhea, such as celiac disease and IBS; therefore, colonic mucosal biopsies are required for diagnosis. Lymphocytic and collagenous colitis are the two subtypes of MC, and they are distinguishable only by histology. The pathophysiology of MC is not well known. In some patients, certain medications (such as NSAIDs and proton pump inhibitors) have been implicated as causative agents. MC is associated with other autoimmune diseases such as diabetes mellitus and psoriasis. The association with celiac disease is of particular clinical importance because the symptoms of these conditions are similar. Therefore, in patients with celiac disease or MC whose symptoms do not respond to appropriate therapy, the other condition must be ruled out.

The diagnosis of MC is made by histologic evaluation of colonic biopsies; the classic finding is intraepithelial lymphocytosis (>20 intraepithelial lymphocytes per 100 epithelial cells). In collagenous colitis, the increase in intraepithelial lymphocytes may be less pronounced than in lymphocytic colitis, and the main histologic feature is thickening of the subepithelial collagen band (usually >10 μm).

Therapy for MC is based on symptom severity. Any potentially causative medication should be stopped if possible. In mild disease, antidiarrheal therapy such as loperamide or diphenoxylate can be used. In moderate disease, bismuth subsalicylate may be beneficial. In severe cases or those that do not respond to antidiarrheal agents or bismuth, budesonide is the treatment of choice. It is highly effective (response rates of ≥80%), but the risk of relapse is high once budesonide is stopped (70%-80%); many patients require long-term maintenance therapy with low-dose budesonide or an immunomodulator such as AZA. The 5-ASA medications are not very effective for MC. For patients who do not respond to or do not tolerate budesonide, treatment with a bile salt binder such as cholestyramine may be effective. In severe cases, treatment with an anti-TNF agent may be needed.

KEY POINTS

- Microscopic colitis accounts for 10% to 15% of patients with chronic, watery diarrhea.
- In contrast to inflammatory bowel disease, microscopic colitis is more common in older persons and does not cause endoscopically visible inflammation.

Constipation

Definition

The clinical definition of constipation (as defined by the Rome III international working group) is a symptom complex that includes at least two of the following: straining during defecation, passage of lumpy or hard stool, sensation of incomplete defecation, use of manual maneuvers to facilitate a bowel movement, and/or frequency of less than three bowel movements per week. Accompanying symptoms may include abdominal cramping, abdominal pain, bloating, abdominal distention, nausea, passage of mucus, and diarrhea (overflow diarrhea). Patients at particular risk for overflow diarrhea are the elderly, especially those who are institutionalized or hospitalized or have altered mental status. An abdominal radiograph can confirm the suspicion of excessive fecal loading.

Constipation has an estimated prevalence of 15% to 30% in the general population and is more common in women, the elderly, and institutionalized patients. Prevalence approaches 50% in nursing homes, with 74% of residents using daily laxative therapy.

KEY POINT

- The Rome III criteria define constipation as a symptom complex that includes at least two of the following: straining during defecation, passage of lumpy or hard stool, sensation of incomplete defecation, use of manual maneuvers to facilitate a bowel movement, and/or frequency of less than three bowel movements per week.

Classification

Constipation is classified as acute or chronic; it is also classified as secondary or functional. Chronic constipation is char-

acterized by the regular presence of symptoms for a minimum of 3 months, with symptom onset at least 6 months prior to diagnosis. If secondary causes of constipation (**Table 22**) are excluded based on history, structural testing, and biochemical testing, constipation is classified as functional. Functional constipation is then further categorized as normal-transit constipation, slow-transit constipation, or dyssynergic defecation based on results of physiologic testing. Dyssynergic defecation represents a functional outlet obstruction that arises from the inability to coordinate the relaxation of the puborectalis and/or external anal sphincter muscles while increasing intraabdominal pressure that results in normal evacuation of stool. Dyssynergic defecation is believed to be an acquired behavioral disorder, resulting from causes such as sexual abuse, obstetric trauma, pelvic/abdominal surgery, or traumatic injury to the pelvis/abdomen. The causes of constipation are frequently multifactorial; medications (particularly narcotic analgesics) are the most common cause.

Evaluation

A careful history and physical examination, including rectal examination, can identify alarm features (**Table 23**) that necessitate colonoscopy, CT scan, and/or further biochemical evaluation. If a secondary cause is identified following an initial clinical assessment (such as a comorbidity, medication(s), or a biochemical or structural cause), it should be addressed, and laxative therapy should be used as needed. If no secondary cause is identified, a positive diagnosis of functional constipation can be made. The diagnosis should be explained to the patient, and therapy should be initiated.

For persistent constipation symptoms despite lifestyle changes, dietary measures, and laxative use, further physiologic evaluation and/or referral to a gastroenterologist should be pursued. Physiologic tests to consider include balloon expulsion testing, anorectal manometry, defecography, and colonic transit testing.

Treatment

Initial lifestyle and dietary measures that should be pursued are increased physical activity and increased dietary fiber. Over-the-counter laxative therapy includes fiber supplements, surfactants, and osmotic and stimulant laxatives. Soluble fibers such as psyllium, methylcellulose, calcium polycarbophil, inulin, and wheat dextrin are better tolerated and more effective than insoluble fiber supplements such as bran, flax seed, and rye. Fiber should be introduced at a low dose, ingested with adequate fluids, and increased gradually as tolerated to a maximum daily ingestion of 25 grams. Surfactants such as docusate sodium or docusate calcium are weak laxatives with an excellent safety profile. As such, they are most appropriate for very mild, intermittent constipation. Osmotic laxatives include magnesium hydroxide, lactulose, sorbitol, and polyethylene glycol (PEG) 3350; clinical trials have demonstrated the superiority and safety of PEG. Stimulant laxatives include anthraquinone, senna, and the diphenylmethanes bisacodyl and sodium

TABLE 22. Secondary Causes of Constipation

Mechanical

Colorectal cancer

Rectocele

Sigmoidocele

Enterocele

Anastomotic stricture

Anal stenosis/stricture

Extrinsic compression from pelvic/abdominal process

Metabolic

Diabetes mellitus

Hypothyroidism

Hypercalcemia

Hypokalemia

Pregnancy

Porphyria

Panhypopituitarism

Pheochromocytoma

Glucagonoma

Heavy metal poisoning (arsenic, lead, mercury)

Neuropathic/Myopathic

Parkinson disease

Systemic sclerosis

Multiple system atrophy

Cerebrovascular accident

Spinal cord injury/spinal cord lesions

Multiple sclerosis

Amyloidosis

Myotonic dystrophy

Dermatomyositis

Shy-Drager syndrome

Autonomic neuropathy

Chagas disease

Intestinal pseudo-obstruction (myopathy and neuropathy)

Hirschsprung disease

Ganglioneuromatosis

Hypoganglionosis

Medications

Narcotic-containing analgesics

Anticholinergic agents (antispasmodics, tricyclic antidepressants, antipsychotics, antiparkinsonian drugs)

Antacids (aluminum and calcium based)

Iron supplements

Antihypertensive agents (calcium channel blockers, β-blockers, diuretics)

NSAIDs

Antidiarrheal agents

TABLE 23. Alarm Features Warranting Immediate Structural Evaluation in Patients with Constipation

Age >50 years (or >45 years in black patients)

New-onset constipation in elderly patients

Severe constipation symptoms

Rectal bleeding

Unexplained weight loss

Family history of colon cancer

History of colonic resection

History of abdominal or pelvic cancer

History of abdominal or pelvic irradiation

Palpable rectal or abdominal mass on examination

picosulfate. The stimulants are the fastest-acting agents (8-12 hours) and are most effective for acute exacerbations of constipation as well as slow-transit constipation. Chronic senna use can lead to benign pigmentation of the colon, known as melanosis coli. Theoretical concerns about the development of cathartic colon with long-term stimulant use remain unproved; recent randomized controlled trials (RCTs) demonstrate safety and efficacy of long-term stimulants with chronic use.

When constipation symptoms do not respond to fiber supplementation or osmotic and stimulatory laxative therapy, prosecretory agents, including the chloride channel activator lubiprostone and the guanylate cyclase-C activator linaclotide, are available by prescription. High-quality RCTs have demonstrated efficacy and safety for both agents. Lubiprostone can cause headache, nausea, diarrhea, and shortness of breath. Linaclotide can cause diarrhea. Agents in development include serotonin receptor activators, bile salt analogues, and bile acid transporter inhibitors. Complementary therapies include probiotics, such as *Bifidobacterium lactis*, *Bifidobacterium animalis*, and *Lactobacillus rhamnosus*, as well as food supplements such as hemp seed and dried plums/prunes. Physical therapy with biofeedback is utilized for the treatment of dyssynergia.

KEY POINT

• Initial lifestyle and dietary measures that should be pursued to improve constipation are increased physical activity and increased dietary fiber.

Irritable Bowel Syndrome

Irritable bowel syndrome (IBS) is a heterogeneous symptom complex characterized by abdominal pain and altered bowel habits. This chronic condition affects 10% to 15% of the general population and lacks a single unifying pathophysiology and disease-defining biomarker. As a result, the diagnosis is made by the fulfillment of symptom-based criteria created by the Rome III international working group (**Table 24**). IBS is further subtyped based on the predominant stool pattern as IBS with constipation (IBS-C), IBS with diarrhea (IBS-D), or mixed IBS

TABLE 24. Rome III Diagnostic Criteria[a] for Irritable Bowel Syndrome and Its Subtypes

IBS

Recurrent abdominal pain or discomfort at least 3 days per month in the last 3 months associated with two or more of the following:
 	
    Improvement with defecation
 	
    Onset associated with a change in frequency of stool
 	
    Onset associated with a change in form (appearance) of stool

IBS with Constipation (IBS-C)
Hard or lumpy stools for >25% of bowel movements
Loose (mushy) or watery stools for <25% of bowel movements
IBS with Diarrhea (IBS-D)
Loose (mushy) or watery stools for >25% of bowel movements
Hard or lumpy stools for <25% of bowel movements
Mixed IBS (IBS-M)
Hard or lumpy stools for >25% of bowel movements
Loose (mushy) or watery stools for >25% of bowel movements

C = constipation; D = diarrhea; IBS = irritable bowel syndrome; M = mixed-type.

[a]Diagnostic criteria fulfilled for the last 3 months with symptom onset at least 6 months prior to diagnosis.

Adapted with permission of Elsevier Science and Technology Journals, from Longstreth GF, Thompson WG, Chey WD, Houghton LA, Mearin F, Spiller RC. Functional bowel disorders. Gastroenterology. 2006 Apr;130(5):1480-91. [PMID: 16678561]; permission conveyed through Copyright Clearance Center, Inc.

TABLE 25. Conditions Associated with Irritable Bowel Syndrome

Functional dyspepsia
Nonerosive gastroesophageal reflux disease
Cyclic vomiting syndrome
Gastroparesis
Anxiety disorder
Depression
Somatoform disorders
Posttraumatic stress disorder
Fibromyalgia and other chronic musculoskeletal pain syndromes
Migraines and nonmigrainous headaches
Chronic pelvic pain
Interstitial cystitis
Dysmenorrhea
Sexual dysfunction

(IBS-M). Additional symptoms that are not part of the diagnostic criteria but are frequently reported in IBS include fewer than three bowel movements per week, more than three bowel movements per day, abnormal stool form, straining, rectal urgency, sensation of incomplete emptying, passage of mucus, and bloating. A variety of other conditions occur in association with IBS, adding to the symptom profile (**Table 25**). IBS occurs in patients of all ages and racial/ethnic groups, but it is more common in women (67% more likely than men) and in younger adults (25% more likely than in those age ≥50 years).

Evaluation

IBS was previously considered a diagnosis of exclusion after eliminating organic causes; however, an accurate diagnosis of IBS can now be made with fulfillment of the diagnostic criteria without further testing in the absence of alarm features (anemia; weight loss; and family history of colorectal cancer, IBD, or celiac disease). Rectal bleeding and nocturnal abdominal pain are poor predictors of organic disease. Therefore, a confident diagnosis of IBS can be made in the absence of alarm symptoms. The routine pursuit of a complete blood count, serum chemistry studies, thyroid function studies, stool studies for ova and parasites, and abdominal imaging is unnecessary in this setting. Testing for celiac disease with serum IgA–based tTG should be considered in patients with IBS-D or IBS-M symptoms. Breath testing for lactase deficiency or SIBO

can be considered based on initial treatment response and/or presence of risk factors. Colonoscopy should be pursued only in patients who meet criteria for colon cancer screening based on age, race, and family history. Random colon biopsies should be obtained at the time of colonoscopy to screen for microscopic colitis in patients with IBS-D. There is no established role for food allergy testing in IBS.

KEY POINT

- Irritable bowel syndrome was previously considered a diagnosis of exclusion after eliminating organic causes; however, an accurate diagnosis can now be made with fulfillment of the diagnostic criteria without further testing in the absence of alarm features (anemia; weight loss; and family history of colorectal cancer, inflammatory bowel disease, or celiac disease).

HVC

Management

An essential initial step in management of IBS is the clear establishment of the diagnosis with explanation of and reassurance regarding the patient's symptoms. A strong clinician-patient relationship should be established using a patient-centered approach that is focused on effective patient and clinician communication. This can be achieved by using open-ended questions, actively listening to the patient, and showing empathy during patient encounters.

Given the growing role of presumed food intolerances in IBS symptoms (more than half of patients report symptom onset following meals), dietary interventions are growing in popularity. Although RCTs are lacking, dietary interventions may include the avoidance of trigger foods (caffeine, carbonated beverages, or fatty foods), increased dietary fiber, and various elimination diets that restrict gluten, lactose, fructose, or FODMAPs (Fermentable Oligosaccharides, Disaccharides,

Monosaccharides, And Polyols). It is best to involve a dietitian when pursuing elimination diets to ensure safety and improve efficacy. These initial management steps may lead to symptom improvement in patients with mild symptoms. For persistent symptoms, directed pharmacologic therapy should be pursued based on the predominant stool pattern.

KEY POINTS

- An essential initial step in managing irritable bowel syndrome is the clear establishment of the diagnosis with explanation of and reassurance regarding the patient's symptoms.
- Given the growing role of presumed food intolerances in irritable bowel syndrome symptoms, dietary interventions are growing in popularity.

Therapy for Irritable Bowel Syndrome with Constipation

The soluble fiber supplement psyllium has demonstrated limited efficacy in IBS, primarily addressing stool frequency and consistency. Insoluble fiber supplements such as bran appear to worsen IBS-C symptoms. Although a variety of surfactant, osmotic, and stimulant laxatives can be used for the constipation symptoms associated with IBS-C, only the osmotic laxative PEG has been tested in IBS. Lubiprostone and linaclotide have demonstrated safety and efficacy in treating the global symptoms of IBS-C in high-quality RCTs. Lubiprostone is FDA approved for women with IBS-C, and linaclotide is FDA approved for the treatment of IBS-C in adults. There is also considerable cost associated with lubiprostone and linaclotide.

Therapy for Irritable Bowel Syndrome with Diarrhea

The antispasmodic agents hyoscyamine and dicyclomine are used for the short-term treatment of abdominal pain in IBS-D or IBS-C, although they can cause constipation. The antidiarrheal agent loperamide is safe and is only effective for the bowel symptoms associated with IBS-D. The nonabsorbable antimicrobial agent rifaximin can be effective for global symptoms and bloating associated with IBS-D, presumably by altering the colonic microbial flora; however, it is not FDA approved for this use. The 5-HT$_3$ antagonist alosetron is available for women with IBS-D whose symptoms have not responded to conventional therapy; however, owing to an increased risk of severe constipation and ischemic colitis with its use, it is restricted by a mandatory prescribing program.

Other Therapies

When the previously mentioned therapies are unsuccessful, central-acting agents such as tricyclic antidepressants and selective serotonin reuptake inhibitors are effective, primarily for overall symptoms and abdominal pain. The use of tricyclic antidepressants is preferred in IBS-D given their constipating side effects, and selective serotonin reuptake inhibitors are preferred in IBS-C.

Complementary Therapy

If pharmacologic therapies are not effective or not desired by the patient, a variety of complementary interventions can be considered. Although RCTs are lacking in most cases, limited clinical evidence supports the use of prebiotics (nondigestible nutrients intended to encourage desirable bacterial growth), probiotics, herbal medicine, cognitive behavioral therapy, hypnotherapy, and acupuncture in IBS.

Diverticular Disease

Diverticulosis is the presence of asymptomatic colonic mucosal outpouchings, known as diverticula. They are usually located in the sigmoid colon, but any part of the colon may be involved. These mucosal protrusions occur through weak areas where the vasa recta penetrate and are facilitated by increased intraluminal pressure, such as with chronic constipation. The prevalence of diverticulosis increases with age; it is present in 10% of patients older than 45 years and in 80% of those older than 85 years.

If a diverticulum becomes blocked, trapped bacteria proliferate, inflaming the diverticulum and surrounding tissues and resulting in diverticulitis. The inflamed diverticulum may perforate, which results in an abscess. The abscess may decompress into adjacent structures and cause fistulas to the bladder, vagina, or skin. It may also decompress into the peritoneum, resulting in peritonitis.

Approximately 20% of patients with diverticula have an episode of diverticulitis. Symptoms include abdominal pain, fever, and altered bowel habits (typically diarrhea). Although the stool may contain some blood, significant bleeding from diverticulitis is very uncommon. Dysuria, urinary frequency, and urinary urgency may reflect bladder irritation. Pneumaturia, fecaluria, or recurrent/polymicrobial urinary tract infections suggest a colovesical fistula. Physical examination findings include fever, left lower quadrant tenderness, and/or a lower abdominal or rectal mass.

The therapeutic approach to diverticulitis is dictated by patient-related factors, the severity of clinical features, and the ability to tolerate oral intake. In a healthy, immunocompetent patient with mild symptoms, outpatient therapy is appropriate and should consist of a liquid diet and oral antimicrobial agents that cover colonic organisms and include anaerobic coverage (such as ciprofloxacin and metronidazole). Close follow-up is warranted to detect any deterioration as soon as possible. For older, frail, sicker patients, hospitalization is recommended for administration of intravenous antimicrobial agents and observation.

If clinical features are highly suggestive of diverticulitis, imaging studies are unnecessary. If the diagnosis is not clear or if an abscess is suspected (severe pain, high fever, palpable mass), CT imaging is indicated. A small abscess may resolve with antimicrobial therapy alone. For larger abscesses, CT-guided drainage can facilitate nonsurgical management and decrease the chance of sepsis. Emergent surgery is

CONT.

required for generalized peritonitis, uncontrolled sepsis, or perforation. Elective surgery is indicated for fistulas and recurrent diverticulitis.

After an acute attack has resolved, a high-fiber diet is generally recommended to facilitate stool passage and decrease intracolonic pressure. When inflammation and the resulting edema have completely resolved, colonoscopy should be performed to exclude cancer or IBD.

Another major complication of diverticulosis is diverticular hemorrhage, which occurs more commonly in the right colon (but can occur anywhere in the colon) and typically resolves spontaneously. For a discussion of diverticular bleeding, see Gastrointestinal Bleeding. **H**

KEY POINTS

- Approximately 20% of patients with diverticula have an episode of diverticulitis.
- Symptoms of diverticulitis include abdominal pain, fever, and altered bowel habits (typically diarrhea).

HVC
- If clinical features are highly suggestive of diverticulitis, imaging studies are unnecessary.

Ischemic Bowel Disease

Acute or chronic alteration of arterial or venous intestinal blood flow may result in intestinal ischemia. The intestinal insult may be mild and reversible, requiring only supportive care, or it may be severe and life threatening, requiring surgery or culminating in intestinal gangrene, sepsis, and death. The most important factor predicting outcome is the presence of bowel infarction.

H Acute Mesenteric Ischemia
Clinical Features and Diagnosis
Acute mesenteric ischemia (AMI) is an uncommon vascular emergency that accounts for less than 1 in 1000 hospital admissions and has a mortality rate of 60%.

Embolism to the mesenteric arteries causes 50% of cases of AMI and usually involves the superior mesenteric artery (SMA). Emboli are usually of cardiac origin and are due to atrial fibrillation or left ventricle thrombus. Arterial thrombosis is more common than venous thrombosis and accounts for one third of cases of AMI. Thrombosis within the mesenteric arteries is usually due to superimposed atherosclerotic disease. Symptoms of chronic mesenteric insufficiency due to atherosclerosis may be elicited in up to 25% of patients before they experience SMA occlusion. Mesenteric vein thrombosis may also lead to AMI and may result from other systemic conditions such as malignancy, hypercoagulable states, abdominal or cardiac surgery, or pancreatitis. It may also result from the use of contraceptive and estrogen-containing medications.

Nonocclusive mesenteric ischemia is caused by decreased mesenteric perfusion in low-flow states such as heart failure, sepsis, profound hypotension, or hypovolemia. It may also occur with use of vasoactive medications (vasopressors, ergots, triptans, cocaine, digitalis).

Patients typically present in the seventh decade of life and often have associated comorbidities (for example, atrial fibrillation, recent myocardial infarction, or heart failure in the case of embolism; mesenteric atherosclerosis in the case of thrombosis). The classic presentation of early AMI is abdominal pain out of proportion to the physical examination findings; however, symptoms may vary depending on the timing of presentation and cause of ischemia.

Early in AMI, laboratory studies may be normal. Leukocytosis, hemoconcentration, anion gap metabolic acidosis, and elevations in lactate dehydrogenase and/or amylase levels may be seen as disease progresses. Abdominal plain radiographs can be used to exclude other causes of pain, and they may detect bowel wall edema or pneumatosis later in the disease course. The usefulness of vascular ultrasound is limited to visualization of the proximal origin of vessels. Splanchnic angiography, once considered the standard for diagnosis and potential treatment of AMI, is increasingly being reserved for patients with nonocclusive mesenteric ischemia in whom medical management is unsuccessful, those who require intra-arterial papaverine infusion, or those who are candidates for a primary percutaneous endovascular approach in the setting of thromboembolic occlusion when peritoneal signs have not yet developed. Endovascular intervention for AMI requires careful patient selection and interventional radiology or vascular surgical expertise. When a patient has signs of peritonitis or a bowel infarction is suspected, experts favor immediate surgery.

CT angiography is considered the standard for diagnosis of AMI because it is fast, noninvasive, widely available, and has a high sensitivity and specificity for diagnosing AMI and excluding other causes of pain. It provides an accurate assessment of mesenteric vessel patency and bowel injury but offers no therapeutic role. Although MR angiography has high accuracy for detecting high-grade stenosis and occlusions in the origin of the celiac artery and SMA, it is a long test, is not quickly available, and has limited ability to detect distal arterial thrombi or emboli and nonocclusive mesenteric ischemia. **H**

KEY POINT

- The classic presentation of early acute mesenteric ischemia is abdominal pain out of proportion to the physical examination findings.

Treatment
Treatment consists of volume resuscitation, correction of acidosis and electrolyte imbalances, broad-spectrum antimicrobial agents, nasogastric decompression, and discontinuation of medications associated with vasoconstriction. Surgery is indicated for patients with peritoneal signs or for those in whom there is a high index of concern for AMI despite negative imaging studies. Necrotic bowel should be resected. Embolectomy or, in the case of thrombosis, thrombectomy

and surgical revascularization or endovascular stenting of the underlying atherosclerotic lesion should be performed. Intra-arterial papaverine is often used as an adjunct to surgery to minimize vasoconstriction, and it is the definitive treatment for nonocclusive mesenteric ischemia. In patients without peritonitis, endovascular or open embolectomy should be performed. Local thrombolysis is recommended in cases of incomplete endovascular embolectomy or distal artery embolization. Thrombosis should be managed with open or endovascular revascularization. Anticoagulants are the appropriate treatment for mesenteric vein thrombosis. ▨

Chronic Mesenteric Ischemia
Clinical Features and Diagnosis
Chronic mesenteric ischemia is estimated to affect 1 in 100,000 individuals. It is almost always associated with atherosclerotic disease. Rare causes include fibromuscular dysplasia, compression of the celiac artery by the median arcuate ligament (also known as median arcuate ligament syndrome), vasculitis, and chronic mesenteric venous thrombosis. Symptoms consist of postprandial pain within 60 minutes after meals, which results in fear of eating and weight loss. Symptoms usually develop when two or more arteries have hemodynamically significant stenoses. Single-vessel involvement may be causative when collateral flow is inadequate. Vascular Doppler ultrasound is a useful screening test for chronic mesenteric ischemia but is limited by the presence of intestinal gas or obesity. Peak systolic velocities greater than 275 cm/s in the SMA and greater than 200 cm/s in the celiac artery correlate to stenoses of greater than 70% in each vessel. CT and MR angiography have high sensitivity and specificity for detecting mesenteric stenosis, but MR angiography may not be as effective for detecting distal stenosis. Conventional angiography may be used to confirm the diagnosis and plan endovascular or open surgical therapy.

> **KEY POINTS**
> - Chronic mesenteric ischemia is almost always associated with atherosclerotic disease.
> - Symptoms of chronic mesenteric ischemia consist of postprandial pain within 60 minutes after meals, which results in fear of eating and weight loss.

Treatment
Surgical revascularization is the most durable treatment for chronic mesenteric ischemia. Periprocedural morbidity and mortality are lower with endovascular stenting, which may be indicated for select patients.

Colonic Ischemia
Clinical Features and Diagnosis
Ischemic colitis is the most common form of intestinal ischemic injury, accounting for 1 in 1000 hospitalizations. Approximately 90% of cases occur in patients older than 60

years. It is most often due to transient alterations in systemic circulation or local mesenteric vasculature, which decreases intestinal blood flow. Conditions that can alter circulation include hypotension, dehydration, strenuous physical activity, medications and illicit drugs, thrombophilia, aortic or cardiac bypass, vasculitis, or an obstructing colon lesion. Symptoms include sudden abdominal pain and diarrhea followed later by rectal bleeding. The diagnosis is based on clinical history. There is no role for angiography. Left colon inflammatory changes may be detected by colonoscopy or abdominal CT. ▨

> **KEY POINT**
> - Ischemic colitis is the most common form of intestinal ischemic injury; symptoms include sudden abdominal pain and diarrhea followed later by rectal bleeding.

Treatment
Treatment depends on the severity of symptoms. Most patients have mild and transient disease and can receive outpatient management. Patients with more severe symptoms require hospitalization for supportive care with bowel rest, intravenous fluids, antimicrobial therapy, and close observation. Most cases resolve; however, up to 20% of patients require colectomy for necrotic bowel or stricturing complications.

Anorectal Disorders
Perianal Disorders
Perianal disorders affect men and women of all ages and range from benign conditions such as hemorrhoids to potentially life-threatening diseases such as anorectal cancer. A thorough history and detailed physical examination (including inspection of the anus, digital rectal examination, and direct visualization with anoscopy or proctoscopy) allow a diagnosis to be made. Patients with alarm features (such as unexplained weight loss, change in bowel movements, iron deficiency anemia, age older than 50 years, or personal or family history of colorectal cancer or IBD) warrant colonoscopy.

Hemorrhoids
Hemorrhoids are arteriovenous communications covered by cushions of connective tissue in the anal canal. Hemorrhoids above the dentate line are internal, and those below it are external. External hemorrhoids produce pain and an acutely tender nodule when thrombosed. Internal hemorrhoids cause most hemorrhoidal symptoms (painless, bright red blood dripping in the toilet bowl or noted on toilet paper; a protrusion of tissue; itching; and pain).

Initial treatment of internal and external hemorrhoids consists of dietary and lifestyle modifications to soften bowel movements and avoid constipation, straining, and prolonged time on the toilet. Increased fiber intake has been shown to reduce symptomatic prolapse and bleeding. Local therapy such as topical anesthetics and glucocorticoids may relieve pain and itching, but data to support their use are scant. Oral micronized, purified flavonoid fraction, a preparation that increases venous vascular tone, has been shown in some studies to improve hemorrhoidal symptoms. Office-based nonoperative therapy with sclerotherapy, rubber band ligation, infrared coagulation, radiofrequency ablation, and cryotherapy is recommended for most symptomatic hemorrhoids. Band ligation has the most durable response. Surgical excision is indicated for patients in whom nonoperative therapy is unsuccessful and in those with large or acutely thrombosed external hemorrhoids.

KEY POINT

- Initial treatment of hemorrhoids consists of dietary and lifestyle modifications to soften bowel movements and avoid constipation, straining, and prolonged time on the toilet.

Anal Fissure

Anal fissures are tears in the anoderm below the dentate line that can be seen on inspection of the perianal area, often unaided by the use of an anoscope. They are usually in the posterior position and are less often in the anterior midline. Lateral fissures should raise suspicion for IBD and infectious or neoplastic causes. The classic symptom is pain with and after defecation, which may be associated with bright red blood on the toilet tissue. Most acute fissures heal spontaneously. Sitz baths, fiber or stool softeners, topical anesthetics, or anti-inflammatory ointments may provide symptomatic relief. Chronic fissures may heal with use of topical calcium channel blockers or 0.2% nitroglycerin, although headache often limits use of nitroglycerin. The evidence to support botulinum toxin injections is limited. Lateral internal sphincterotomy is the treatment of choice for refractory fissures.

KEY POINT

- Most acute anal fissures heal spontaneously; sitz baths, fiber or stool softeners, topical anesthetics, or anti-inflammatory ointments may provide symptomatic relief.

Fecal Incontinence

Fecal incontinence is the involuntary loss of stool. Prevalence increases with age and is 16% in adults older than 70 years. Urinary incontinence, obesity, neurologic disorders, pelvic surgery, or obstetric trauma are additional risk factors. Lifestyle and dietary modification should be initiated using specific toileting regimens, fiber and antidiarrheal medications to normalize stool consistency, and biofeedback if other therapies are unsuccessful. Endoanal ultrasound is used to identify sphincter defects, and anorectal manometry assesses sphincter function, rectal sensation, and compliance. If conservative measures are unsuccessful, submucosal injection of a bulking agent in the anal canal or implantation of a device for electrostimulation of the sacral nerves have been shown to decrease fecal incontinence in patients with weak sphincters. Either sacral nerve stimulation or surgery is indicated for patients with sphincter defects.

KEY POINT

- Prevalence of fecal incontinence increases with age and is 16% in adults older than 70 years.

Anal Cancer

Anal carcinoma is a rare but increasing cause of cancer and accounts for approximately 2% of gastrointestinal cancers. Most anal cancers are squamous cell carcinomas and are associated with human papillomavirus (HPV) infection, particularly HPV 16 and HPV 18. HPV vaccine is approved for and has been shown to prevent anal HPV infection and anal intraepithelial neoplasia, precursors of anal cancer.

Risk factors for anal cancer include HPV infection; sexually transmitted infections; multiple sex partners; men having sex with men; receptive anal intercourse; history of vaginal, cervical, or vulvar cancer; smoking; immunosuppression due to hematologic malignancy; solid organ transplantation; or HIV infection.

Most patients present with a perianal lesion or mass associated with rectal bleeding or anal discomfort. Twenty percent of patients may be asymptomatic.

When anal carcinoma is suspected, biopsy is essential to establish the diagnosis. Once confirmed, the clinical examination is critical for staging. Staging is based on lesion size, local invasion, and status of regional lymph nodes. Digital rectal examination, anoscopy, inguinal lymph node palpation (with biopsy or fine-needle aspiration if enlarged), and CT scan of the pelvis, abdomen, and chest are recommended.

For treatment, follow-up, and prognosis of anal cancer, see MKSAP 17 Hematology and Oncology.

KEY POINTS

- Anal carcinoma is a rare but increasing cause of cancer and accounts for approximately 2% of gastrointestinal cancers.
- Most patients with anal cancer present with a perianal lesion or mass associated with rectal bleeding or anal discomfort.

Colorectal Neoplasia
Epidemiology

Colorectal cancer is the second most common cause of cancer and cancer-related mortality in men and women in the United States. The cumulative lifetime risk of developing colorectal cancer is 1 in 19 in men and 1 in 20 in women. More than 50% of patients are diagnosed with stage III and IV cancer, which is associated with 5-year survival rates of approximately 65% and 10%, respectively. The incidence of colorectal cancer has steadily declined over the past 30 years. The annual rate of decline between 1998 and 2009 was 2.6% in men and 2.1% in women. Since 1975, a decrease in mortality of more than 30% has been noted; this is attributable largely to the use of colorectal cancer screening. Despite this evidence, 35% of eligible Americans have not been screened for colorectal cancer with fecal occult blood testing, flexible sigmoidoscopy, or colonoscopy.

KEY POINTS

- Colorectal cancer is the second most common cause of cancer and cancer-related mortality in men and women in the United States.

HVC
- Despite a decrease in colorectal cancer mortality that is largely attributable to the use of screening, 35% of eligible Americans have not been screened for colorectal cancer with fecal occult blood testing, flexible sigmoidoscopy, or colonoscopy.

Pathogenesis

Colorectal cancer is a heterogeneous genetic disease that arises from three well-characterized molecular pathways: chromosomal instability (CIN), microsatellite instability (MSI), and the CpG island methylator phenotype (CIMP).

CIN results from gains or losses of whole or portions of chromosomes, which can result in an imbalance in chromosome number (aneuploidy) or loss of paired genomic regions on complementary chromosomes (heterozygosity), leaving only one copy of certain genes. Progressive accumulation of mutations in tumor suppressor genes and oncogenes leads to subsequent development of malignancy. Seventy percent of colorectal cancers arise from adenomatous polyps through the CIN pathway.

Microsatellites are repetitive noncoding nucleotide sequences scattered throughout the human genome. The fidelity of microsatellites during DNA replication is maintained by the enzyme products of the mismatch repair (MMR) genes (*MLH1*, *MSH2*, *MSH6*, and *PMS2*). Alterations in MMR gene function are associated with defective replication error repair and resultant changes in length of microsatellite sequences in a tumor; when present in a tumor, this is known as MSI. Five percent of colon cancers arise from adenomas in patients with a germline mutation in the MMR genes, which are an essential component of Lynch syndrome. These tumors are characterized by high levels of MSI (MSI-H).

A third genetic molecular pathway involved in colorectal neoplasia does not involve disruption of the genetic sequence but instead involves disruption of normal gene function by the addition of a methyl group (methylation) within the promoter region of specific genes (most commonly at the 5'-CG-3' [CpG] dinucleotide) and silences their function (known as an epigenetic change). Patients with a tendency to excessively methylate (hypermethylate) certain genes are designated as having CIMP. When hypermethylation occurs with different genes that normally suppress tumor development, colorectal neoplasia may result. These tumors tend to be poorly differenti-

ated and have a high degree of MSI and other genetic abnormalities. Clinically, the precursor lesions for CIMP-associated tumors are sessile serrated polyps; up to 30% of colon cancers develop from this type of polyp.

Risk Factors
Modifiable Factors

Modifiable factors associated with colorectal polyps and cancer include high dietary fat or red meat, low dietary fiber, smoking, excess alcohol ingestion, obesity, type 2 diabetes mellitus, and low physical activity.

KEY POINT

- Modifiable factors associated with colorectal polyps and cancer include high dietary fat or red meat, low dietary fiber, smoking, excess alcohol ingestion, obesity, type 2 diabetes mellitus, and low physical activity.

Predisposing Factors

Nonmodifiable risk factors include male gender, acromegaly, older age (with a peak incidence of cancer after the eighth decade of life), and black ethnicity (which is associated with a higher cancer incidence and stage-adjusted mortality compared with other ethnicities).

The risk for colorectal cancer is elevated in the presence of chronic colorectal inflammation from ulcerative colitis or Crohn disease of the colon. This increased risk is dependent on the proximal extent of mucosal involvement; patients with pancolitis are at highest risk, whereas risk is negligible in patients with proctitis. Risk is also increased with longer duration of disease, greater severity of inflammation, and the presence of coexistent primary sclerosing cholangitis. After a decade of disease, the cancer risk increases yearly by 0.5% to 1%.

Ureterosigmoidostomy also increases the risk for colon cancer. The mechanism is unknown but may be related to chronic colonic inflammation.

A personal history of adenomatous polyps or colorectal cancer increases the risk for metachronous colorectal cancer (multiple primary tumors developing at different time intervals).

KEY POINT

- Predisposing factors for colorectal cancer include male gender, acromegaly, older age, black ethnicity, ulcerative colitis or Crohn disease of the colon, ureterosigmoidostomy, and history of adenomatous polyps or colorectal cancer.

Nonsyndromic Family History

Individuals with a first-degree relative with colorectal cancer have a two- to threefold increased risk for colorectal cancer. The risk is increased with a greater number of relatives affected and an earlier age of cancer onset (defined as younger than age 60 years).

- Individuals with a first-degree relative with colorectal cancer have a two- to threefold increased risk for colorectal cancer.

Hereditary Colon Cancer Syndromes

Patients with the highest risk of colorectal cancer are those who have a hereditary colorectal cancer syndrome (**Table 26**). Recognition of a hereditary colon cancer syndrome requires an accurate and comprehensive family history, which should include the ages and causes of death of relatives in three generations, any diagnosis of cancer and age of onset, birth defects, and other inherited conditions. The family history should be confirmed with medical records when possible and should be updated periodically to ensure proper surveillance recommendations.

- Patients with the highest risk of colorectal cancer are those who have a hereditary colorectal cancer syndrome.

Hereditary Nonpolyposis Colon Cancer

Hereditary nonpolyposis colon cancer (HNPCC) is the term that describes families that satisfy the Amsterdam I or II criteria. The Amsterdam I and II criteria are similar with one notable exception: Amsterdam I criteria include only colorectal cancer. The Amsterdam II criteria are as follows:

- Three or more relatives with HNPCC-related cancers (colorectal cancer or cancer of the endometrium, small intestine, ureter, or renal pelvis)
- One relative a first-degree relative of the other two
- At least two successive generations affected
- One cancer diagnosed before age 50 years
- Familial adenomatous polyposis excluded
- Tumors verified histologically

Lynch syndrome is the term used to describe patients who meet the Amsterdam II criteria for HNPCC and have an identified germline mutation in one of the four MMR genes or the epithelial cell adhesion molecule (*EPCAM*) gene (which codes for a transmembrane glycoprotein that plays a role in tumorigenesis and metastasis). Colon cancer occurs in up to 80% of individuals with Lynch syndrome, usually at a mean age of 44 years. The colon cancer is often right-sided and has particular pathologic features that include tumor-infiltrating lymphocytes, a Crohn-like lymphocytic reaction, and mucin or signet cell histology. Lynch syndrome is associated with an increased risk for extracolonic tumors (endometrial [40%-60%], followed much less commonly by ovarian, urothelial, gastric, brain, small bowel, hepatobiliary tract, sebaceous, and pancreatic). The cumulative lifetime cancer risk and age of cancer onset vary according to the specific germline mutation present.

Familial colorectal cancer type X is the term used to identify patients and families who meet the Amsterdam criteria for HPNCC but have no molecular evidence of a MMR deficiency. Patients with familial colorectal cancer type X have a much lower lifetime risk of colon cancer, later age of onset, and no increased risk of extracolonic cancers compared with patients with Lynch syndrome. Recommendations state that patients with colorectal cancer should undergo molecular testing of their tumor to determine if it has evidence of defective MMR (also known as universal testing). This can be done by MSI testing or immunohistochemistry for expression of the MMR proteins in the tumor.

- Colon cancer occurs in up to 80% of individuals with Lynch syndrome, usually at a mean age of 44 years.

Adenomatous Polyposis Syndromes

The adenomatous polyposis syndromes include familial adenomatous polyposis (FAP) and *MYH*-associated polyposis (MAP).

FAP is caused by a mutation of the adenomatous polyposis coli (*APC*) gene, a tumor suppressor gene that normally attenuates cell proliferation. Classic FAP results in the development of hundreds to thousands of colorectal adenomas that

TABLE 26.	Hereditary Colorectal Cancer Syndromes		
Syndrome	**Prevalence**	**Inheritance**	**Polyp Type**
Lynch syndrome	1 in 440	AD	Adenoma
Familial adenomatous polyposis	1 in 10,000	AD	Adenoma
MYH-associated polyposis	1 in 20,000	AR	Adenoma
Peutz-Jeghers syndrome	1 in 120,000	AD	Hamartoma
Juvenile polyposis syndrome	1 in 100,000	AD	Hamartoma
PTEN hamartoma tumor syndrome	1 in 200,000	AD	Hamartoma, adenoma, ganglioneuroma, serrated
Serrated polyposis syndrome	1 in 3000	Familial	Serrated

AD = autosomal dominant; AR = autosomal recessive.

often manifest by the second decade of life. Without treatment, colorectal cancer typically develops in all patients by the age of 40 years. Gastric fundic gland polyposis and duodenal adenomas are also present in most patients. Gastric cancer is rare, but duodenal and periampullary cancers are the second leading cause of cancer death in this group (2.5%-30%, depending on duodenal polyposis stage). Papillary carcinoma of the thyroid is increasingly recognized as accompanying FAP.

A milder form of FAP has also been identified and is known as attenuated FAP (AFAP); patients with AFAP have fewer colorectal polyps, generally less than 100. AFAP has a later age of onset and a lower cumulative lifetime risk of colorectal cancer than classic FAP. The colorectal polyps are often right-sided.

Gardner syndrome is a phenotypic variant of FAP that is characterized by colonic polyposis, benign soft tissue tumors (including sebaceous cysts and lipomas), osteomas, supernumerary teeth, desmoid tumors, and congenital hypertrophy of the retinal pigment epithelium. Turcot syndrome is another variant of FAP that includes polyposis associated with brain tumors, including cerebellar medulloblastoma, astrocytoma, and ependymoma.

Biallelic mutations in the base excision repair gene *MYH* cause MAP. MAP is an autosomal recessive syndrome that has similar colonic and extraintestinal features as AFAP, at least a 50% lifetime risk of cancer, and a mean age of cancer onset of 52 years.

Peutz-Jeghers Syndrome

Peutz-Jeghers syndrome (PJS) is caused by a mutation in a gene that encodes for threonine kinase (*STK11*) gene. PJS results in development of diffuse intestinal hamartomatous polyps (which often cause small-bowel obstruction by the age of 20 years) and mucocutaneous pigmentation that is most obvious on the vermilion border of the lips. Diagnostic criteria for PJS consist of two or more of the following: two or more small-bowel hamartomas, mucocutaneous pigmentation, or a family history of PJS. There is a 90% cumulative lifetime risk for intestinal and extraintestinal cancer in PJS. The cumulative lifetime risk for specific sites is as follows: breast, 55%; colon, 38%; pancreas, 38%; gastric, nearly 30%; ovary, 20%; lung, 18%; small intestine, 12%; uterus and cervix, 10%; unusual gonadal neoplasms of the ovary, 20%; and unusual gonadal neoplasms of the testes, 10%.

Juvenile Polyposis Syndrome

Patients with juvenile polyposis syndrome (JPS) develop numerous hamartomatous polyps, known as juvenile polyps, in the colon. Germline mutations are detected in 50% of patients with JPS and are either in the *BMPR1A* or *SMAD4* gene. Although most patients develop symptoms by the age of 20 years, the name "juvenile" refers to the histology of the polyp, not the age of the affected individual. The clinical criteria for this syndrome consist of (1) more than three juvenile polyps of the colon, (2) juvenile polyps throughout the gastro-

intestinal tract, or (3) one or more juvenile polyps combined with a family history of juvenile polyposis syndrome. Juvenile polyposis syndrome usually presents with gastrointestinal bleeding, diarrhea, gastric outlet obstruction, or protein-losing enteropathy from massive gastric polyposis. There is an increased risk for colon cancer (39%), gastric cancer (25%), and more rarely small-bowel and pancreatic cancer.

Solitary juvenile polyps are one of the most commonly found colorectal polyps, particularly in children under the age of 10 years; they confer no future health risk once the polyp is removed, and follow-up surveillance colonoscopy is not required.

PTEN Hamartoma Tumor Syndrome

PTEN hamartoma tumor syndrome (including Cowden syndrome and Bannayan-Riley-Ruvalcaba syndrome) is caused by a mutation in the *PTEN* gene, which functions as a tumor suppressor gene. Macrocephaly and intestinal polyposis are primary features. There is an increased risk of thyroid, breast, endometrial, colon, and renal cell cancers.

Serrated Polyposis Syndrome

Serrated polyposis syndrome is a familial polyposis syndrome characterized by multiple, large, proximal hyperplastic polyps or serrated adenomas without a known genetic cause. It is diagnosed using the World Health Organization criteria of (1) five or more serrated polyps proximal to the sigmoid colon, two or more of which are 10 mm in diameter or greater; (2) any number of serrated polyps proximal to the sigmoid colon in an individual with a first-degree relative who has serrated polyposis syndrome; or (3) more than 20 serrated polyps distributed throughout the colon. Serrated polyposis syndrome is associated with an increased risk of colorectal but not extraintestinal cancer. The mean age of colon cancer diagnosis is 56 years, and metachronous colon cancer occurs in up to 7% of patients at 5 years of follow-up. Surveillance is recommended.

Screening

For a discussion of screening in patients at average risk for colorectal cancer, see MKSAP 17 General Internal Medicine.

Patients with a greater-than-average risk for colorectal cancer should undergo colonoscopic surveillance, which should be customized according to the patient's risk factors.

Patients with a family history of an adenoma or colorectal cancer in a first-degree relative prior to age 60 years, or in two or more first-degree relatives at any age, should undergo colonoscopy every 5 years beginning at age 40 years (or at an age 10 years younger than the earliest age of the case in the immediate family). Patients with a family history of an adenoma or colorectal cancer in a first-degree relative age 60 years or older or with two second-degree relatives with colorectal cancer at any age should undergo colorectal cancer screening with any average-risk strategy; however, colonoscopy every 10 years is recommended by some experts. For these patients, the U.S. Multi-Society Task Force (MSTF) on Colorectal Cancer recommends starting screening at age 40 years, whereas the American College of Gastroenterology recommends beginning at age 50 years. The MSTF recommends stopping colonoscopy surveillance when the risk of the procedure outweighs the benefit to the high-risk patient. At ages 75 to 85 years, the potential benefit of surveillance is higher than for average-risk patients. At ages older than 85 years, patients with high-risk adenomas are at higher risk for metachronous advanced neoplasia than average-risk patients; continued surveillance should be individualized based on medical comorbidities and life expectancy, but routine screening should not be continued.

KEY POINTS

- Patients with a greater-than-average risk for colorectal cancer should undergo colonoscopic surveillance, which should be customized according to the patient's risk factors.
- Patients with a family history of an adenoma or colorectal cancer in a first-degree relative prior to age 60 years, or in two or more first-degree relatives at any age, should undergo colonoscopy every 5 years beginning at age 40 years (or at an age 10 years younger than the earliest age of the case in the immediate family).

Chemoprevention

Epidemiologic studies have demonstrated an association between high consumption of folate, fruits, vegetables, and fiber with a lower risk of colorectal neoplasia; however, these findings have not been confirmed in randomized controlled trials.

Chemoprevention is not indicated for patients at average risk for colorectal neoplasia. However, there is increasing evidence that a number of agents, particularly NSAIDs, may be beneficial in preventing colorectal neoplasia. Long-term aspirin use substantially reduces the risk of benign and malignant colorectal neoplasms and colorectal cancer deaths by up to 60%. These results have been confirmed in cohort, case control, and randomized controlled trials in low- and very-high-risk populations, including patients with Lynch syndrome. Strong data demonstrate that celecoxib, rofecoxib, and sulindac (in combination with difluoromethylornithine) effectively reduce recurrent adenomas in patients who have undergone polypectomy. Celecoxib promotes the regression of adenomas in adult and pediatric patients with FAP. Additionally, a significant decrease in metachronous adenomas was observed in patients taking 1200 mg of calcium carbonate daily. However, routine use of these agents for chemoprevention is not recommended owing to the increased risk of vascular and bleeding complications with NSAIDs, the cardiovascular risk associated with exogenous calcium supplementation, the lack of consensus on the optimal dosing of these agents, and the balance of risks and benefits of aspirin use, especially in patients at low risk.

KEY POINT

- Chemoprevention is not indicated for patients at average risk for colorectal neoplasia, and it is not routinely recommended for patients at high or very high risk for colorectal neoplasia.

Clinical Presentation

The majority of colon polyps and colon cancers are asymptomatic until they are advanced. Gastrointestinal bleeding is the most common sign and may be revealed by positive fecal occult blood testing, iron deficiency anemia, or hematochezia. Unexplained anorexia, change in bowel habits, abdominal pain, weight loss, or symptoms of bowel obstruction may occur when tumors are advanced.

Diagnosis and Staging

The diagnosis of colorectal neoplasia is most often made by colonoscopy performed for gastrointestinal symptoms, screening, or surveillance.

Polyps are typically described by their appearance: sessile (in which the entire base is attached to the colonic wall), flat (in which the diameter of the lesion is at least twice as great as the height), or pedunculated (where a mucosal stalk exists between the colonic wall and the polyp).

The histologic types of polyps are noted in **Table 27**. Screening colonoscopy studies demonstrate that polyps are detected in approximately 60% of average-risk individuals. The prevalence of polyps on average-risk screening colonoscopy is 22% to 25% for adenomas, 12% for hyperplastic polyps, and 0.6% for sessile serrated polyps. The degree of dysplasia in a polyp is also reported as high, intermediate, or low.

TABLE 27. Classification of Colorectal Polyps
Adenomatous Polyps[a]
Tubular adenoma
Tubulovillous adenoma
Villous adenoma
Serrated Polyps
Hyperplastic polyp
Sessile serrated polyp with or without cytologic dysplasia
Traditional serrated adenoma
Other
Hamartomatous polyp
Inflammatory polyp

[a]With or without high-grade dysplasia.

Adenomatous polyps are neoplastic lesions and therefore have malignant potential; most colorectal cancers arise from adenomatous polyps. Adenomatous polyps are further defined by their glandular architecture: tubular, villous, or a combination of both. The most common pattern is tubular, then tubulovillous, and the least common pattern is primarily villous.

Serrated polyps are classified into three histologic types: hyperplastic polyps, sessile serrated polyps, and traditional serrated adenomas. Hyperplastic polyps are the most common type of serrated polyp. They are non-neoplastic and are composed of normal mucosal elements; small hyperplastic polyps, often found in the rectosigmoid colon, are believed to have no clinical significance. Sessile serrated polyps (also known as sessile serrated adenomas) and traditional serrated adenomas are both neoplastic and are precursors to colorectal cancer; they should be completely excised. Substantial variability has been demonstrated in the ability of a pathologist to differentiate a hyperplastic polyp from a sessile serrated polyp; therefore, some experts recommend managing large (>10 mm) hyperplastic polyps as if they are sessile serrated polyps.

If colorectal cancer is diagnosed, staging provides a uniform description of the depth of tumor invasion into the colon wall and other structures, as well as the spread to lymph nodes and distant organs. There are two types of staging for colorectal cancer: a clinical stage and a pathologic stage. Clinical staging includes findings on physical examination, results of colonoscopic biopsy, and pretreatment CT imaging of the chest, abdomen, and pelvis. If an indeterminate liver mass is detected, MRI of the abdomen with and without gadolinium-based contrast enhancement is suggested. MRI of the pelvis is recommended for patients with rectal cancer. Pathologic staging is performed after the tumor is removed and reports the tumor type and differentiation, depth of invasion, lymph node involvement, distant metastasis, margin status, perineural and angiolymphatic invasion, and many other clinically validated factors.

For treatment of colorectal cancer, see MKSAP 17 Hematology and Oncology.

Surveillance

History of Adenomatous and Serrated Polyps

After neoplastic polyps (adenomas, sessile serrated polyps, or traditional serrated adenomas) are removed, postpolypectomy colonoscopy should be performed; the surveillance interval depends on the size, number, and pathology of the polyps (**Table 28**). Colonoscopy intervals are as short as 3 to 6 months in patients with removal of large (>2 cm) sessile polyps, more than 10 adenomas, piecemeal removal of adenomas or sessile serrated polyps, or adenomas with invasive cancer and favorable prognostic features.

Invasive adenocarcinoma arising in a pedunculated or sessile polyp may be adequately treated by endoscopic polypectomy alone if the lesion is removed en bloc, invades only the submucosa, possesses no adverse histologic features

TABLE 28. Postpolypectomy Surveillance	
Adenomatous Polyps	**Interval to Next Colonoscopy**
1-2 <10-mm tubular adenomas	5-10 years
3-10 adenomas, ≥10 mm, villous histology, or high-grade dysplasia	3 years
≥10 adenomas on single examination	<3 years; a genetic cause of disease should be investigated
Serrated Polyps	
<10-mm rectosigmoid hyperplastic polyps	10 years
SSP <10 mm	5 years
SSP ≥10 mm or SSP with dysplasia or TSA	3 years
Serrated polyposis syndrome	1 year

SSP = sessile serrated polyps; TSA = traditional serrated adenomas.

(poorly differentiated, lymphovascular invasion), and has clear margins. These polyps containing invasive cancer should be followed up with colonoscopy 3 to 6 months after removal.

KEY POINT

- After neoplastic polyps (adenomas, sessile serrated polyps, or traditional serrated adenomas) are removed, postpolypectomy colonoscopy should be performed; the surveillance interval depends on the size, number, and pathology of the polyps.

History of Colorectal Cancer

Patients who undergo a complete perioperative colonoscopy with clearing of synchronous neoplasia and curative surgical resection for colon cancer should have a subsequent surveillance colonoscopy within 1 year. If the colonoscopy is normal, a repeat examination is recommended at 3 years, and, if normal, every 5 years thereafter. If neoplasms are detected during any follow-up examination, then the surveillance interval should be adjusted based on polyp size, number, and histology (see Table 28). Owing to the heightened risk of early local recurrence after rectal cancer therapy, patients with rectal cancer should undergo a flexible sigmoidoscopy evaluation of the anastomosis every 3 to 6 months for the first 3 years.

KEY POINT

- Patients who undergo a complete perioperative colonoscopy with clearing of synchronous neoplasia and curative surgical resection for colon cancer should have a subsequent surveillance colonoscopy within 1 year.

Hereditary Nonpolyposis Colon Cancer

Patients who meet the Amsterdam criteria for HNPCC should receive genetic counseling and should be offered genetic testing.

Individuals who have or are at risk for Lynch syndrome should undergo colonoscopy every 1 to 2 years beginning at age 20 to 25 years, or 2 to 5 years earlier than the youngest age at diagnosis of colorectal cancer if the affected relative was less than 25 years old. Although the evidence is low, consideration should be given to yearly urinalysis (to check for microscopic hematuria) or upper endoscopy every 2 to 3 years beginning at age 30 to 35 years (to screen for upper gastrointestinal cancer). Prophylactic hysterectomy and bilateral salpingo-oophorectomy is a risk-reducing option that should be considered in women who have completed childbearing. Annual endometrial sampling and transvaginal ultrasonography may be considered in women with Lynch syndrome who are older than 25 years.

Familial Adenomatous Polyposis and *MYH*-Associated Polyposis

Patients with FAP and MAP should receive genetic counseling and should be offered genetic testing. Because MAP is autosomal recessive, both parents must be carriers of an *MYH* mutation in order for a child to inherit the syndrome.

Beginning at age 10 to 15 years, *APC* gene carriers or those with indeterminate status for FAP should undergo yearly flexible sigmoidoscopy or colonoscopy. Individuals who have or who are at risk for MAP should undergo colonoscopy every 2 to 3 years beginning at age 25 to 30 years. After colectomy is performed, lifelong yearly surveillance of the rectum or ileal pouch is required to manage recurrent polyposis and decrease the risk of rectal or pouch adenocarcinoma. Upper endoscopy for surveillance of duodenal cancer is indicated every 1 to 5 years at an interval based on the stage of the duodenal polyposis.

Ulcerative or Crohn Colitis

Patients with long-standing colitis are at increased risk for colon cancer and should undergo surveillance colonoscopy every 1 to 2 years beginning after 8 to 10 years of disease. This recommendation applies to patients with ulcerative colitis involving more than the rectum and those with Crohn colitis involving at least one third of the colon.

KEY POINT

- Patients with ulcerative colitis or Crohn colitis should receive surveillance colonoscopy every 1 to 2 years beginning after 8 to 10 years of disease.

Peutz-Jeghers Syndrome

For patients with Peutz-Jeghers syndrome, surveillance of the small bowel with capsule endoscopy or CT or magnetic resonance enterography is recommended every 2 to 3 years starting at age 8 to 10 years. Colonoscopy and upper endoscopy should be performed every 2 to 3 years beginning in the late teenage years. MRI or endoscopic ultrasound of the pancreas should be performed every 1 to 2 years beginning at age 30 to 35 years. Patients should also receive early and aggressive surveillance for cancer of the breast, ovary, cervix, uterus, and testis.

Other Syndromes

For patients with juvenile polyposis syndrome, colonoscopy and upper endoscopy are recommended every 2 to 3 years beginning at age 15 years.

For patients with *PTEN* hamartoma tumor syndrome, colonoscopy is recommended every 5 years beginning at age 35 years. Annual surveillance of the breasts and thyroid should begin at age 25 and 18 years, respectively.

Patients with serrated polyposis syndrome should undergo colonoscopy yearly.

Disorders of the Liver

Approach to the Patient with Abnormal Liver Chemistry Studies

Approximately 13% of patients undergoing medical evaluation have abnormal liver test results; 5% of patients have persistent abnormalities of one or more liver enzyme levels.

Typical serum elevations and clinical features of common liver diseases are shown in **Table 29**.

Disorders that cause liver disease are considered hepatocellular when the predominant elevation is of the serum alanine aminotransferase (ALT) and aspartate aminotransferase (AST) levels. Disorders are considered cholestatic when the predominant elevation is of serum alkaline phosphatase (ALP). Elevations in ALT are more specific for liver injury than AST elevations; however, severe muscle injury can produce elevations of both enzymes. An elevated ALP level accompanied by elevations in other liver enzymes is nearly always due to liver or biliary disease; an isolated elevation in the ALP can be secondary to an elevation in bone fraction. Measurement of γ-glutamyl transpeptidase may be used to confirm a liver origin of an elevated ALP level.

Liver function is assessed by measuring prothrombin time and serum albumin level, which depend on the liver's synthetic ability.

Bilirubin is also a useful marker of liver function for hepatocellular diseases. Liver diseases generally cause an increase in both conjugated (direct) and unconjugated (indirect) bilirubin. Gilbert syndrome is a benign condition characterized by mild unconjugated hyperbilirubinemia, which is caused by a congenital decrease in hepatic uridine diphosphate glucuronyl transferase.

Imaging of the liver with ultrasound, CT, and MRI can assess for parenchymal changes and vascular flows. Ultrasound is useful because it does not require intravenous access, but its usefulness may be limited in obese patients and it has the lowest sensitivity for the detection of liver masses. MRI is useful because it does not expose the patient to radiation and allows for assessment of the biliary tree using magnetic resonance cholangiopancreatography (MRCP). Histologic assessment will often require a liver biopsy; however, serologic markers and ultrasound- or

TABLE 29. Typical Liver Chemistry Studies in Common Hepatobiliary Disorders

Disease	AST	ALT	ALP	Bilirubin	Other Features
Acute viral hepatitis	↑↑↑	↑↑↑	Normal to ↑	Normal to ↑↑↑	Exposure history, fatigue, nausea
Chronic viral hepatitis	↑	↑↑	Normal to ↑	↑ if advanced	History of exposure to infected blood or body fluids
Nonalcoholic steatohepatitis	↑	↑	Normal to ↑	Normal	Metabolic syndrome
Alcoholic hepatitis	↑↑	Normal or ↑	↑	Normal to ↑↑↑	Excess alcohol intake
Acute autoimmune hepatitis	↑↑↑	↑↑↑	Normal to ↑	Normal to ↑↑	Autoantibodies
Chronic autoimmune hepatitis	↑	↑↑	Normal to ↑	Normal	Autoantibodies
Wilson disease	↑	↑	Low	↑ and often unconjugated	Hemolysis if acute, neurologic symptoms if chronic
α₁-Antitrypsin deficiency	↑	↑	Normal	↑ if advanced	May have pulmonary disease
Hemochromatosis	Normal	Normal	Normal	Normal	Joint symptoms, family history, other organ involvement
Primary biliary cirrhosis	↑	↑	↑↑↑	↑ if advanced	Female, sicca symptoms, antimitochondrial antibody
Primary sclerosing cholangitis	↑	↑	↑↑↑	↑ if advanced or dominant stricture is present	Ulcerative colitis, abnormal cholangiogram
Large duct obstruction	↑ (↑↑ if acute)	↑ (↑↑ if acute)	↑↑	↑↑	Pain if acute, dilated ducts on imaging
Infiltrative liver disease	↑	↑	↑↑↑	Normal	Features of malignancy, sarcoid, amyloid, or mycobacterial or fungal infection
Hepatic ischemia	↑↑↑	↑↑↑	Normal	Normal	AST >5000 U/L, history of hypotension
Celiac disease	Normal or ↑	Normal or ↑	Normal or ↑	Normal	Usually other features of celiac disease

ALP = alkaline phosphatase; ALT = alanine aminotransferase; AST = aspartate aminotransferase.

magnetic resonance–based elastography are increasingly used to assess for fibrosis. Elastography uses the velocity at which waves pass through the liver to provide an assessment of liver tissue stiffness, which correlates with fibrosis. For patients with obvious clinical features of cirrhosis, such as splenomegaly or other complications of portal hypertension, liver biopsy is unnecessary.

KEY POINT

- Disorders that cause liver disease are considered hepatocellular when the predominant elevation is of the serum alanine aminotransferase and aspartate aminotransferase levels; disorders are considered cholestatic when the predominant elevation is of serum alkaline phosphatase.

Viral Hepatitis

Hepatitis A

The burden of hepatitis A virus (HAV) infection correlates with socioeconomic indicators, especially income levels and quality of sanitation. In areas with lower incomes and poorly developed sanitation systems, more than 90% of children have evidence of previous HAV infection by the age of 10 years. Areas with relatively higher incomes and better-developed sanitation systems such as the United States have a lower prevalence of HAV infection.

The incubation period of HAV is 2 to 6 weeks. Symptoms of acute HAV are jaundice, fatigue, mild abdominal pain, fever, and diarrhea. Patients older than 30 years are more likely than younger individuals to have jaundice with an acute HAV infection, and acute liver failure (ALF) may rarely occur. Transmission from an infected patient occurs during the incubation period or within 1 week after jaundice develops. Acute HAV is diagnosed with detection of serum IgM antibodies to HAV. The presence of IgG antibodies to HAV is a marker of immunity due to either previous exposure or vaccination.

The majority of patients with acute HAV infection have resolution of symptoms and liver test abnormalities within 3 months. A relapsing or prolonged course can occur in up to 10% of individuals, but chronic infection does not occur. The clinical course of relapsing HAV is characterized by clinical recovery with near normalization of the serum liver tests, followed several weeks later by biochemical and sometimes clinical relapse. No specific treatment is available for HAV.

HAV infection is prevented by administration of hepatitis A vaccine (see MKSAP 17 General Internal Medicine). Postexposure prophylaxis with hepatitis A vaccine is effective in preventing infection and obviates the need for administration of immune globulin in most patients. The administration of immune globulin can be considered for postexposure prophylaxis in patients who are immunocompromised (such as those who have undergone organ transplantation) or were previously unvaccinated and are traveling to an endemic area if departure is within 2 weeks.

KEY POINT

- The majority of patients with acute hepatitis A virus infection have resolution of symptoms and liver test abnormalities within 3 months.

Hepatitis B

Hepatitis B virus (HBV) is a DNA virus that can cause both acute and chronic hepatitis. Worldwide, chronic infection with HBV is common, with about 350 million persons infected. Transmission occurs following exposure to blood or body fluids from an infected patient. Because resolution of infection is less common when infection is acquired at a young age, as opposed to an older age, most chronically infected patients were infected perinatally or in early childhood. The incubation period of HBV infection is 4 to 24 weeks. In the United States, chronic HBV infection is encountered clinically much more frequently than acute infection. Extrahepatic manifestations of HBV infection, such as arthritis, polyarteritis nodosa, and kidney disease, are rarely encountered in clinical practice.

Relatively simple blood tests are widely available to diagnose HBV and help determine disease activity (**Table 30**).

Acute HBV infection will resolve (defined as clearance of hepatitis B surface antigen within 6 months) in 90% of adult patients. Serial monitoring of liver enzymes and markers of liver synthetic function is the most appropriate management strategy. Antiviral therapy can be considered for prolonged and severe cases.

Chronic HBV infection is characteristically divided into phases of disease (**Figure 25**). Not all patients go through each phase. Patients who acquire HBV infection at birth (vertical transmission) often go through the immune tolerant phase, which is characterized by a normal ALT level despite a positive hepatitis B e antigen (HBeAg) and very high HBV DNA level. This phase may persist until the age of 30 years. Liver biopsy will show little injury, presumably owing to an absence of immunologic damage to the infected hepatocytes. In cross-sectional studies, approximately 60% of patients with chronic HBV infection are in the inactive carrier, or "immune control," phase that is characterized by a normal ALT level and an HBV DNA level less than 10,000 IU/mL. Patients in the HBeAg-positive ("immune active") or HBeAg-negative ("reactivation") chronic HBV phases have an elevated ALT level and an HBV DNA level above 10,000 IU/mL. When liver biopsy is performed, lymphocytic inflammation and variable degrees of fibrosis are identified.

HBV treatment is not advised in patients in the immune tolerant or inactive carrier (immune control) phases; however,

TABLE 30. Interpretation of Hepatitis B Test Results							
Clinical Scenario	HBsAg	Anti-HBs	IgM anti-HBc	IgG anti-HBc	HBeAg	Anti-HBe	HBV DNA (IU/mL)
Acute hepatitis B; occasionally reactivation of chronic hepatitis B	+	–	+	–	+	–	>20,000
Resolved previous infection	–	+	–	+	–	+/–	Undetected
Immunity due to previous vaccination	–	+	–	–	–	–	Undetected
False positive anti-HBc or resolved previous infection	–	–	–	+	–	–	Undetected
Immune tolerant (HBeAg-positive chronic hepatitis B) (perinatally acquired, age <30 years)	+	–	–	+	+	–	>1 million
Immune control (chronic hepatitis B inactive carrier)	+	–	–	+	–	+	<10,000
Immune active (HBeAg-positive chronic hepatitis B)	+	–	–	+	+	–	>10,000
Reactivation (HBeAg-negative chronic hepatitis B)	+	–	–	+	–	+	>10,000

Anti-HBc = hepatitis B core antibody; anti-HBe = hepatitis B e antibody; anti-HBs = hepatitis B surface antibody; HBeAg = hepatitis B e antigen; HBsAg = hepatitis B surface antigen; HBV = hepatitis B virus.

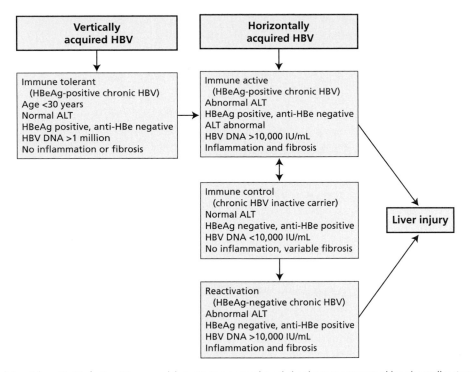

FIGURE 25. Phases of chronic hepatitis B infection. It is assumed that patients progress through the phases in sequence, although not all patients will develop HBeAg-negative chronic hepatitis B, and only patients with vertical transmission of hepatitis B will have a clinically recognized immune tolerant phase. All phases have positive HBsAg, negative anti-HBs, and positive IgG anti-HBc. ALT = alanine aminotransferase; anti-HBc = hepatitis B core antibody; anti-HBe = hepatitis B e antibody; anti-HBs = hepatitis B surface antibody; HBeAg = hepatitis B e antigen; HBsAg = hepatitis B surface antigen; HBV = hepatitis B virus; HBV DNA = hepatitis B virus DNA.

monitoring with ALT measurement is necessary to detect transitions to other phases. For patients with HBV, treatment is recommended for those who (1) have ALF, (2) have chronic infection with an elevated ALT level and an HBV DNA level greater than 10,000 IU/mL, or (3) are receiving immunosuppressive therapy. Treatment usually consists of entecavir or tenofovir. For most patients, chronic treatment is necessary unless seroconversion of HBeAg or hepatitis B surface antigen (HBsAg) is observed. Lamivudine, adefovir, and telbivudine are used less often because of development of resistance with chronic use. Pegylated interferon may be used for patients without cirrhosis who have high ALT levels, relatively low HBV DNA levels, and ability to tolerate the side effects of pegylated interferon. The treatment goal is normalization of the ALT level and a decline in HBV DNA level to <50 IU/mL. Only a few patients will become HBsAg negative with treatment; therefore, cure of HBV is an unrealistic goal for most chronically infected patients.

In approximately 50% of untreated patients with chronic HBV infection in the United States, HBV will contribute to the cause of death (from hepatocellular carcinoma [HCC] or other complications of end-stage liver disease, such as cirrhosis). Patients who respond to treatment have a decreased risk of liver-related complications of HBV. The following characteristics are associated with an increased risk for HCC in patients with HBV and are indications for surveillance with ultrasound or other imaging every 6 months: (1) patients with cirrhosis, (2) Asian men older than 40 years, (3) Asian women older than 50 years, (4) African patients older than 20 years, (5) patients with persistent inflammatory activity (defined as an elevated ALT level and HBV DNA levels greater than 10,000 IU/mL for at least a few years), and (6) patients with a family history of HCC.

Population-based studies have shown that widespread use of HBV vaccination decreases the incidence and prevalence of HBV. This has also been demonstrated to result in fewer cases of HCC in endemic areas. See MKSAP 17 General Internal Medicine for a discussion of vaccinations.

KEY POINTS

- Treatment is recommended for patients with hepatitis B virus infection who (1) have acute liver failure, (2) have chronic infection with an elevated alanine aminotransferase level and a hepatitis B virus DNA level greater than 10,000 IU/mL, or (3) are receiving immunosuppressive therapy.

- Population-based studies have shown that widespread use of hepatitis B virus vaccination decreases the incidence and prevalence of hepatitis B virus infection.

Hepatitis C

Hepatitis C virus (HCV) is the most common bloodborne infection in the United States, with an estimated 4 million patients infected. Globally, approximately 180 million patients are infected. Because patients with HCV infection are often asymptomatic and unaware of their infection, screening is recommended by the U.S. Preventive Services Task Force for individuals born between 1945 and 1965 (see MKSAP 17 General Internal Medicine). Transmission occurs with exposure to blood; most patients acquire HCV from illicit drug use. Although the risk of transmission of HCV from needle-stick exposure is low, transmission of HCV in the health care setting is well documented. Sixty percent to 85% of patients who acquire HCV infection remain chronically infected. Over a period of 25 to 30 years, approximately 30% of patients with chronic HCV infection develop cirrhosis and are at risk for liver failure or HCC. Although the number of new HCV infections in the United States is decreasing, the number of patients with liver failure and HCC continues to increase owing to the propensity of HCV to result in chronic infection and the long lag time between infection and development of liver complications. In contrast to HBV, HCV rarely causes HCC in the absence of cirrhosis.

Symptomatic acute HCV infection is unusual. Patients with chronic HCV infection are often asymptomatic, but fatigue and vague right upper quadrant pain are sometimes reported. Those with cirrhosis may present with complications of portal hypertension. Cryoglobulinemic vasculitis, membranoproliferative glomerulonephritis, and porphyria cutanea tarda are extrahepatic manifestations of HCV infection.

The diagnosis of HCV is established by the presence of HCV RNA in serum. Patients with spontaneous resolution of acute HCV or who have been treated successfully for HCV will have clearance of HCV RNA but usually remain positive for antibody to HCV. Liver biopsy findings consistent with HCV are lymphocytic portal inflammation with nodular lymphoid aggregates, steatosis, and variable fibrosis. With the advent of more successful HCV treatment and the use of less invasive ways to assess fibrosis, liver biopsy is now done in a minority of patients with HCV. HCV RNA level does not influence disease progression, and serial monitoring of HCV RNA level is not recommended (except during HCV treatment). HCV genotyping should be performed at the time of diagnosis to help choose a treatment regimen.

The goal of HCV treatment is sustained virologic response (SVR), defined as undetectable HCV RNA 6 months after completion. SVR results in improved patient outcomes, including a decrease in all-cause mortality. Patients with cirrhosis are less likely to achieve SVR than those without cirrhosis. The treatment of HCV continues to evolve rapidly. SVR rates in excess of 90% are now achieved in most patient groups. Approved options for therapy in patients with HCV genotype 1 (the most prominent genotype in the United States) include the direct-acting antivirals sofosbuvir and ledipasvir (available as a combination tablet), which has been shown to result in SVR in 95% of treated patients. Other treatment regimens for genotype 1 include the combination of the direct-acting antivirals ombitasvir and paritaprevir and the protease inhibitor

ritonavir (available in a single tablet), which is packaged and coadministered with an additional tablet, the direct-acting antiviral dasabuvir; these drugs may be administered with or without concurrent ribavirin. A third option not approved by the FDA for this indication is the combination of the protease inhibitor simeprevir and the direct-acting antiviral sofosbuvir, with or without concurrent ribavirin; these agents are not available as a combined preparation. Patients with genotype 2 are usually treated with sofosbuvir and ribavirin for 12 weeks, whereas those with genotype 3 are treated with sofosbuvir and ribavirin for 24 weeks. Sofosbuvir and ledipasvir, combined with ribavirin, may have a role in the treatment of patients with genotype 3 who do not achieve SVR with other regimens. Patients with genotype 4 are currently treated with pegylated interferon, ribavirin, and sofosbuvir.

Patients with cirrhosis should undergo surveillance for HCC. Patients with HCV who have decompensated disease or localized HCC are candidates for liver transplantation. Posttransplant hepatitis C viremia occurs in nearly all patients and has a variable natural history. Treatment with antiviral agents can be effective for patients with recurrent HCV after liver transplantation.

A vaccine against HCV has not been developed, likely related to the ability of the virus to mutate. For patients exposed to HCV, prophylactic therapy to prevent disease acquisition is not yet advised. For patients with recognized acute infection, a period of monitoring for 3 months is worthwhile to document the 15% to 40% chance for spontaneous resolution prior to initiating treatment. Patients whose disease does not resolve after 3 months are generally treated.

Patients infected with HCV are advised to avoid blood exposures (includes avoidance of sharing dental and shaving appliances). For monogamous heterosexual couples, the risk of sexual transmission is 0.07% per year, and therefore condom use is not generally recommended. Men who have sex with men are likely at increased risk of transmission of HCV compared with those in heterosexual relationships.

Owing to shared risk factors, infection with HCV is seen in 15% to 30% of individuals with HIV infection. Coinfection leads to more rapid progression of liver disease than in patients with HCV alone. Treatment of patients with coinfection is similar to that for patients with HCV alone, but careful attention to potential drug interactions is necessary.

KEY POINT

- Because patients with hepatitis C virus infection are often asymptomatic and unaware of their infection, screening is recommended by the U.S. Preventive Services Task Force for individuals born between 1945 and 1965.

Hepatitis D

Hepatitis D virus (HDV) is a defective RNA virus that requires the presence of HBV to replicate. HDV infection is most common in South America and Mediterranean countries. HDV can be acquired simultaneously with HBV (coinfection) or subsequently in a patient already infected with HBV (superinfection). Patients with HBV infection should be tested for HDV, especially in the presence of an otherwise unexplained acute hepatitis in a patient with chronic HBV. HDV is typically diagnosed with antibody tests, but HDV RNA testing is available at specialized laboratories. Treatment for HDV is with pegylated interferon; however, response rates are only approximately 25% to 30%. Therefore, treatment is pursued only in patients with progressive liver injury despite treatment of HBV.

Hepatitis E

Hepatitis E (HEV) is an RNA virus that most commonly causes epidemics in India, parts of Asia, and Central America. The disease presents similarly to HAV and is diagnosed by the presence of an IgM antibody to HEV.

A second genotype of the virus is increasingly recognized in more developed countries, including the United States. Population-based studies suggest that up to 20% of the U.S. population has serologic evidence of a prior HEV infection; however, acute HEV is rarely encountered. HEV in developed countries may be acquired from an animal reservoir.

Other Viruses

Epstein-Barr virus (EBV), cytomegalovirus (CMV), and other herpesviruses can cause liver injury that is usually mild and self-limited.

Patients with an infectious mononucleosis syndrome due to EBV may have a serum ALT level up to ten times the upper limit of normal, but they are not usually jaundiced. Other typical symptoms of EBV infection, such as fever, fatigue, and sore throat, are usually present.

CMV infection may cause acute hepatitis, especially in immunocompromised patients. Detection of CMV in blood by polymerase chain reaction is more specific than serologic tests.

Hepatitis due to herpesviruses (either herpes simplex viruses or varicella zoster virus) may cause serum aminotransferase levels greater than 5000 U/L, but jaundice is unusual. Most patients with severe herpes hepatitis are immunocompromised or pregnant and have features of encephalitis. The typical herpetic rash is not always present. Antiviral therapy is advised in patients with herpes hepatitis.

Alcohol-Induced Liver Disease

The earliest histologic change in alcoholic liver disease is macrovesicular steatosis. Fatty liver can be caused by binge drinking or chronic alcohol abuse. Patients are usually asymptomatic and may or may not have mild elevations in ALT, AST, γ-glutamyltransferase, or mean corpuscular volume. Abstinence from alcohol results in resolution of fatty liver in 4 to 6 weeks, whereas continued alcohol consumption over many years can result in cirrhosis.

Hepatic steatosis with inflammation is called alcoholic steatohepatitis (ASH). Mild forms of ASH are common, are usually asymptomatic, and are associated with mild elevations in aminotransferase levels.

The most severe form of ASH is called alcoholic hepatitis (AH) and is distinguished from alcohol-induced steatosis and steatohepatitis by the presence of symptoms. AH is the clinical syndrome of jaundice, anorexia, and tender hepatomegaly with or without fever in patients with high-dose (>100 g/d) alcohol intake. Severe AH may be accompanied by hepatic encephalopathy (HE), variceal bleeding, ascites, or hepatorenal syndrome. Laboratory evaluation may demonstrate elevated aminotransferase levels (<300-400 U/L), an AST to ALT ratio greater than 2, conjugated hyperbilirubinemia, elevated γ-glutamyltransferase level, elevated mean corpuscular volume, leukocytosis, and coagulopathy.

Severity of AH is determined by the Maddrey discriminant function (MDF) score, which is calculated as follows:

$$MDF = 4.6 \text{ (prothrombin time [s]}$$
$$- \text{control prothrombin time [s])}$$
$$+ \text{total bilirubin (mg/dL)}$$

Patients with mild disease (MDF <32) should be treated with supportive measures. All patients with alcoholic liver disease should be (1) counseled about abstinence from alcohol and monitored for signs of withdrawal, (2) assessed for thiamine and fat-soluble vitamin deficiencies, and (3) monitored for ongoing malnutrition. Enteral feedings are required in patients with prolonged periods of poor caloric intake.

The presence of HE or an MDF score of 32 or greater signifies a high risk of death and warrants treatment with prednisone or pentoxifylline. Prednisone is the first-line treatment unless contraindications such as infection, variceal hemorrhage, or acute kidney injury are present. If the serum bilirubin level does not improve by day 7, then prednisone should be discontinued. Changing therapy to pentoxifylline thereafter is not beneficial. Portal hypertensive complications should be managed according to usual practice.

Cirrhosis develops in up to 25% of patients with chronic alcohol abuse. Sustained abstinence can stabilize liver function and even resolve portal hypertensive complications.

KEY POINTS

- Abstinence from alcohol results in resolution of fatty liver in 4 to 6 weeks, whereas continued alcohol consumption over many years can result in cirrhosis.

- All patients with alcoholic liver disease should receive counseling about abstinence from alcohol and should be monitored for signs of withdrawal.

Drug-Induced Liver Injury

Drug-induced liver injury (DILI) can be caused by prescription or over-the-counter medications, herbs, or supplements. Clinical manifestations range from an asymptomatic elevation in liver chemistry studies to ALF. The annual incidence of DILI is estimated to be 19 per 100,000 persons. DILI can be categorized as idiosyncratic or intrinsic (predictable). Intrinsic DILI has a short duration from drug ingestion to liver injury (latency), is dose related, and is most common, whereas idiosyncratic DILI is unpredictable, has longer latency, and is less common. Acetaminophen hepatotoxicity is the classic example of intrinsic DILI and is the most common cause of ALF. The following discussion refers to idiosyncratic DILI.

The most common agents that cause idiosyncratic DILI are antimicrobial agents (particularly amoxicillin-clavulanate), antiepileptic drugs (phenytoin, valproate), antituberculosis drugs (isoniazid, rifampin), NSAIDs, and azathioprine. The most common drugs that cause ALF in the United States are antituberculosis drugs, sulfa-containing antimicrobial agents, and antifungal agents. Statins can cause ALF, but this is exceedingly rare. It is safe to continue statins in most patients with mild liver test elevations if no jaundice or symptoms are present. Supplements account for approximately 10% of DILI in the United States.

Diagnosis and management of DILI are described in **Figure 26**.

Diagnosis of DILI requires a history of drug or supplement exposure within 6 to 12 months, a biochemical pattern that fits the hepatotoxicity profile of the causative agent, improvement after drug removal (dechallenge), and the absence of underlying liver or biliary diseases.

Liver biochemistry studies and clinical features can be used to help determine the causative agent, as certain drugs tend to produce typical liver test patterns. Hepatocellular liver test abnormalities (with elevated aminotransferases) are typical of liver injury caused by allopurinol, diclofenac, isoniazid, phenytoin, and valproate. A cholestatic pattern (with elevated ALP) is seen with amoxicillin-clavulanate, carbamazepine, erythromycin, and sulfonamides. A mixed pattern (with elevated aminotransferases and ALP) is typical when azathioprine, enalapril, and ibuprofen are the causative agents.

Hypersensitivity reactions may present with fever, rash, and eosinophilia. Autoimmune-like hepatitis may present with a hepatocellular profile and elevated antinuclear antibody or anti-smooth muscle antibody titers. Minocycline and nitrofurantoin are the most common causes of autoimmune-like hepatitis.

A liver biopsy is rarely necessary but is helpful in cases of uncertainty or suspected drug-induced autoimmune hepatitis. Zone 3 necrosis and eosinophilia are classic histologic findings in DILI, but other findings may include hepatitis, cholestasis, steatosis, or granulomas.

The prognosis for most forms of idiosyncratic DILI is good after removal of the drug and supportive care. However, the mortality rate is as high as 10% when jaundice develops; such patients should be referred to a hepatologist.

Patients with suspected acetaminophen-related DILI should have acetaminophen serum concentrations measured at 4 and 16 hours after ingestion. Patients with levels above 150 μg/mL (at 4 hours after ingestion) or 18.8 μg/mL (at 16 hours after ingestion) should be treated with N-acetylcysteine (NAC)

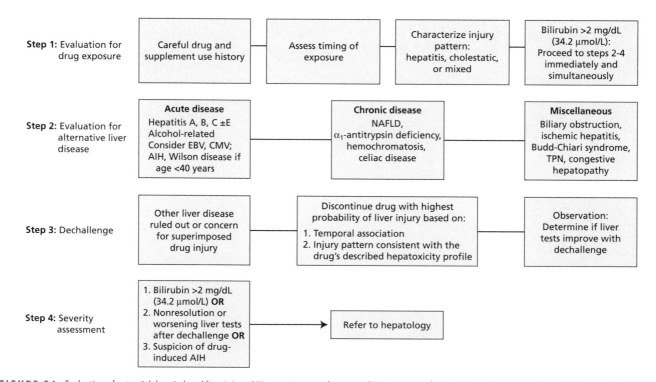

FIGURE 26. Evaluation of potential drug-induced liver injury. AIH = autoimmune hepatitis; CMV = cytomegalovirus; EBV = Epstein-Barr virus; NAFLD = nonalcoholic fatty liver disease; TPN = total parenteral nutrition.

CONT. (Rumack-Matthews nomogram). This strategy is not effective for determining the need for treatment in at-risk patients (such as those with alcoholism or those who are malnourished) with multiple smaller overdoses. If a patient with presumed or known acetaminophen-related DILI develops HE, jaundice, and coagulopathy, this represents ALF in the absence of known chronic liver disease and should be managed accordingly. See Acute Liver Failure for a discussion of management strategies for ALF secondary to acetaminophen. **H**

KEY POINTS

- Acetaminophen is the most common cause of intrinsic drug-induced liver injury; the most common causes of idiosyncratic drug-induced liver injury are antimicrobial agents (particularly amoxicillin-clavulanate), antiepileptic drugs (phenytoin, valproate), antituberculosis drugs (isoniazid, rifampin), NSAIDs, and azathioprine.
- The prognosis for most forms of idiosyncratic drug-induced liver injury is good after removal of the drug and supportive care.

Acute Liver Failure

Acute liver failure (ALF) is defined by the onset of HE, jaundice, and coagulopathy (INR ≥1.5) in patients without a history of chronic liver disease. Liver injury is distinct from ALF and presents with elevated liver test results and/or jaundice in the absence of evidence of liver function failure. The most common cause of ALF in the United States is acetaminophen overdose, followed by indeterminate causes, idiosyncratic DILI, and HBV infection.

A diagnosis of ALF necessitates immediate contact with a liver transplant center, regardless of the cause. Transfer is optimal early in the process when the patient has low-grade HE and can be safely transported.

Patients with ALF require frequent monitoring for hypoglycemia, hypophosphatemia, acute kidney injury, infections, and progressive HE, which can be accompanied by cerebral edema and intracranial hypertension. Patients with grade II HE (**Table 31**) should receive management in the ICU. Many patients with grade III HE and all with grade IV HE require endotracheal intubation and mechanical ventilation. The risk of cerebral edema and intracranial hypertension increases as HE worsens. Intracranial hypertension may manifest as cranial nerve palsies, papilledema, and Cushing triad, which consists of systemic hypertension, bradycardia, and irregular respiration. The initial treatment of intracranial hypertension is with mannitol, followed by hyperventilation.

Specific treatments for ALF include oral antiviral agents for HBV, penicillin G or silymarin for *Amanita* mushroom poisoning, intravenous acyclovir for herpes simplex hepatitis, and urgent delivery of the fetus in acute fatty liver of pregnancy. Other general measures include maintenance of euvolemia, close monitoring for infection, nutritional support, and peptic ulcer disease prophylaxis. In patients requiring renal replace-

TABLE 31. Hepatic Encephalopathy Classification

Grade	Intellectual Function	Neuromuscular Abnormality
0	Normal	Normal
Minimal	Normal examination; subtle changes in driving/work	Minor abnormalities on psychometric tests
I	Personality changes, attention deficits, irritability, depressed state	Tremor and incoordination
II	Sleep-wake cycle alterations, behavioral changes, cognitive dysfunction, fatigue	Asterixis, ataxia, slow speech
III	Altered level of consciousness (somnolence), confusion, disorientation, and amnesia	Muscular rigidity, nystagmus, clonus, plantar extensor response, hyporeflexia
IV	Stupor and coma	Unresponsiveness to noxious stimuli

Adapted from Nevah MI, Fallon MB. Hepatic Encephalopathy, Hepatorenal Syndrome, Hepatopulmonary Syndrome, and Systemic Complications of Liver Disease. In: Sleisenger and Fordtran's Gastrointestinal and Liver Diseases. 9th Ed. Philadelphia, PA: Saunders; 2010. Copyright Elsevier 2010.

ment therapy, continuous venovenous hemofiltration is usually better tolerated than intermittent hemodialysis.

Patients with ALF secondary to acetaminophen toxicity typically present with aminotransferase levels in the thousands after ingestion of greater than 10 g in 24 hours. If the ingestion of acetaminophen occurred within 3 to 4 hours of presentation, activated charcoal can be administered. NAC should be given as soon as possible and is probably effective even up to 48 hours after acetaminophen ingestion. The interval from ingestion to administration of NAC is very important; mortality rates were 0.4%, 6%, 13%, and 19% when the time interval was less than 12 hours, greater than 12 hours, greater than 24 hours, and greater than 48 hours, respectively. Even in patients with non–acetaminophen-related ALF with grades I to II HE, NAC has been shown in a randomized controlled trial to improve transplant-free survival. **H**

KEY POINTS

- The most common cause of acute liver failure in the United States is acetaminophen overdose.
- A diagnosis of acute liver failure necessitates immediate contact with a liver transplant center.

Autoimmune Hepatitis

Autoimmune hepatitis is a chronic inflammatory liver disease that is usually seen in women (female to male ratio is 4 to 1) and can be associated with other autoimmune diseases (most commonly autoimmune thyroiditis, synovitis, or ulcerative colitis) in 38% of patients. The disease presentation ranges from asymptomatic to ALF. Serum aminotransferase levels are elevated and range from mild elevations to greater than 1000 U/L. Serum IgG levels are also elevated. The ALP is normal to mildly elevated but may be more than two to three times the upper limit of normal in overlap syndromes with primary biliary cirrhosis (PBC) or primary sclerosing cholangitis (PSC). There is no single test to diagnose autoimmune hepatitis; rather, diagnosis requires a constellation of clinical, biochemical, serologic, and histologic findings. Viral hepatitis, Wilson disease (especially in young adults), and alcohol- and/or drug-induced liver injury must be ruled out. Anti-smooth muscle or antinuclear antibodies are typically present; higher antibody titers strengthen the diagnosis. Liver biopsy is usually necessary to confirm the diagnosis. Classic histologic findings are interface hepatitis and lymphoplasmacytic infiltrates.

Absolute indications for treatment are: (1) an AST level greater than 10 times the upper limit of normal, (2) an AST level greater than five times the upper limit of normal with an IgG level greater than two times the upper limit of normal, or (3) bridging necrosis on liver biopsy. Treatment with glucocorticoids and azathioprine normalizes the ALT and IgG levels in most patients and should be continued for at least 24 months. Relapse occurs after stopping treatment in most patients, underscoring the need for long-term ALT/AST surveillance. The decision to stop treatment for autoimmune hepatitis should be made in conjunction with a hepatologist. **H**

Metabolic Liver Disease

Nonalcoholic Fatty Liver Disease

Nonalcoholic fatty liver disease (NAFLD) is the most common cause of abnormal liver test results in the United States. Approximately 30% of individuals in the U.S. have NAFLD, some of whom have normal liver enzyme levels. Most patients with NAFLD have insulin resistance–associated obesity, hypertriglyceridemia, and/or type 2 diabetes mellitus. Approximately 20% of patients with NAFLD have nonalcoholic steatohepatitis (NASH), which is characterized by hepatic steatosis accompanied by inflammation and often fibrosis. Of patients with NASH, approximately 10% have progression to advanced fibrosis. Markers for a higher risk of advanced fibrosis include age older than 50 years, BMI greater than 28, serum triglyceride level greater than 150 mg/dL (1.7 mmol/L), and an ALT level greater than twice the upper limit of normal. Low platelet count and an AST to ALT ratio greater than 1 are clues to the presence of advanced fibrosis. Many cases of "cryptogenic" cirrhosis are likely due to NAFLD, as steatosis may regress as cirrhosis progresses. Although the risk of death from liver disease in patients with NASH is increased compared with patients without NAFLD, the more common causes of death are not liver related. The presence of NAFLD may be an independent predictor of cardiovascular disease.

Although NASH requires a liver biopsy for accurate diagnosis, a presumptive diagnosis can be made in a patient with mild abnormalities of aminotransferase levels, risk factors for NAFLD (such as diabetes, obesity, and hyperlipidemia), and imaging features consistent with hepatic steatosis. Because other liver diseases may also result in hepatic steatosis, patients with elevated liver chemistry studies suspected to have NASH should be evaluated to exclude other causes of chronic liver disease.

Treatment for NAFLD generally consists of controlling risk factors for insulin resistance. Loss of 5% of body weight improves steatosis. One randomized controlled trial showed that vitamin E results in biochemical and histologic improvement in patients without diabetes who have NASH; however, this therapy has not yet been widely accepted. Weight loss after bariatric surgery improves the histologic features of NAFLD and can also be considered if portal hypertension is not present. Statins are not contraindicated in patients with NASH.

Patients with advanced liver disease or HCC due to NAFLD represent an increasing percentage of all liver transplant recipients. NASH commonly recurs after transplantation but rarely causes significant graft dysfunction.

KEY POINTS

- Nonalcoholic fatty liver disease is the most common cause of abnormal liver test results in the United States.
- Treatment for nonalcoholic fatty liver disease generally consists of controlling risk factors for insulin resistance.

Hereditary Hemochromatosis

Hereditary hemochromatosis is often diagnosed based on abnormal iron test results detected during a presymptomatic phase. Hemochromatosis may be discovered during an evaluation for chronic liver disease. Although the serum ferritin level is often elevated in patients with acute liver disease, hemochromatosis is not a cause of acute liver disease. Patients with cirrhosis due to hereditary hemochromatosis are at increased risk for HCC.

The most appropriate initial test for hemochromatosis is a fasting serum transferrin saturation level. Ferritin is not typically used as an initial study because it is nonspecific for hereditary hemochromatosis as a cause of liver disease; it is most effective as a follow-up study for those with an elevated transferrin saturation level. Ferritin is elevated in patients with organ iron overload but can be normal in patients with early disease. Abnormal iron test results can also result from liver disease of any cause, particularly NAFLD and HCV. Patients who require multiple transfusions or have long-standing ineffective erythropoiesis can also have secondary iron overload and can develop symptoms compatible with tissue iron overload. Advanced liver disease of any cause commonly leads to an elevated serum ferritin level, but the iron saturation is usually normal.

A definitive diagnosis of hereditary hemochromatosis is established on the basis of homozygosity for the *C282Y* polymorphism of the *HFE* gene. A liver biopsy is only rarely required to make the diagnosis. Biopsy to assess for cirrhosis is recommended (unless cirrhosis is clinically apparent) for a patient with hemochromatosis and a serum ferritin level greater than 1000 ng/mL (1000 µg/L).

Hemochromatosis is discussed further in MKSAP 17 Hematology and Oncology.

KEY POINTS

- The most appropriate initial test for hereditary hemochromatosis is a fasting serum transferrin saturation level.
- A definitive diagnosis of hereditary hemochromatosis is established on the basis of homozygosity for the *C282Y* polymorphism of the *HFE* gene.

α_1-Antitrypsin Deficiency

Patients with α_1-antitrypsin deficiency can present with lung disease and liver disease. The spectrum of liver diseases includes neonatal hepatitis, hepatomegaly with elevated aminotransferase levels, cirrhosis, and HCC. Patients with two copies of the Z allele (ZZ), which produces a deficient amount of α_1-antitrypsin, are at highest risk for developing liver disease. Patients who have a deficient allele in combination with a normal α_1-antitrypsin allele (MZ) also have an increased risk of liver disease, but usually there is another contributor such as viral hepatitis or NAFLD. Infusions of α_1-antitrypsin do not help the liver disease associated with α_1-antitrypsin deficiency because the liver disease is related to hepatic accumulation of the abnormal protein and not the loss of protease activity that contributes to lung disease. Liver transplantation is the definitive treatment for the liver consequence of the metabolic defect.

Wilson Disease

Wilson disease is a rare congenital disorder of copper excretion that affects approximately 1 in 30,000 live births. Young patients with Wilson disease tend to present with ALF; older patients present with chronic liver disease and/or neurologic manifestations. Wilson disease should be considered in all patients younger than 40 years of age who have unexplained liver disease. When Wilson disease causes an acute hepatitis, usually in young patients, the sudden release of copper from liver cells can also induce hemolytic anemia. Kayser-Fleischer rings are most common in patients with neurologic manifestations and are usually only visualized with slit-lamp examination. Biochemically, Wilson disease is generally characterized by a low or low-normal serum ALP level, relatively modest increases of aminotransferase levels, low or low-normal ceruloplasmin level, and urine copper level greater than 250 µg/24 h (3.9 µmol/d) (normal range, 15-60 µg/24 h [0.2-0.9 µmol/d]). Molecular genetic studies that test for mutations in the *ATP7B* gene can be helpful when the diagnosis is uncertain.

Treatment consists of trientine or penicillamine. Trientine is generally preferred because of the side effects associated with penicillamine. Zinc is also beneficial because it decreases intestinal absorption of copper, but it should not be used alone until copper has been depleted with a chelating agent.

Cholestatic Liver Diseases

Primary Biliary Cirrhosis

Primary biliary cirrhosis (PBC) is a slowly progressive disorder that involves the immune-mediated destruction of the small intralobular bile ducts; it is more common in women than in men. Symptoms are generally more common in patients with advanced fibrosis and include fatigue, pruritus, jaundice, and/or complications of portal hypertension. Patients may have features of hyperpigmentation, xanthelasma, xanthomas, or hepatomegaly on physical examination.

The diagnosis of PBC is generally made on the basis of a cholestatic liver enzyme profile in the setting of a positive antimitochondrial antibody test. The predominant liver enzyme abnormality is an increase in serum ALP levels, but a mild to moderate increase in aminotransferase levels is also seen. Ten percent of patients with PBC have a negative antimitochondrial antibody test and require liver biopsy for diagnosis. Histologic changes of PBC include granulomatous inflammation centered on the septal bile duct.

Treatment of pruritus associated with PBC and other liver diseases is challenging. Antihistamines such as hydroxyzine can be helpful for sedation in patients who have itching that is most troublesome at night. Cholestyramine, rifampin, naltrexone, and sertraline may also be beneficial, but responses are widely variable. Patients with PBC should be assessed for consequences of long-term decreased bile acid secretion, including fat-soluble vitamin deficiencies and metabolic bone disease, with appropriate treatment as indicated.

Ursodiol slows disease progression and may prevent or delay advanced disease and the need for liver transplantation. Forty percent to 50% of patients with PBC treated with ursodiol continue to have a serum ALP level greater than 1.5 times the upper limit of normal and have a worse outcome than those with treatment response. Nonresponse is more common in younger patients with PBC. Outcomes with liver transplantation for PBC are excellent. Disease recurrence after transplantation occurs in 20% of patients but only rarely causes graft failure.

KEY POINTS

- Symptoms of primary biliary cirrhosis are generally more common in patients with advanced fibrosis and include fatigue, pruritus, jaundice, and/or complications of portal hypertension.
- Ursodiol slows disease progression of primary biliary cirrhosis and may prevent or delay advanced disease and the need for liver transplantation.

Primary Sclerosing Cholangitis

Primary sclerosing cholangitis (PSC) is a fibroinflammatory disorder of the bile ducts. Most patients have large-duct changes that can be identified on MRCP or endoscopic retrograde cholangiopancreatography (ERCP). Eighty percent of patients with PSC have inflammatory bowel disease, usually ulcerative colitis; however, only 4% of patients with ulcerative colitis have PSC. In patients with ulcerative colitis, the pattern of disease most highly associated with PSC is right-sided colon involvement, rectal sparing, backwash ileitis, and a quiescent clinical course. These patients also have a greater risk of colon cancer and greater risk of pouchitis after colectomy with an ileal pouch–anal anastomosis than other patients with ulcerative colitis. The risk of colon cancer in patients with PSC and inflammatory bowel disease is high enough that surveillance is recommended, regardless of duration or extent of disease.

Most patients with PSC are asymptomatic and present with a cholestatic liver enzyme profile. Diagnosis is usually established with a characteristic cholangiogram on MRCP (**Figure 27**). Patients without large-duct disease require liver biopsy for diagnosis.

There is no effective medical therapy for PSC. Endoscopic dilatation of biliary strictures and removal of stones may be necessary in patients with progressive cholestasis or symptoms of cholangitis. PSC is generally a progressive disease that often requires liver transplantation. Cholangiocarcinoma is a complication that occurs in approximately 10% of patients with PSC. Up to half of patients are diagnosed with cholangiocarcinoma within 2 years of the diagnosis of PSC. For patients with PSC, surveillance for cholangiocarcinoma is recommended by some experts using liver chemistry studies, CA 19-9 measurement, and an imaging study at 12-month intervals. A subspecialty guideline recommends an annual ultrasound of the gallbladder to screen for gallbladder cancer. Liver transplantation is effective for patients with PSC and for highly selected patients with cholangiocarcinoma.

KEY POINTS

- Eighty percent of patients with primary sclerosing cholangitis have inflammatory bowel disease, usually ulcerative colitis; however, only 4% of patients with ulcerative colitis have primary sclerosing cholangitis.
- Cholangiocarcinoma is a complication that occurs in approximately 10% of patients with primary sclerosing cholangitis.

Determining Prognosis

The Model for End-Stage Liver Disease (MELD) score predicts short-term prognosis for cirrhosis. The MELD score is used to prioritize the allocation of deceased-donor livers for transplantation. It has also demonstrated usefulness in prognosticating survival in patients with acute alcoholic hepatitis and ALF, as well as in those with cirrhosis who are undergoing surgery. A MELD score calculator and a guide to using the score for specific clinical indications may be found at www.mayoclinic.org/meld/.

The Child-Turcotte-Pugh (CTP) score is another model commonly used to classify cirrhosis (**Table 32**). The 1- and 2-year survival rates for patients with CTP class A, B, and C cirrhosis are 100% and 85%, 80% and 60%, and 45% and 35%, respectively.

Complications of Advanced Liver Disease

Chronic liver disease from a variety of causes may ultimately progress to cirrhosis if left undiagnosed or untreated. Patients

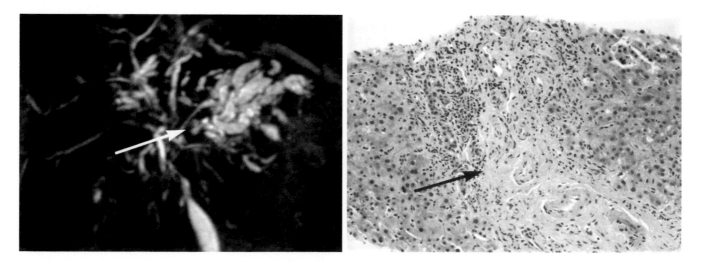

FIGURE 27. Magnetic resonance cholangiopancreatography (*left panel*) revealing upstream intrahepatic bile duct dilatation involving the left hepatic lobe (*arrow*) with stricturing of the left hepatic duct. Liver histology (*right panel*) demonstrates portal tract expansion, edema, and ductular proliferation with lymphocytic cholangitis (*arrow*) consistent with primary sclerosing cholangitis.

TABLE 32. Child-Turcotte-Pugh Score[a]

	1 Point	2 Points	3 Points
Encephalopathy	None	Grade I-II	Grade III-IV
Ascites	None	Mild/moderate	Severe
Bilirubin	<2 mg/dL (34.2 µmol/L)	2-3 mg/dL (34.2-51.3 µmol/L)	>3 mg/dL (51.3 µmol/L)
Albumin	>3.5 g/dL (35 g/L)	2.8-3.5 g/dL (28-35 g/L)	<2.8 g/dL (28 g/L)
Prothrombin time/INR	<4 s/<1.7	4-6 s/1.7-2.3	>6 s/>2.3

[a]5-6 points = Child-Turcotte-Pugh class A; 7-9 points = Child-Turcotte-Pugh class B; 10-15 points = Child-Turcotte-Pugh class C.

with cirrhosis but no complications are referred to as having compensated cirrhosis; they may be asymptomatic or may have nonspecific symptoms such as fatigue, poor sleep, muscle cramps, feeling cold, or itching. Patients with complications of cirrhosis (HE, variceal hemorrhage, ascites, spontaneous bacterial peritonitis, hepatorenal syndrome, jaundice, or HCC) are referred to as having decompensated cirrhosis. Portal hypertension is responsible for the majority of these complications, which are a major cause of mortality. Portal hypertension also causes splenomegaly and hypersplenism with resultant consumption of platelets, which may also be accompanied by consumption of leukocytes and erythrocytes. Loss of hepatic synthetic function leads to coagulopathy and hypoalbuminemia, as the liver manufactures the majority of clotting factors and albumin.

For a discussion of HCC, see Hepatic Tumors, Cysts, and Abscesses.

Portal Hypertension

Portal hypertension can be divided into prehepatic, intrahepatic, and posthepatic causes. The most common cause of portal hypertension is cirrhosis, an intrahepatic form. Examples of pre- and posthepatic portal hypertension are portal vein thrombosis and Budd-Chiari syndrome, respectively.

Portal hypertension develops in cirrhosis owing to mechanical factors of fibrosis and regenerative liver nodules as well as increased intrahepatic vascular resistance and increased portal inflow. The high pressure in the portal vein is decompressed through collateral portosystemic shunts that occur predictably in the mucosa of the distal esophagus and proximal stomach.

Esophageal Varices

The prevalence of esophageal varices is 85% in patients with CTP class C (decompensated) cirrhosis and 40% in those with CTP class A cirrhosis. Risk factors for variceal hemorrhage are CTP class B and C cirrhosis, large varices (>5 mm), and the endoscopic finding of red markings on varices. Approximately 15% to 20% of patients die within 6 weeks of hemorrhage.

All patients with cirrhosis should undergo screening for esophageal varices with upper endoscopy. The CTP class,

variceal size, and variceal appearance on endoscopy are the features that determine the need for primary prophylaxis with nonselective β-blockers (for example, nadolol, propranolol) or esophageal variceal band ligation. **Figure 28** shows a management and surveillance algorithm for patients with nonbleeding esophageal varices. Patients who receive nonselective β-blockers for primary prophylaxis do not require further upper endoscopy unless bleeding occurs. Band ligation requires indefinite endoscopic surveillance, which should be repeated every 2 to 4 weeks until varices are obliterated, then at 3 months, and every 6 to 12 months thereafter to assess for variceal recurrence. If no varices are seen on initial endoscopy, then endoscopy should be performed 3 years later, or sooner if hepatic decompensation develops.

Management of esophageal variceal bleeding includes placement of two large-bore intravenous lines, fluid resuscitation, and erythrocyte transfusion to a goal hemoglobin level of 7 g/dL (70 g/L). More liberal blood transfusion thresholds lead to increased portal pressures and risk of further bleeding. No data exist to guide specific thresholds at which fresh frozen plasma or platelets should be transfused. Up to 50% of patients with cirrhosis and gastrointestinal bleeding develop infections within 1 week, and prophylactic antimicrobial agents improve mortality rates. Oral norfloxacin or intravenous ciprofloxacin is recommended for 7 days. Ceftriaxone is preferred in patients with CTP class B and C cirrhosis, in those already receiving fluoroquinolone prophylaxis, or in geographic areas with high rates of fluoroquinolone resistance. Antimicrobial prophylaxis should be administered even if ascites is absent because it significantly reduces the risk of other infections, including urinary tract infection, pneumonia, and bacteremia; it also reduces rebleeding rates and mortality rates. A splanchnic vasoconstrictor such as octreotide is recommended for 3 to 5 days. Upper endoscopy with band ligation should be performed within 12 hours followed by addition of a nonselective β-blocker after stabilization. Upper endoscopy should be repeated every 2 to 4 weeks until varices are obliterated, then at 3 months, and every 6 to 12 months thereafter. For the 10% to 20% of patients with uncontrolled bleeding and those with early rebleeding, a transjugular intrahepatic portosystemic shunt (TIPS) should be placed.

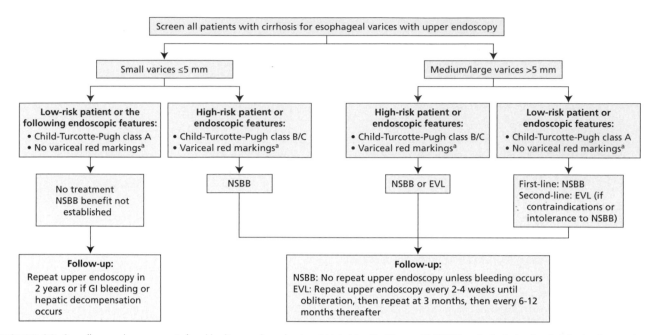

FIGURE 28. Surveillance and management of nonbleeding esophageal varices. A high-risk patient is one with Child-Turcotte-Pugh class B or C cirrhosis, whereas a low-risk patient has Child-Turcotte-Pugh class A cirrhosis. EVL = endoscopic variceal ligation; GI = gastrointestinal; NSBB = nonselective β-blockers.

ªVariceal red markings are longitudinal red streaks on the surface of esophageal varices.

KEY POINT

HVC
- Management of esophageal variceal bleeding includes placement of two large-bore intravenous lines, fluid resuscitation, and erythrocyte transfusion to a goal hemoglobin level of 7 g/dL (70 g/L); more liberal blood transfusion thresholds lead to increased portal pressures and risk of further bleeding.

Gastric Varices and Portal Hypertensive Gastropathy

Gastric varices are present in 20% of patients with cirrhosis. Limited data are available on the efficacy of nonselective β-blockers for primary prophylaxis of gastric varices. Hemodynamic resuscitation, antimicrobial agents, and octreotide should be initiated for bleeding gastric varices. Gastric varices that are extensions of esophageal varices into the lesser curvature of the stomach can be treated successfully with band ligation during an acute event. All other types of bleeding gastric varices respond poorly to band ligation, with high rates of rebleeding. Cyanoacrylate (glue) injection is recommended by the major societies for these other types of bleeding gastric varices. However, glue is only available in the United States under exceptional circumstances and is not FDA approved. If glue is not available, band ligation can be attempted despite its shortcomings. A TIPS should be placed for uncontrolled bleeding or rebleeding. Splenectomy is the best treatment for bleeding isolated fundic gastric varices caused by a splenic vein thrombosis in the absence of liver disease.

Portal hypertensive gastropathy (PHG) is a congestive gastropathy that occurs as a result of portal hypertension. It typically manifests as chronic gastrointestinal bleeding and rarely can result in significant acute bleeding. Despite a lack of data on efficacy, most specialists treat chronic gastrointestinal bleeding from PHG with nonselective β-blockers and iron supplementation.

Hepatic Encephalopathy

Hepatic encephalopathy (HE) is a neuropsychiatric syndrome that develops in patients with hepatic dysfunction. Symptoms range from barely perceptible cognitive changes to coma. HE is graded 0 to IV according to severity (see Table 31) and can be characterized as episodic, persistent, or minimal. Because it is clinically difficult to distinguish between grade 0 (minimal) and grade I HE, new terminology has been proposed that refers to grade 0 to I as covert HE and grades II through IV as overt HE. Grade II HE is typically associated with disorientation to time and asterixis.

Diagnosis of HE is made based on the history and physical examination. The plasma ammonia level can be helpful in cases of diagnostic uncertainty; however, monitoring serial ammonia values in patients with HE is not useful. Head CT is overutilized and is warranted only in patients with unwitnessed falls or head trauma, or in cases of diagnostic uncertainty. The diagnosis of HE indicates a poor prognosis, and liver transplantation should be considered.

Management of HE depends on its acuity and severity and focuses on treatment of significant (≥grade II, also known as overt) episodes of HE followed by maintenance of remission (secondary prophylaxis). Overt episodic HE of grade II or greater usually requires hospitalization. Up to 80% of patients have a precipitating factor, most commonly infection or gastrointestinal bleeding. Other precipitants include opioids, benzodiazepines, electrolyte abnormalities, hypoglycemia, hypoxia, TIPS placement, inappropriate lactulose dosing, or dehydration. All patients with overt episodic HE should undergo screening for infections, including diagnostic paracentesis when ascites is present. Lactulose is first-line treatment and should be titrated to three stools per day. Rifaximin (off label) or neomycin can be added as adjunctive therapy in patients who do not respond to lactulose. Neomycin carries a risk of ototoxicity and nephrotoxicity. Rifaximin is not FDA approved for overt, episodic HE, but recent data suggest a significant benefit in patients with grades III and IV HE when added to lactulose as compared with lactulose alone. Albumin dialysis is FDA approved for medically refractory, severe HE.

Secondary prophylaxis (maintenance of remission) is warranted in most patients who recover from overt episodic HE. Lactulose is first-line maintenance therapy. Patients should receive instruction on titrating the dose to achieve three stools per day. Taking fixed doses of lactulose without monitoring stool frequency commonly precipitates overt episodes of HE. Discharging patients without secondary prophylaxis or with inadequate instructions for titrating lactulose may result in hospital readmissions. In patients with recurrent overt HE while on lactulose, the addition of rifaximin can prevent further recurrences of overt HE and hospitalizations. Dietary protein restriction is no longer recommended.

The best diagnostic test for covert HE is an active area of investigation. Historically, the diagnosis of minimal HE (now included in the term covert HE) was made by neuropsychometric testing. However, this is not widely available. Empiric treatment with lactulose is reasonable when the diagnosis is suspected, with continuation of the drug if a favorable response occurs and discontinuation if no improvement is observed.

KEY POINTS

- There is no utility in monitoring serial ammonia values in patients with hepatic encephalopathy; head CT is warranted only in patients with unwitnessed falls or head trauma, or in cases of diagnostic uncertainty.
- Lactulose is first-line treatment of overt episodic hepatic encephalopathy, and it should be titrated to three stools per day.
- In patients with recurrent overt episodes of hepatic encephalopathy while on lactulose, rifaximin should be added, as it has been shown to reduce recurrence and need for hospitalization.

Hepatopulmonary Syndrome

Hepatopulmonary syndrome (HPS) is defined by hypoxemia and intrapulmonary vascular dilatation in the presence of liver disease with portal hypertension. It is present in 4% to 32% of pretransplant patients with variable severity. Patients with HPS usually have a preexisting diagnosis of liver disease and present with shortness of breath. Classic features are platypnea (worsening shortness of breath in the upright position) and orthodeoxia (worsening arterial oxygen saturation in the upright position). The diagnosis is made by demonstrating an arterial oxygen tension less than 80 mm Hg (10.6 kPa) breathing ambient air, or an alveolar-arterial gradient of 15 mm Hg (2 kPa) or greater, along with evidence of intrapulmonary shunting on echocardiography with agitated saline or macroaggregated albumin study. Clinically significant HPS is treated with supplemental oxygen and liver transplantation.

KEY POINT

- Patients with hepatopulmonary syndrome usually have a preexisting diagnosis of liver disease and present with shortness of breath; classic features are platypnea (worsening shortness of breath in the upright position) and orthodeoxia (worsening arterial oxygen saturation in the upright position).

Portopulmonary Hypertension

Portopulmonary hypertension (PoPH) is pulmonary hypertension in the presence of chronic liver disease with portal hypertension. It is less common than HPS, with a prevalence of 5% to 9% in liver transplant candidates. The typical presentation of PoPH is dyspnea on exertion in a patient with known liver disease. Patients with typical symptoms or those being evaluated for liver transplantation should undergo transthoracic echocardiography. Those with a right ventricular systolic pressure greater than 50 mm Hg on echocardiogram require investigation for causes of pulmonary hypertension, including right heart catheterization.

Patients with moderate PoPH with a mean pulmonary artery pressure greater than 35 mm Hg at the time of diagnosis should be treated with medical therapy, which may include prostacyclin analogues, endothelin antagonists, or phosphodiesterase inhibitors. Those who respond to therapy and have satisfactory right ventricular function can benefit from liver transplantation. Survival at 1 and 3 years after liver transplantation is 83% and 76%, respectively. The effect of liver transplantation on the symptoms of pulmonary hypertension is unpredictable; 40% to 50% of patients may be weaned from medical therapy after transplantation.

KEY POINT

- Portopulmonary hypertension is pulmonary hypertension in the presence of chronic liver disease with portal hypertension.

Ascites

Ascites is the most common complication of cirrhosis and develops in approximately 50% of patients within 10 years. Ultrasound is the most cost-effective study to detect the presence of ascites. Ultrasound should be followed by diagnostic paracentesis when ascites is present. Ascitic fluid analysis should include measurement of albumin and total protein; cell count and bacterial cultures should be checked when infection is suspected. The serum-ascites albumin gradient (SAAG) should be calculated by subtracting the ascitic fluid albumin level from the serum albumin level. A differential diagnosis can be formulated based on the SAAG and ascites total protein (Table 33).

In patients with ascites associated with cirrhosis, management consists of sodium restriction (<2 g/d) and spironolactone with furosemide. Spironolactone is more effective for mobilization of ascites than furosemide, and the combination allows for effective natriuresis while maintaining potassium homeostasis. Serum creatinine and electrolyte levels should be checked approximately 1 week after initiation of treatment and with dose increases. Patients who cannot tolerate diuretics (such as those with kidney dysfunction or hyponatremia) or in whom diuretics are ineffective can be treated with large-volume paracentesis. If more than 5 L of ascitic fluid is removed, 8 g of 25% albumin should be given for each liter removed; this is done to prevent postparacentesis circulatory dysfunction. A meta-analysis of 1225 patients receiving 25% albumin after large-volume paracentesis reported decreased postparacentesis circulatory dysfunction, hyponatremia, and mortality. All patients should discontinue ACE inhibitors, angiotensin receptor blockers, and NSAIDs, which can exacerbate ascites. Nonselective β-blockers should be used with caution in patients with refractory ascites because there is an association with decreased survival. Midodrine can be used as adjunctive therapy for refractory ascites, especially in patients with hypotension. A TIPS can be considered for patients with refractory ascites in the absence of HE, heart failure, and pulmonary hypertension when the serum bilirubin level is less than 4 mg/dL (68.4 μmol/L) and the MELD score is less than 15 to 18. The presence of ascites should prompt consideration for liver transplantation. **H**

TABLE 33. Differential Diagnosis of Ascites Based on the Serum-Ascites Albumin Gradient

Total Protein	SAAG	
	≥1.1 g/dL (11 g/L)	<1.1 g/dL (11 g/L)
<2.5 g/dL (25 g/L)	Cirrhosis	Nephrotic syndrome, myxedema
≥2.5 g/dL (25 g/L)	Cardiac ascites, Budd-Chiari syndrome	Infections, malignancy, pancreatic ascites

SAAG = serum-ascites albumin gradient.

Mayo Clinic Gastroenterology and Hepatology Board Review, 4th Edition, edited by Hauser (2011). Adapted Table 28.2 from Chapter "Ascites, Hepatorenal Syndrome and Encephalopathy" by Hay, page 318, by permission of Oxford University Press, USA.

KEY POINTS

- Ascites is the most common complication of cirrhosis and develops in approximately 50% of patients within 10 years.
- Ultrasound is the most cost-effective diagnostic test for ascites.
- Management of ascites consists of sodium restriction (<2 g/d) and spironolactone with furosemide.

Spontaneous Bacterial Peritonitis

Spontaneous bacterial peritonitis (SBP) is an infection of the ascitic fluid in patients with portal hypertension that carries a 10% to 20% risk of mortality. It can present with abdominal pain, fever, HE, or acute kidney injury. A polymorphonuclear cell count greater than 250/μL in the ascitic fluid is diagnostic of SBP. A polymorphonuclear cell count less than 250/μL with positive ascitic fluid cultures is diagnostic in symptomatic patients.

Treatment of SBP is with intravenous cefotaxime (or a similar third-generation cephalosporin), which covers the most common pathogens (*Escherichia coli*, *Klebsiella pneumoniae*, and *Streptococcus pneumoniae*). Patients who acquire SBP in the hospital or have recent exposure to β-lactams should receive broader-spectrum antimicrobial agents as determined by local microbial and resistance patterns. For culture-positive SBP, antimicrobial agents can be tailored to the susceptibility pattern. Follow-up paracentesis should be performed only in patients with nosocomial SBP, recent β-lactam exposure, infection with an atypical organism, or worsening clinical status. Patients with a serum creatinine level greater than 1 mg/dL (88.4 μmol/L), a serum bilirubin level greater than 4 mg/dL (68.4 μmol/L), or a blood urea nitrogen level greater than 30 mg/dL (10.7 mmol/L) should receive 1.5 g/kg of albumin on the day of the diagnosis of SBP and 1 g/kg of albumin on day 3; this practice has demonstrated a survival benefit.

Patients with SBP should receive indefinite prophylaxis with norfloxacin or ciprofloxacin (preferred), or trimethoprim-sulfamethoxazole. Long-term primary prophylaxis with norfloxacin is beneficial for patients at high risk for SBP. Criteria for patients at high risk for SBP include an ascitic fluid total protein level less than 1.5 g/dL (15 g/L) in conjunction with any of the following: serum sodium level less than or equal to 130 mEq/L (130 mmol/L), serum creatinine level greater than or equal to 1.2 mg/dL (106.1 μmol/L), blood urea nitrogen level greater than or equal to 25 mg/dL (8.9 mmol/L), serum bilirubin level greater than or equal to 3 mg/dL (51.3 μmol/L), or CTP class B or greater cirrhosis. **H**

KEY POINT

- Spontaneous bacterial peritonitis is an infection of the ascitic fluid in patients with portal hypertension that carries a 10% to 20% risk of mortality.

Hepatorenal Syndrome

Approximately 20% of hospitalized patients with cirrhosis develop acute kidney injury. Of this group, approximately two thirds have a prerenal cause. Although most of these patients will respond to volume expansion, approximately 30% of this group will have hepatorenal syndrome. Therefore, hepatorenal syndrome accounts for a minority of patients who develop acute kidney injury.

Hepatorenal syndrome diagnostic criteria consist of (1) an increase in the serum creatinine level to greater than 1.5 mg/dL (132.6 µmol/L) over days to weeks, (2) lack of response to an albumin challenge of 1 g/kg/d for 2 days, and (3) the absence of shock, nephrotoxic drugs, active urine sediment, proteinuria greater than 500 mg/d, and ultrasound evidence of parenchymal kidney disease or obstruction. Type 1 hepatorenal syndrome is more severe, with a doubling of the serum creatinine level in excess of 2.5 mg/dL (221 µmol/L) in less than 2 weeks. Type 2 hepatorenal syndrome is less severe, with a more gradual increase in the creatinine level; it is usually associated with diuretic-refractory ascites.

The creatinine level is one of the most important predictors of death in patients with cirrhosis. An increase in creatinine of 1.5 times baseline or the presence of acute kidney injury should increase suspicion for infections, blood loss, and fluid loss. Diuretics and any potential nephrotoxic agents should be stopped. A fluid challenge with albumin at 1 g/kg of body weight should be given over 24 hours. Patients who do not respond to these strategies and who meet criteria for hepatorenal syndrome should be treated for hepatorenal syndrome.

Patients with type 1 hepatorenal syndrome should be treated with a vasoconstrictor and albumin. Terlipressin has been shown to improve kidney outcomes but is not available in the United States. Therefore, recommendations state that patients in the ICU with type I hepatorenal syndrome should be treated with norepinephrine and albumin, whereas patients on the general ward should be treated with midodrine, octreotide, and albumin. Patients with type I hepatorenal syndrome who do not respond to medical therapy and are suitable candidates should undergo liver transplantation with or without simultaneous kidney transplantation, depending on the duration of kidney dysfunction. Patients with type 1 hepatorenal syndrome who do not receive therapy usually die within weeks. ▣

Health Care Maintenance of the Patient with Chronic Liver Disease

Hepatic Osteodystrophy

Hepatic osteodystrophy encompasses osteoporosis, osteopenia, and rarely osteomalacia in the context of liver disease. Diagnostic criteria for these diseases are the same as in the general population. There is a fourfold increase in risk of osteoporosis in patients with PBC. Concomitant inflammatory bowel disease increases the risk of osteoporosis in patients with PSC. Cirrhosis of any cause is a risk factor for osteoporosis, with a prevalence of approximately 25%. Women (especially those who are postmenopausal) are at higher risk than men. Standard evaluation should include measurement of serum calcium, phosphate, and vitamin D levels. Up to two thirds of patients with cirrhosis are deficient in vitamin D. Dual-energy x-ray absorptiometry is recommended for patients with cirrhosis or PBC (even if noncirrhotic) and before liver transplantation. Patients with a previous fragility fracture, postmenopausal women, and those with glucocorticoid use for longer than 3 months should also receive dual-energy x-ray absorptiometry. Osteopenia should be treated according to standard guidelines. Osteoporosis should be managed with a bisphosphonate (after vitamin D repletion), which should be an intravenous formulation in patients with esophageal varices.

KEY POINT

- Dual-energy x-ray absorptiometry is recommended for patients with cirrhosis or primary biliary cirrhosis (even if noncirrhotic) and before liver transplantation.

Immunizations

Patients with cirrhosis who develop an infection have a 30% mortality rate at 1 month, and another 30% die within 12 months; this underscores the importance of prevention of infection. Immunizations lose their effectiveness as the severity of liver disease worsens. Immunizations should ideally be provided before the patient develops cirrhosis. Inactivated vaccines are safe in patients with cirrhosis, whereas attenuated live virus vaccines should be avoided. **Table 34** describes the recommended vaccinations in patients with chronic liver disease and/or cirrhosis. Limited data exist regarding the efficacy and safety of vaccines against tetanus and diphtheria; *Haemophilus influenzae* type b; measles, mumps and rubella; herpes zoster; and human papillomavirus in patients with cirrhosis.

KEY POINT

- Inactivated vaccines are safe in patients with cirrhosis, whereas attenuated live virus vaccines should be avoided.

Avoidances

Oysters and other raw shellfish should be avoided in patients with cirrhosis because there is a risk of potentially lethal infection with *Vibrio vulnificus*. All NSAIDs should be avoided owing to the risk of precipitating acute kidney injury and gastrointestinal bleeding. Occasional doses of acetaminophen are well tolerated in patients with cirrhosis but should never be used with alcohol. Complete cessation of alcohol use is recommended in all forms of chronic liver disease. All supplements should be reviewed with a physician before initiation given the risk of DILI with some agents. Medications with significant risk of hepatoxicity, such as antituberculosis drugs

TABLE 34. Immunizations in Patients with Cirrhosis

Immunization	Recommendation	Schedule	Notes
Inactivated influenza	Yes	Yearly	Less effective than in healthy individuals; may prevent hepatic decompensation
23-Valent pneumococcal polysaccharide vaccine (PPSV-23)	Yes	Dose 1 given at time of diagnosis if ≥19 years Dose 2 given 5 years later Dose 3 given at age 65 years (if ≥5 years or more since previous vaccination)	Probably less effective than in healthy individuals
13-Valent pneumococcal conjugate vaccine (PCV-13)	No	—	—
Hepatitis A	Yes	Dose 1 given at time zero Dose 2 given at 6-12 months	Lower rates of seroprotection in decompensated cirrhosis
Hepatitis B	Yes	Dose 1 given at time zero Dose 2 given at 1 month Dose 3 given at 6 months	Patients with cirrhosis should receive a double dose (40 μg) with the standard schedule
Herpes zoster	No	—	Limited data for safety and efficacy in cirrhosis

and antiepileptic drugs, should be reviewed by a hepatologist before initiation. Opioid pain medications and anxiolytics should be avoided in patients with cirrhosis, if possible, given the risk of precipitating HE. Patients with cirrhosis and HE are at increased risk for traffic accidents and should be advised not to drive.

Cirrhosis increases the risk of complications and decompensation from surgery. Many patients with CTP class A cirrhosis or a MELD score less than 10 can tolerate low-risk surgeries. Patients with CTP class A and B cirrhosis should be evaluated by a hepatologist before considering surgery. Patients with CTP class C cirrhosis or a MELD score greater than 15 should not undergo elective surgeries.

Nutrition

Patients with cirrhosis are catabolic and may exhibit muscle wasting. Protein consumption is crucial to maintain muscle and should not be reduced. Daily protein intake should be 1.2 g/kg/d in compensated cirrhosis and 1.5 g/kg/d in decompensated cirrhosis. Sodium restriction (<2 g/d) is necessary in patients with fluid retention. Fluid restriction is necessary in those with hypervolemic hyponatremia (serum sodium level of 125 mEq/L [125 mmol/L] or greater). Coffee may be beneficial for liver health, but data are insufficient to make any specific recommendations. Probiotics have demonstrated some efficacy in the management of HE, but further studies are necessary.

KEY POINT

- Patients with cirrhosis are catabolic and may exhibit muscle wasting; protein consumption is crucial to maintain muscle and should not be reduced.

Hepatic Tumors, Cysts, and Abscesses

Most benign liver masses are discovered incidentally on abdominal imaging and only rarely result in symptoms. Lesions that are most likely to result in symptoms include abscesses or lesions larger than 5 cm, especially if subcapsular. The diagnosis of liver lesions can usually be made using imaging, but biopsy is generally safe, even for vascular lesions.

KEY POINT

- Most benign liver masses are discovered incidentally on abdominal imaging and only rarely result in symptoms.

Hepatic Cysts

Hepatic cysts are frequently identified in patients undergoing abdominal imaging and can be multiple. Ultrasound shows an anechoic structure with smooth, thin walls and posterior shadowing. Occasionally, cysts can have thin septations or even exhibit hemorrhage. Nodular wall thickening can suggest a cystic neoplasm. Patients with autosomal dominant polycystic kidney disease may also have multiple liver cysts that can cause symptomatic hepatomegaly. Incidentally discovered cysts require no follow-up. Only large, symptomatic cysts require surgical treatment.

Focal Nodular Hyperplasia

Focal nodular hyperplasia (FNH) is a hyperplastic reaction of the liver to long-standing aberrant arterial blood flow that is most likely congenital. On contrast-enhanced imaging, FNH usually demonstrates enhancement on the arterial phase with a central "scar." The central scar may not be identified in small lesions. The main differential diagnosis for FNH is hepatic adenoma. FNH rarely causes bleeding, and estrogen does not affect growth. Unless a patient is definitely symptomatic from FNH, further imaging and therapy are not required.

Hepatocellular Adenoma

Hepatocellular adenomas are generally seen in women because they can be dependent on estrogen for growth. They may be also associated with NAFLD. Adenomas may be subclassified depending on β-catenin (a proto-oncogene) nuclear reactivity on histologic specimens. Although malignant transformation of adenomas is unusual, those lesions that exhibit β-catenin nuclear reactivity are more likely to become malignant than those that are β-catenin negative. Adenomas larger than 5 cm have a risk of bleeding that can occasionally cause hemodynamic compromise. Regression of hepatic adenomas may be seen with withdrawal of estrogen therapy. Treatment with surgical resection or radiofrequency ablation is advised for lesions that are larger than 5 cm (or larger than 3 cm when pregnancy is anticipated) or that exhibit β-catenin nuclear reactivity.

Hepatic Hemangioma

Hepatic hemangiomas are identified in 5% of patients undergoing abdominal imaging. Hemangiomas of the liver generally have a characteristic enhancing pattern on contrast-enhanced CT or MRI, with peripheral nodular enhancement filling in toward the center of the lesion on later phases. These lesions are not estrogen dependent and do not have premalignant potential. Only hemangiomas larger than 10 cm cause symptoms and, if so, require surgery.

Hepatic Abscesses

Pyogenic liver abscesses are usually due to peritonitis and biliary tract infections. Most patients present with fever and symptoms owing to the underlying cause of the abscess. Liver abscesses are usually polymicrobial. Image-guided aspiration can be both diagnostic and therapeutic, in combination with antimicrobial agents, for small abscesses. Larger abscesses, especially if solitary, require percutaneous tube drainage in addition to antimicrobial agents. Surgery is only rarely required.

Amebiasis

Hepatic amebic cysts are due to portal vein spread of intestinal infection to the liver. Patients with amebic cysts have either lived in or traveled to endemic areas such as India, Africa, or Central or South America. Typical symptoms are right upper quadrant pain, fever, and sometimes cough. The diagnosis is usually established with compatible imaging and serologic testing. Treatment of the systemic infection with metronidazole or another appropriate agent should be following by a luminal agent such as paromomycin.

Hepatocellular Carcinoma

The incidence of HCC in the United States is increasing; it is currently the ninth most common cancer. The highest incidence occurs in sub-Saharan Africa, China, Taiwan, and Hong Kong. Liver diseases associated with the highest risk of HCC are HBV, HCV, and hemochromatosis. The most important preventive measure for HCC is HBV vaccination. Approximately 80% of HCC occurs in patients with cirrhosis, but it can develop in the absence of cirrhosis in patients with HBV infection. All patients with cirrhosis from any cause should undergo liver ultrasound every 6 months. Serum α-fetoprotein measurement is no longer recommended for HCC surveillance.

Hepatic lesions identified on screening that are smaller than 1 cm on ultrasound warrant a repeat ultrasound in 3 months. For lesions larger than 1 cm, a four-phase CT scan or contrast-enhanced MRI is recommended. A diagnosis of HCC can be made in lesions larger than 1 cm that enhance in the arterial phase and have washout of contrast in the venous phase. The vast majority of patients can be diagnosed by radiology and do not require a biopsy. If the imaging characteristics in a lesion larger than 1 cm are atypical, the alternative imaging modality (MRI or CT) may be used to attempt to confirm a radiologic diagnosis, or a liver biopsy can be performed. A negative liver biopsy can be falsely reassuring, and continued follow-up is recommended.

HCC should be managed according to the Barcelona Classification for Liver Cancer Treatment System (**Figure 29**). Small, singular lesions in patients with cirrhosis but without portal hypertension and hyperbilirubinemia should be managed with surgical resection. Patients with cirrhosis within the Milan criteria (2-3 tumors ≤3 cm or 1 tumor ≤5 cm without vascular invasion or extrahepatic spread) are best treated with liver transplantation. Transarterial chemoembolization should be used in patients with CTP class A and B cirrhosis who have large or multiple lesions confined to the liver without vascular invasion. Radiofrequency ablation is best suited for solitary, 2- to 3-cm lesions in patients with CTP class A and B cirrhosis. Either transarterial chemoembolization or radiofrequency ablation can be used in patients after approval for liver transplantation as a bridge to transplant. Patients with CTP class A and B cirrhosis, good performance status, and evidence of vascular, lymphatic, or extrahepatic spread have a survival benefit from sorafenib. Common side effects of sorafenib are hypertension, gastrointestinal symptoms, and hand-foot (rash) syndrome.

KEY POINTS

- Approximately 80% of hepatocellular carcinoma occurs in patients with cirrhosis, but hepatocellular carcinoma can arise in the absence of cirrhosis in patients with hepatitis B virus infection.

- All patients with cirrhosis should undergo liver ultrasound every 6 months to evaluate for hepatocellular carcinoma.

- The vast majority of hepatocellular carcinoma can be diagnosed by radiology and does not require a biopsy.

HVC

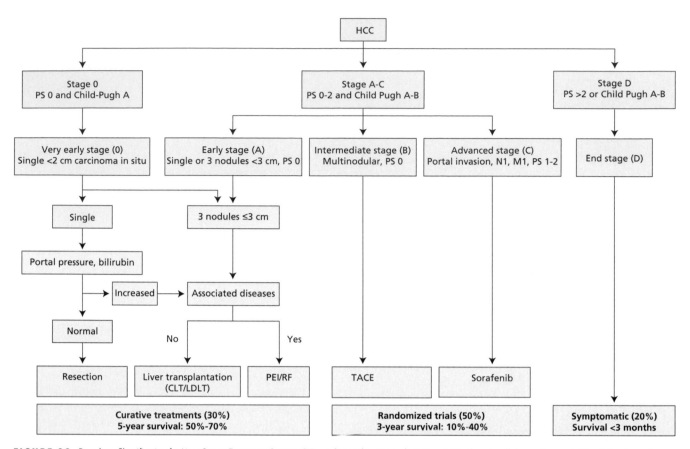

FIGURE 29. Barcelona Classification for Liver Cancer Treatment System. CLT = cadaveric liver transplantation; HCC = hepatocellular carcinoma; LDLT = living donor liver transplantation; PEI = percutaneous ethanol injection; PS = physical status; RF = radiofrequency (ablation); TACE = transarterial chemoembolization.

Llovet JM, Di Bisceglie AM, Bruix J, et al; Panel of Experts in HCC-Design Clinical Trials. Design and endpoints of clinical trials in hepatocellular carcinoma. J Natl Cancer Inst. 2008;100(10):698-711. [PMID: 18477802], by permission of Oxford University Press.

Liver Transplantation

In the United States, deceased and living-donor liver transplantation are options for selected candidates. Referral to a transplant center is indicated for patients with ALF or for patients with cirrhosis with a MELD score of 15 or greater or decompensation. The MELD score accurately predicts 3-month survival and is the basis for organ allocation. Decompensation is defined by the development of HE, variceal hemorrhage, ascites, hepatorenal syndrome, or HCC.

Contraindications for liver transplantation include severe cardiopulmonary disease, uncontrolled infections, ongoing or recent history of certain extrahepatic malignancies, a severe psychiatric disorder or untreated chemical dependency, inability to comply with medical management, lack of social support, and advanced age.

Liver transplantation provides a survival advantage for patients with MELD scores of 15 or greater. One- and 5-year survival with transplantation is approximately 87% and 73%, respectively.

Most liver transplant recipients receive tacrolimus or cyclosporine, which are metabolized by CYP3A enzymes and pose a risk for drug-drug interactions (**Table 35**). Liver

TABLE 35. Drug Interactions with Calcineurin Inhibitors		
Drugs that Increase Levels of CNIs		
Antimicrobials	**Calcium Channel Blockers**	**Others**
Caspofungin	Diltiazem	Danazol
Azoles	Verapamil	Grapefruit juice
Macrolides	Amlodipine (less)	Diazepam, alprazolam
Chloroquine	Felodipine (less)	Allopurinol
Protease inhibitors	Nicardipine	Sertraline
Ofloxacin		
Drugs that Decrease Levels of CNIs		
Antimicrobials	**Anticonvulsants**	**Others**
Rifampin	Carbamazepine	Orlistat
Rifabutin	Phenobarbital	St. John's wort
	Phenytoin	
CNIs = calcineurin inhibitors.		

CONT.

transplant recipients are at higher risk of diabetes, hypertension, hyperlipidemia, kidney disease, and malignancy.

KEY POINTS

- Referral to a transplant center is indicated for patients with acute liver failure or for patients with cirrhosis with a Model for End-Stage Liver Disease score of 15 or greater or decompensation.

- Contraindications for liver transplantation include severe cardiopulmonary disease, uncontrolled infections, ongoing or recent history of certain extrahepatic malignancies, a severe psychiatric disorder or untreated chemical dependency, inability to comply with medical management, lack of social support, and advanced age.

Pregnancy-Related Liver Disease

Pregnancy-related liver disease can be divided into acute liver diseases that incidentally occur in a pregnant patient, liver diseases unique to pregnancy, and coincident chronic liver diseases in a pregnant patient.

Patients who are pregnant may acquire viral hepatitis in any trimester. Pregnant patients who acquire HEV have a high risk of ALF. Pregnant patients are also at increased risk for herpes hepatitis and Budd-Chiari syndrome.

The liver diseases associated with pregnancy are shown in **Table 36**. Patients with preeclampsia, HELLP (Hemolysis, Elevated Liver tests, and Low Platelets) syndrome, and acute fatty liver of pregnancy may have continuation or even worsening of their course for up to several days after delivery, so careful monitoring is necessary.

Newborns of mothers who are hepatitis B surface antigen positive should receive hepatitis B immune globulin and HBV vaccine. Patients who are not otherwise candidates for HBV treatment but have levels of HBV DNA greater than 10^8 IU/mL

should be offered antiviral therapy with tenofovir during the late second or third trimester to help decrease risk of transmission to the newborn. Pregnant patients with HCV transmit infection to the newborn in less than 5% of cases; however, infants born to HCV-positive mothers should be tested for HCV at age 6 months.

Vascular Diseases of the Liver
Portal Vein Thrombosis

Portal vein thrombosis (PVT) is uncommon in patients with compensated cirrhosis, but it occurs in 8% to 25% of patients with decompensated cirrhosis. The presentation may be asymptomatic or symptomatic with variceal hemorrhage and ascites. Ultrasound with Doppler studies is the most cost-effective diagnostic test. Differentiating acute from chronic PVT is important. Chronic PVT does not require treatment. Patients with acute PVT can be considered for anticoagulation therapy after assessment and prophylaxis for esophageal varices. No formal recommendation for or against anticoagulation in acute PVT in patients with cirrhosis can be made owing to limited data. Patients with extension of PVT into the superior mesenteric vein should receive anticoagulation to prevent intestinal infarction. Evaluation for a hypercoagulable state is generally not recommended or cost effective in patients with cirrhosis. Occasionally, PVT may represent a tumor thrombus, and this should be considered in the setting of a liver mass.

KEY POINT

- Portal vein thrombosis is uncommon in patients with compensated cirrhosis, but it occurs in 8% to 25% of patients with decompensated cirrhosis; evaluation for a hypercoagulable state is not cost effective in patients with cirrhosis.

HVC

TABLE 36.	Liver Diseases Unique to Pregnancy					
Disease	**Trimester**	**Clinical Features**	**Laboratory Studies**	**Bilirubin Level**	**Management**	**Recurrence**
Hyperemesis gravidarum	First	Severe vomiting	ALT elevated in 50% of patients, may be 20 times ULN	Normal	Hydration	Variable
Intrahepatic cholestasis of pregnancy	Second or third	Pruritus	ALT normal to 10-fold increase, elevated serum bile acids	Usually normal	Ursodiol	45%-70%
Preeclampsia	Third	Hypertension, edema, and proteinuria	Mild increase in ALT	Normal	Delivery	5%-25%
HELLP syndrome	Third	Features of preeclampsia	Hemolysis, elevated ALT, thrombocytopenia	Usually normal	Delivery	5%-25%
Acute fatty liver of pregnancy	Third	Features of preeclampsia, features of liver failure	ALT 200-1000 U/L, hemolysis, low platelets, high ammonia	Normal unless severe	Delivery	20%-70%

ALT = alanine aminotransferase; HELLP = Hemolysis, Elevated Liver tests, Low Platelets; ULN = upper limit of normal.

Budd-Chiari Syndrome

Budd-Chiari syndrome (BCS) refers to obstruction of the hepatic venous outflow tract by thrombus. The classic presentation is severe right upper quadrant pain, hepatomegaly, ascites, and jaundice, but BCS may present with ALF. Diagnosis can be made by ultrasound with Doppler studies of the hepatic veins and inferior vena cava; CT or MRI should be reserved for patients in whom Doppler studies are negative but suspicion remains high. BCS is associated with an underlying risk factor for thrombosis in more than 85% of patients; assessment for paroxysmal nocturnal hemoglobinuria, myeloproliferative neoplasms, and hypercoagulable disorders is appropriate. Oral contraceptives and pregnancy are also associated with BCS. Management consists of immediate and indefinite anticoagulation unless a contraindication exists. Hepatic vein angioplasty, stenting, or TIPS should be attempted in patients with acute or symptomatic BCS as determined by anatomy and local expertise. Liver transplantation is reserved for patients with ALF or those in whom attempts at hepatic vein decompression have been unsuccessful. Chronic BCS with collateral vein formation and compensated liver function may be managed with anticoagulation alone.

KEY POINTS

- Budd-Chiari syndrome refers to obstruction of the hepatic venous outflow tract by thrombus.

- The classic presentation of Budd-Chiari syndrome is severe right upper quadrant pain, hepatomegaly, ascites, and jaundice, but it may present with acute liver failure.

Disorders of the Gallbladder and Bile Ducts

Asymptomatic Gallstones

Gallstones are classified as cholesterol, pigment, or mixed types. Risk factors for cholesterol or mixed gallstones are female gender, advancing age, and North or South American Indian ethnicity. Risk factors for pigment gallstones include chronic hemolysis (such as occurs in hereditary spherocytosis), cirrhosis, and terminal ileal disease or resection (such as might accompany Crohn disease).

Eighty percent of patients with asymptomatic gallstones remain asymptomatic over a 15-year period, and most serious complications of gallbladder stone disease are preceded by an episode of biliary colic. Therefore, cholecystectomy is not generally advised in asymptomatic patients. Prophylactic cholecystectomy should be performed in asymptomatic patients with gallbladder polyps larger than 1 cm or those with polyps of any size with gallbladder stones or primary sclerosing cholangitis.

KEY POINTS

- Eighty percent of patients with asymptomatic gallstones remain asymptomatic over a 15-year period, and most serious complications of gallbladder stone disease are preceded by an episode of biliary colic.

- Cholecystectomy is not generally advised in asymptomatic patients with gallstones.

Biliary Colic and Acute Cholecystitis

Clinical Manifestations

Biliary colic is the relatively acute onset of fairly severe, steady upper abdominal pain that occurs in the epigastrium or the right upper quadrant. Episodes generally last 15 minutes to several hours and are often accompanied by nausea, possibly with vomiting. Fever, leukocytosis, and elevated liver chemistry studies are only seen in the presence of acute cholecystitis or obstruction of the common bile duct. Fatty food intolerance is a nonspecific symptom that is not usually related to gallbladder disease and therefore does not warrant cholecystectomy.

Patients with acute cholecystitis have more severe and prolonged pain along with abdominal tenderness. In patients with acute cholecystitis, deep palpation of the gallbladder may cause the patient to arrest inspiration owing to contact of the gallbladder wall with the examiner's fingers (Murphy sign). Ninety percent of cases of acute cholecystitis occur in the setting of obstruction of the cystic duct by gallstones.

KEY POINT

- Ninety percent of cases of acute cholecystitis occur in the setting of obstruction of the cystic duct by gallstones.

Diagnosis

Gallbladder stones are generally diagnosed with gallbladder ultrasound. Clues to gallbladder inflammation include a thickened gallbladder wall and the presence of pericholecystic fluid. Air within the gallbladder wall suggests severe inflammation with possible necrosis.

KEY POINT

- Ultrasound is the diagnostic test of choice for gallbladder stones, and findings include a thickened gallbladder wall and the presence of pericholecystic fluid.

Management

Treatment of gallbladder disease is with laparoscopic cholecystectomy. Open cholecystectomy may be necessary for patients with unfavorable anatomy, extensive upper abdominal adhesions, or severe acute inflammation of the gallbladder and surrounding tissues. Patients with acute cholecystitis should be given an intravenous antibiotic such as a β-lactam/β-lactamase inhibitor or a third-generation cephalosporin plus metronidazole. Patients who improve should undergo cholecystectomy during the same hospitalization; urgent cholecystectomy can be considered for patients who do not improve with antibiotics. Percutaneous or endoscopically placed cholecystostomy tubes can be used in patients with acute cholecystitis who are not improving or who are at unacceptably high risk for cholecystectomy. Laparoscopic cholecystectomy can be safely performed during pregnancy, particularly in the second trimester.

KEY POINTS

- Treatment of acute cholecystitis includes intravenous antibiotics and a cholecystectomy during the same hospitalization; urgent cholecystectomy can be considered for patients who do not improve with antibiotics.

- Cholecystostomy tubes can be used in patients with acute cholecystitis who are not improving or who are at unacceptably high risk for cholecystectomy.

Acalculous Cholecystitis

Ill patients (generally those who are hospitalized) can have acute cholecystitis without gallbladder stones. This is known as acalculous cholecystitis and is thought to reflect either bacterial seeding of the gallbladder wall or gallbladder wall ischemia. An elevation of temperature accompanying abdominal pain in a critically ill patient should prompt assessment for cholecystitis. Diagnosis is usually made with ultrasound findings of acute cholecystitis or a radionuclide biliary scan that fails to visualize the gallbladder. Treatment for acute cholecystitis, as described above, is advised; however, these ill patients more often require percutaneous cholecystectomy or endoscopic drainage owing to contraindications to cholecystectomy.

Common Bile Duct Stones and Cholangitis

Common bile duct stones are most often due to the passage of gallbladder stones. Approximately 10% to 20% of patients with gallbladder stones will have a clinical manifestation of a common bile duct stone that could include a transient elevation of serum AST or ALT up to 1000 U/L, cholangitis, or pancreatitis. A small percentage of common bile duct stones develop in patients with biliary strictures (such as those with primary sclerosing cholangitis) or infections and are known as primary duct stones. Common bile duct stones are most reliably diagnosed with magnetic retrograde cholangiopancreatography (MRCP) or endoscopic ultrasound, but they can occasionally be seen on abdominal CT or ultrasound. Management of known common bile duct stones consists of removal, usually with endoscopic retrograde cholangiopancreatography;

however, experienced surgeons may be able to remove common bile duct stones at the time of laparoscopic cholecystectomy. Open common bile duct exploration is rarely required.

Patients with common bile duct stones who have cholangitis may have Charcot triad (fever, right upper quadrant pain, and jaundice) or Reynolds pentad (Charcot triad plus hypotension and mental status change). Patients with cholangitis should receive immediate broad-spectrum antimicrobial therapy similar to that for acute cholecystitis and, if not improving rapidly, urgent endoscopic stone removal. Those who improve with antibiotics can undergo elective stone removal.

Biliary stone disease is a common cause of acute pancreatitis. It should be suspected as the cause when gallbladder stones are noted or when there is a transient rise in liver chemistry studies at presentation. Patients with acute pancreatitis presumed to be from gallbladder stones should undergo cholecystectomy.

KEY POINTS

- Common bile duct stones are most reliably diagnosed with magnetic retrograde cholangiopancreatography or endoscopic ultrasound, but they can occasionally be seen on abdominal CT or ultrasound.

- Cholangitis should be treated with immediate broad-spectrum antimicrobial therapy and, if rapid improvement is not seen, urgent endoscopic stone removal with endoscopic retrograde cholangiopancreatography.

Gallbladder Cancer

Gallbladder cancer is the most common biliary cancer in the United States, but it is rare, with less than 5000 cases yearly. Risk factors for gallbladder cancer include cholelithiasis, gallbladder polyps, porcelain gallbladder, anomalous pancreaticobiliary junction, chronic *Salmonella typhi* carriage, and obesity.

Presenting symptoms may include right upper quadrant pain, nausea, vomiting, weight loss, or jaundice for more advanced cancers and biliary colic for early cancers. The diagnosis may be suspected after cross-sectional imaging to evaluate symptoms. Early gallbladder cancer is most commonly diagnosed incidentally on pathology at the time of cholecystectomy performed for biliary colic. Less than 10% of patients with symptoms and less than 20% of patients with incidentally discovered cancer are found to have early-stage tumors. Diagnosis at a late stage contributes to the poor prognosis of gallbladder cancer.

Incidental tumors found to invade the lamina propria (stage T1a) are treated with cholecystectomy, whereas more advanced lesions require repeat surgery for extended cholecystectomy. Surgery is the treatment of choice for resectable cancers identified preoperatively. Unresectable disease without metastasis can be treated with chemotherapy, with or without radiation, or with palliative care.

Prophylactic cholecystectomy is recommended for patients with an anomalous pancreaticobiliary duct junction, gallbladder polyps 1 cm or larger, gallbladder polyp(s) with concomitant gallstones, or polyps of any size in the setting of primary sclerosing cholangitis. Prophylactic cholecystectomy can also be considered in patients with a porcelain gallbladder or with gallstones larger than 3 cm.

KEY POINTS

- Gallbladder cancer is the most common biliary cancer in the United States, but it is rare, with less than 5000 cases yearly.

- Gallbladder cancer is commonly diagnosed at a late stage, which contributes to its poor prognosis.

Cholangiocarcinoma

Cholangiocarcinoma, or bile duct cancer, is the second most common primary malignancy of the liver after hepatocellular carcinoma. The incidence of cholangiocarcinoma is rising. Established risk factors include primary sclerosing cholangitis, choledochal cysts, the liver flukes *Clonorchis* and *Opisthorchis*, previous exposure to thorium dioxide contrast media, and hepatolithiasis.

Presenting symptoms may include right upper quadrant pain, constitutional symptoms, or jaundice.

Tumors can be broadly classified by their location on the biliary tree. Intrahepatic cholangiocarcinoma typically presents as a mass lesion within the liver, perihilar cholangiocarcinoma arises from the confluence of the right and left hepatic ducts (Klatskin tumor), and distal cholangiocarcinoma arises from the common bile duct, below the cystic duct insertion. Perihilar cholangiocarcinoma is the most common. Intrahepatic tumors are usually asymptomatic until late-stage disease, which may present with right upper quadrant pain, constitutional symptoms, or an elevated serum alkaline phosphatase level. Perihilar and distal tumors commonly present with jaundice and are associated with a mass or dilated bile ducts above the lesion on imaging.

Diagnosis of extrahepatic bile duct cancers usually requires endoscopic retrograde cholangiopancreatography with bile duct brushings or biopsy in combination with MRCP or contrast-enhanced CT. Intrahepatic cholangiocarcinoma can be evaluated with MRCP or contrast-enhanced CT, and the diagnosis can be made with percutaneous biopsy. The serum CA 19-9 level may be elevated in patients with cholangiocarcinoma. However, CA 19-9 may also be elevated in patients with bacterial cholangitis and other malignancies, and it may be negative in some patients. Therefore, its diagnostic role in possible cholangiocarcinoma is supportive only, as it is not able to confirm or exclude the diagnosis.

Surgical resection is the treatment of choice when possible. Distal cholangiocarcinoma has the highest resectability rates. Perihilar and intrahepatic cholangiocarcinoma are less likely to be resectable. Chemotherapy is reserved for patients with nonresectable cholangiocarcinoma. Some patients with hilar and distal cholangiocarcinoma require endoscopic stent placement to decompress the biliary system before chemotherapy can be given. Liver transplantation is an option for nonresectable perihilar cholangiocarcinoma that is 3 cm or smaller without extrahepatic spread. Percutaneous biopsy of perihilar cholangiocarcinoma is an exclusion criterion for liver transplantation owing to the risk of tumor seeding. H

KEY POINTS

- Cholangiocarcinoma, or bile duct cancer, is the second most common primary malignancy of the liver after hepatocellular carcinoma.

- Surgical resection, when possible, is the treatment of choice for cholangiocarcinoma.

Gastrointestinal Bleeding
Overview

Gastrointestinal bleeding (GIB) is defined as upper or lower according to whether the bleeding source is proximal or distal to the ligament of Treitz, respectively. Upper GIB is more common.

Upper Gastrointestinal Bleeding H

Patients with upper GIB may present with hematemesis (bright-red or "coffee-ground" emesis), melena (black, tarry-appearing stool), or hematochezia (bright red blood per rectum). Hematochezia is typically from a lower GIB source but may also be seen with a briskly bleeding upper source, the latter of which is associated with increased mortality. H

KEY POINT

- Patients with upper gastrointestinal bleeding may present with hematemesis (bright-red or "coffee-ground" emesis), melena (black, tarry-appearing stool), or hematochezia (bright red blood per rectum).

Causes H

Table 37 summarizes causes of upper GIB. Approximately 80% is due to four causes: peptic ulcer disease, esophagogastric varices, esophagitis, and Mallory-Weiss tear. Bleeding typically stops spontaneously; however, 20% of patients have persistent or recurrent bleeding, which increases mortality. Slow and/or chronic bleeding may be suggested by history and iron deficiency and is typical of erosive disease, tumor, esophageal ulcer, portal hypertensive gastropathy, Cameron lesion (erosions found within 5% of large hiatal hernias), and angiodysplasia.

Table 38 summarizes causes of brisk and/or severe upper GIB that increase mortality. A history of chronic alcohol abuse is a clue to the possibility of variceal bleeding. Although rare, a Dieulafoy lesion is a large, tortuous, submucosal arteriole that erodes and bleeds dramatically; it is most commonly

TABLE 37. Causes and Prevalence of Upper Gastrointestinal Bleeding

Cause	Prevalence
Peptic ulcer	33.9%
Esophagogastric varices	32.8%
Erosive esophagitis	8.1%
Mallory-Weiss tear	6.4%
Erosion	5.1%
Tumor	5.1%
Esophageal ulcer	2.1%
Portal gastropathy	1.0%
Dieulafoy lesion	0.9%
Cameron lesion	0.7%
Other	2.7%

Adapted by permission from Lippincott Williams & Wilkins: Kim JJ, Sheibani S, Park S, Buxbaum J, Laine L. Causes of Bleeding and Outcomes in Patients Hospitalized With Upper Gastrointestinal Bleeding. J Clin Gastroenterol. 2013 May 16. [PMID: 23685847]

TABLE 38. Causes of Brisk and/or Severe Upper Gastrointestinal Bleeding

Peptic ulcer

Esophagogastric varices

Dieulafoy lesion

Aortoenteric fistula

Hemobilia

Hemosuccus pancreaticus (pseudoaneurysm/aneurysm)

Neoplasm
  Esophageal
  Gastric
  GIST

GIST = gastrointestinal stromal tumor.

CONT.

found in the gastric cardia. Hemobilia is usually due to a liver or biliary procedural complication but can also rarely be caused by gallstone complications, tumors, and angiodysplasia. Hemosuccus pancreaticus (blood emerging from the pancreas) is typically associated with pancreatic pseudocysts and pseudoaneurysm; it may also occur as a complication of endoscopic procedures, including sphincterotomy, insertion of pancreatic duct stents, endoscopic cystogastrostomy, and pancreatic fine needle aspiration or biopsy. An aortic aneurysm repair raises concerns for an aortoenteric fistula.

KEY POINT

- Approximately 80% of upper gastrointestinal bleeding is due to four causes: peptic ulcer disease (34%), esophagogastric varices (33%), esophagitis (8%), and Mallory-Weiss tear (6%).

Evaluation

Evaluation of acute GIB involves assessing severity, determining the need for interventions, and differentiating between upper and lower GIB sources. Predictors of severe GIB are hematemesis, comorbidities (such as cirrhosis or malignancy), hemodynamic instability, and a hemoglobin level less than 8 g/dL (80 g/L). Outpatient management is usually appropriate when the following criteria are met: blood urea nitrogen level less than 18.2 mg/dL (6.5 mmol/L), normal hemoglobin level, systolic blood pressure greater than 109 mm Hg, pulse rate less than or equal to 100/min, and absence of melena, syncope, liver disease, and cardiac failure.

The International Consensus Upper Gastrointestinal Bleeding Conference Group, the American College of Gastroenterology Practice Guidelines, and others recommend using risk-stratification tools to guide decisions regarding urgent endoscopy (within 12 hours), hospital admission and nonurgent endoscopy (within 24 hours), and discharge home from the emergency department. Among the tools, the best validated and most useful is the Glasgow-Blatchford score (range 0-23), which is composed of nine variables: blood urea nitrogen (0-6 points), hemoglobin (0-6 points), systolic blood pressure (0-3 points), pulse rate (0-1 point), melena (0-1 point), syncope (0-2 points), hepatic disease (0-2 points), and cardiac failure (0-2 points). The Glasgow-Blatchford score is particularly useful when the score is 0, which is present in up to 22% of patients and has a nearly 100% negative predictive value for severe GIB and the need for hospital-based intervention (defined as treatment with blood transfusion, endoscopic therapy, transcatheter arterial embolization, surgery, and in some studies identification of cancer at upper endoscopy).

By meta-analysis, upper GIB is most reliably predicted by four individual variables: melena, nasogastric lavage with blood or "coffee grounds," blood urea nitrogen to serum creatinine ratio greater than 30, and absence of blood clots in the stool. It is not established whether multiple variables confer an incremental likelihood of upper GIB, but it is likely.

KEY POINT

- Evaluation of acute gastrointestinal bleeding involves assessing severity, determining the need for interventions, and differentiating between upper and lower gastrointestinal bleeding sources.

Management

Upper GIB management involves (1) pre-endoscopic care (resuscitation, hemodynamic monitoring, proton pump inhibitor [PPI] therapy, and attention to coagulopathy); (2) early endoscopic evaluation (with excellent endoscopic vision) and treatment; and (3) postendoscopic care and risk reduction.

Pre-endoscopic Care

Patients should be resuscitated with crystalloids to reach physiologic endpoints (pulse rate <100/min, systolic blood pressure >100 mm Hg, and resolution of orthostasis). Blood transfusion should be performed for patients with (1) hemodynamic instability and ongoing bleeding or susceptibility to complications from oxygen deprivation (for example, ischemic heart disease) and (2) a hemoglobin level less than 7 g/dL (70 g/L) if hemodynamically stable with no active or massive bleeding; the latter approach imparts a 6-week survival benefit (number needed to treat=25), based on a recent landmark study. Early (pre-endoscopic) PPI therapy does not improve clinical outcomes (bleeding, surgery, mortality) but is safe and reduces the likelihood of detecting ulcers with high-risk stigmata and the need for endoscopic therapy compared with treatment with H$_2$ blockers or placebo. Coagulopathy (defined as an INR >1.5) should be corrected with fresh frozen plasma rather than vitamin K (which has a delayed full therapeutic effect) in actively bleeding patients who are receiving anticoagulation. It remains uncertain whether uncorrected drug-induced coagulopathy (INR 1.5-2.5) adversely affects endoscopic treatment outcomes (rebleeding, surgery, mortality); consensus recommendations are to not delay endoscopy unless the INR is supratherapeutic (INR >3.0). Octreotide and antibiotics should be administered before endoscopy for suspected variceal bleeding. Nasogastric tube placement is not required for diagnosis, prognosis, visualization, or therapeutic effect. Routine use of prokinetic agents is not recommended except when patients are suspected of having large amounts of blood in the upper gastrointestinal tract; in such cases, erythromycin can be given prior to upper endoscopy.

For a discussion of variceal bleeding, see Disorders of the Liver.

Endoscopic Evaluation and Treatment

Guidelines recommend upper endoscopy within 24 hours of presentation in patients with features of upper GIB. Endoscopy within 12 hours is generally recommended only for those with suspected variceal GIB. **Table 39** summarizes peptic ulcer management based on rebleeding risk.

Low-risk ulcers are clean-based or have a nonprotuberant pigmented spot (**Figure 30**). Oral PPI therapy should be

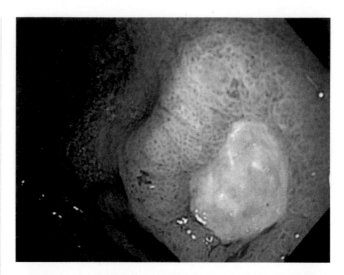
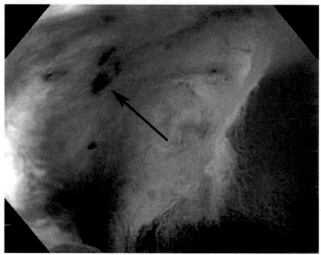
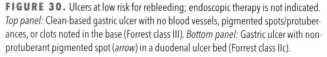

FIGURE 30. Ulcers at low risk for rebleeding; endoscopic therapy is not indicated. *Top panel:* Clean-based gastric ulcer with no blood vessels, pigmented spots/protuberances, or clots noted in the base (Forrest class III). *Bottom panel:* Gastric ulcer with nonprotuberant pigmented spot (*arrow*) in a duodenal ulcer bed (Forrest class IIc).

Courtesy of Louis M. Wong Kee Song M.D., Mayo Clinic.

TABLE 39. Forrest Classification of Peptic Ulcers by Prevalence, Rebleeding Rates, and Treatment

Category	Description	Prevalence	Rebleeding[a]	Endotherapy	PPI Therapy
Ia	Active arterial bleeding	12%	56%	Yes	IV[b]
Ib	Active oozing bleeding	12%	56%	Yes	IV[b]
IIa	Nonbleeding visible vessel	8%	43%	Yes	IV[b]
IIb	Adherent clot	8%	22%	+/−[c]	IV[b]
IIc	Flat pigmented spot	16%	10%	No	Oral
III	Clean ulcer base	55%	5%	No	Oral

IV = intravenous; PPI = proton pump inhibitor.

[a]Rebleeding without endotherapy

[b]IV PPI therapy consists of an intravenous bolus followed by continuous infusion of a high-dose PPI for 72 hours.

[c]Endotherapy of adherent clots is controversial; continuous IV PPI may be sufficient.

Adapted by permission from Macmillan Publishers Ltd: American Journal of Gastroenterology (Laine L, Jensen DM. Management of patients with ulcer bleeding. 107(3):345-60; quiz 361. [PMID: 22310222]), copyright 2012.

CONT.

initiated, and patients should be allowed to eat. Early hospital discharge should be arranged.

Intermediate-risk ulcers have adherent clots (**Figure 31**). They should be vigorously irrigated to dislodge the clot and guide treatment. With successful dislodgment, ulcers should be treated according to recommendations for low-risk ulcers (see previous paragraph) or high-risk ulcers (see next paragraph). For persistent clots, however, the benefit of mechanically removing the clot is unclear but is possibly greater when patients have risk factors for rebleeding, as defined later. After endoscopy, patients with persistent clots should remain hospitalized and should receive continuous intravenous PPI therapy for 72 hours, as for high-risk ulcers.

High-risk ulcers have active arterial spurting or a non-bleeding visible vessel (**Figure 32**). They should be treated endoscopically with hemoclips, thermal therapy, or injection of sclerosants, which are all equally effective at achieving hemostasis. Local injection of the vasoconstrictor epinephrine may be used adjunctively to aid immediate hemostasis for optimizing visibility for subsequent and more durable endoscopic therapy; however, epinephrine injection alone is inadequate for durable hemostasis.

Following endoscopic therapy, the strongest predictors of recurrent bleeding are hemodynamic instability, active bleeding at endoscopy, ulcer size greater than 2 cm, and ulcer location (posterior duodenal or high lesser gastric curvature). Additional predictors may also include age 60 years or older, comorbid illness, and postendoscopy hemoglobin level less than 10 g/dL (100 g/L).

After endoscopic hemostasis, continuous intravenous PPI infusion for 72 hours reduces recurrent bleeding, need for surgery, and mortality. Hospital stay is generally 3 days after endoscopy, assuming clinical stability.

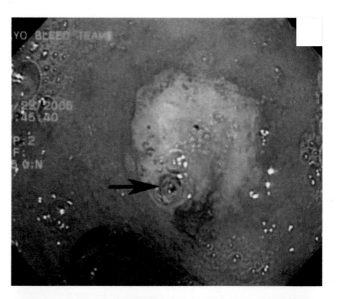

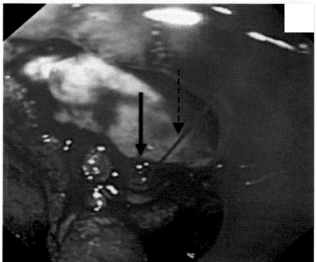

FIGURE 32. Duodenal ulcers at high risk of rebleeding that must be treated endoscopically. *Top panel:* Nonbleeding visible vessel (*arrow*) (Forrest class IIa). *Bottom panel:* Ulcer (*solid arrow*) with active arterial spurting (*dotted arrow*) (Forrest class Ia).

Courtesy of Louis M. Wong Kee Song M.D., Mayo Clinic.

Routine second-look endoscopy in all patients is not recommended, but a second attempt at endoscopic therapy is recommended for rebleeding and when the initial examination was incomplete. Repeat endoscopy can be considered for gastric ulcers after 8 to 12 weeks of PPI therapy if (1) symptoms are persistent despite therapy, (2) ulcers have an endoscopic appearance that is concerning for underlying malignancy, (3) visualization of the stomach was incomplete, or (4) biopsies were not taken at the time of the index upper endoscopy.

Consultation with surgery and interventional radiology (for embolization) may be helpful for patients with severe upper GIB, particularly with active bleeding and hemodynamic instability, and/or when endoscopic therapy fails to achieve hemostasis of a high-risk lesion. H

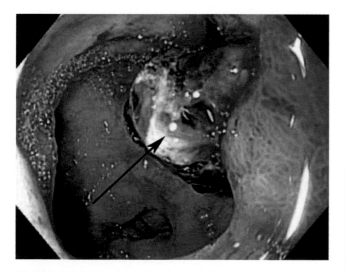

FIGURE 31. Duodenal ulcer with adherent clot (*arrow*) that is at risk for rebleeding (Forrest class IIb). This can be treated medically, or by clot removal and endoscopic therapy in addition to standard medical therapy.

Courtesy of Louis M. Wong Kee Song M.D., Mayo Clinic.

- Guidelines recommend upper endoscopy within 24 hours of presentation in patients with features of upper gastrointestinal bleeding; endoscopy within 12 hours is generally recommended only for patients with suspected variceal bleeding.

- Low-risk ulcers are clean-based or have a nonprotuberant pigmented spot; intermediate-risk ulcers have adherent clots and should be vigorously irrigated to dislodge the clot and reclassified based on appearance; high-risk ulcers have active arterial spurting or a nonbleeding visible vessel and require endoscopic treatment.

HVC
- Routine second-look endoscopy is not required after upper gastrointestinal bleeding unless rebleeding occurs or the initial examination was incomplete.

Postendoscopic Care and Risk Reduction

CONT.

All patients with upper GIB due to peptic ulcer disease should be tested for *Helicobacter pylori* (see Disorders of the Stomach and Duodenum) in the acute setting. If testing is positive, treatment should be initiated and eradication should be confirmed. If initial testing for *H. pylori* is negative, patients should undergo retesting with an alternative modality owing to the possibility of false-negative test results in the setting of bleeding, PPI therapy, or concomitant antibiotic therapy.

The choice of whether to discontinue or withhold antiplatelet agents in patients with clear indications for treatment should balance the risk of rebleeding with the risk of thrombosis. Aspirin should be resumed within 3 to 5 days for patients with established cardiovascular disease. Aspirin reduces mortality rates tenfold over 30 days while increasing rebleeding rates only twofold. Patients taking aspirin and clopidogrel for coronary stents should continue aspirin, but clopidogrel should be temporarily withheld for high-risk ulcers. In situations in which dual antiplatelet therapy is indicated (such as following placement of a drug-eluting stent), clopidogrel should be resumed immediately for low-risk ulcers and as soon as possible for high-risk ulcers.

Long-term, daily PPI therapy should be offered to aspirin users who are *H. pylori* negative or those who use concomitant NSAIDs, anticoagulants, glucocorticoids, or other antiplatelet agents. Long-term PPI therapy may not be necessary for aspirin users who undergo *H. pylori* testing and eradication.

Patients with high thrombotic risk should receive reanticoagulation but only after evaluating thromboembolic risk against rebleeding risk. Criteria for high thrombotic risk are chronic atrial fibrillation with a previous embolic event, CHADS$_2$ score of 3 or greater, recent acute coronary syndrome, mechanical heart valve, deep venous thrombosis, pulmonary embolism, or hypercoagulable state. There are limited data for resuming anticoagulation after major GIB, particularly for patients with endoscopically treated high-risk ulcers; however, available data support

beginning with (1) a bridging treatment (such as low-molecular-weight or unfractionated heparin) and careful observation or (2) beginning oral anticoagulation 7 days after the bleeding event. The latter approach, according to a retrospective study, reduces mortality and risk of thromboembolism (in patients with atrial fibrillation) without increasing GIB risk compared with withholding anticoagulation for 30 days.

Lower Gastrointestinal Bleeding

Lower gastrointestinal bleeding typically occurs in older individuals and presents as acute bright red blood per rectum or red- or maroon-colored stool (hematochezia). Hemodynamic instability is less common but, if present, raises the possibility of a briskly bleeding upper gastrointestinal source.

Causes

Hematochezia is usually from a colonic source, but in approximately 25% of patients the source is in the upper gastrointestinal tract, the small intestine, or an obscure location. **Table 40** summarizes the most common causes of lower GIB. Almost 80% of lower GIB is due to diverticulosis, colitis, hemorrhoids, and postpolypectomy bleeding. **Table 41** summarizes causes of severe lower GIB.

Diverticula represent herniation of mucosa/submucosa through the muscular layers of the colon, typically at the entry site of vasa recta (small arteries), which are a source for bleeding. Diverticula are most commonly left sided, but colonic diverticular bleeding occurs in either side of the colon. For unclear reasons, individual studies report different anatomic distributions of diverticular bleeding based on the diagnostic method; bleeding is most commonly right-sided

TABLE 40. Causes and Prevalence of Lower Gastrointestinal Bleeding

Cause	Prevalence
Diverticulosis	30%
Colitis	24%
Ischemic	12%
IBD	9%
Radiation	3%
Hemorrhoids	14%
Postpolypectomy	8%
Colon polyps or cancer	6%
Rectal ulcer	6%
Angiodysplasia	3%
Other	6%

IBD = inflammatory bowel disease.

Adapted with permission of Current Science, Inc., from Ghassemi KA, Jensen DM. Lower GI bleeding: epidemiology and management. Curr Gastroenterol Rep. 2013 Jul;15(7):333. [PMID: 23737154]; permission conveyed through Copyright Clearance Center, Inc.

TABLE 41. Causes of Severe Lower Gastrointestinal Bleeding

Diverticulosis
Aortoenteric fistula
Colonic or rectal varices
Dieulafoy lesions
Neoplasm
Colitis
Ischemic
IBD
Infectious
Intussusception
Meckel diverticulum
Angiodysplasia

IBD = inflammatory bowel disease.

when diagnosed by angiography and is most commonly left-sided when diagnosed by colonoscopy.

The presence of abdominal pain raises the possibility of neoplasia or colitis from ischemia (12%), inflammatory bowel disease (9%), radiation (3%), and less commonly infectious gastroenteritis (*Campylobacter*, *Salmonella*, *Clostridium difficile*) or drugs (NSAIDs).

Hemorrhoidal bleeding is typically small volume with bright red blood, but it is occasionally large volume. Postpolypectomy bleeding is typically associated with use of electrocautery methods for polypectomy and may have a delayed presentation. The prevalence of angiodysplasia increases with age and can be overlooked during colonoscopy if bleeding has stopped.

KEY POINT

- Almost 80% of lower gastrointestinal bleeding is due to diverticulosis (30%), colitis (24%), hemorrhoids (14%), and postpolypectomy bleeding (8%).

Evaluation

The initial steps in the evaluation of lower GIB are similar to those for upper GIB. They include assessing bleeding severity, determining the need for hospital-based interventions (defined as treatment with blood transfusion, endoscopic therapy, transcatheter arterial embolization, surgery), and differentiating between upper and lower GIB sources (see Upper Gastrointestinal Bleeding, Evaluation).

Management

Initial management of lower and upper GIB is similar in that it focuses on resuscitation and hemodynamic monitoring (see Upper Gastrointestinal Bleeding, Management). Evidence supporting a specific, initial assessment of lower GIB is limited. According to the 2008 Scottish Intercollegiate Guidelines Network (www.sign.ac.uk/pdf/sign105.pdf), clinicians may consider

nonadmission with outpatient follow-up or early hospital discharge when four criteria are present: age less than 60 years, no hemodynamic instability, no evidence of gross rectal bleeding, and identification of an obvious anorectal source of bleeding on rectal examination/sigmoidoscopy. Conversely, hospitalization should be considered in patients with any of five criteria predictive of severe bleeding, including age greater than 60 years, comorbid illnesses (particularly when two or more are present), hemodynamic instability, gross rectal bleeding (or early rebleeding), or exposure to antiplatelet drugs and anticoagulants.

Direct evidence is lacking to define a clear blood transfusion strategy for colonic bleeding. A restrictive blood transfusion strategy (based on a threshold hemoglobin level of 7 g/dL [70 g/L]) imparts a 6-week survival benefit for patients with upper GIB, but the landmark study that resulted in these findings excluded patients with colonic or massive bleeding. According to expert opinion, the blood transfusion threshold for patients with colonic bleeding is a hemoglobin value less than 9 to 10 g/dL (90 to 100 g/L); the higher cutoff should be used when cardiovascular comorbidities (including ischemic heart disease, peripheral vascular surgery, or heart failure) are present.

Lower GIB typically stops within 24 hours. Patients with suspected left-sided bleeding may undergo anoscopy or sigmoidoscopy as an initial evaluation (particularly for colitis, rectal ulcer, and postpolypectomy bleeding from polyps removed from the left colon); anoscopy or sigmoidoscopy can be performed following enemas or in an unprepped colon. Most patients require colonoscopy, however, even if a distal bleeding source is suspected. Colonoscopy identifies a source of bleeding in two thirds of patients.

Colonoscopy performed early is more likely to identify a bleeding source and allow for treatment, which may shorten length of hospitalization; however, the optimal timing of colonoscopy is not established, in part owing to time required for resuscitation and bowel cleansing. According to expert opinion, patients hospitalized for lower GIB should undergo semi-elective inpatient evaluation approximately 24 hours after initial presentation. Early rebleeding is common, however, and should prompt further resuscitation, triage to an appropriate level of care, and more urgent endoscopic evaluation within 12 to 18 hours (after a rapid purge).

Endoscopic treatments for active bleeding are similar to techniques for upper GIB and include multipolar electrocoagulation, hemoclips, and submucosal epinephrine injection. Submucosal epinephrine injection should be combined with thermal or mechanical hemostatic techniques. Data are limited for predicting outcomes based on endoscopic findings; a single center reported that diverticular bleeding associated with major stigmata of hemorrhage (active bleeding, visible vessel, and adherent clot) has a high rate of rebleeding (65%) and emergent surgery (43%) when endoscopic hemostasis is not performed.

For failed endoscopic hemostasis or recurrent bleeding, the next therapeutic step is consultation with interventional radiology for arterial embolization of the bleeding source.

CONT. Major complications include contrast dye reactions, acute kidney injury, transient ischemic attacks, bowel ischemia, hematoma formation, and femoral artery thrombosis. Salvage therapy for recurrent bleeding may require surgery, but this is not frequently necessary because bleeding is typically self-limited and management with endoscopic or angiographic techniques may be effective. Partly because of these factors, overall mortality from colonic bleeding is low (<4%); however, mortality increases in association with age greater than 70 years, two or more comorbidities, and intestinal ischemia. **H**

KEY POINTS

- Lower gastrointestinal bleeding typically stops within 24 hours and can be evaluated semi-electively 24 hours after initial presentation.
- Most patients with suspected lower gastrointestinal bleeding require colonoscopy, even if a distal bleeding source is suspected; colonoscopy identifies a source of bleeding in two thirds of patients.

H Obscure Gastrointestinal Bleeding

Obscure gastrointestinal bleeding (OGIB) is gastrointestinal bleeding of an unknown cause. The initial evaluation includes a negative upper endoscopy and colonoscopy. Overt OGIB is defined as bleeding that is visible, such as with melena or hematochezia. Occult OGIB has no signs of gross blood, but unexplained iron deficiency anemia is present. Approximately 5% of gastrointestinal bleeding has an obscure cause occurring somewhere between the papilla and the ileocecal valve (also known as midgastrointestinal bleeding). **H**

KEY POINTS

- Overt obscure gastrointestinal bleeding is defined as bleeding that is visible, such as with melena or hematochezia.
- Occult obscure gastrointestinal bleeding has no signs of gross blood, but unexplained iron deficiency anemia is present.

Causes

Causes of OGIB are described in **Table 42**. Angiodysplasia is the most common cause (**Figure 33**). It is responsible for up to 40% of cases and is often seen in the elderly. Other causes include NSAID enteropathy, inflammatory bowel disease, tumors (leiomyoma, carcinoid, lymphoma, and adenocarcinoma), Meckel diverticulum (typically seen in younger patients) (**Figure 34**),

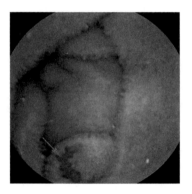

FIGURE 33. Capsule endoscopy image of angiodysplasia. The lesion (*arrow*) has a fernlike pattern and is red in color. Angiodysplasia can have no bleeding or active bleeding.

Courtesy of David J. Hass, MD.

TABLE 42.	Causes of Obscure Gastrointestinal Bleeding		
Location	**Differential Diagnosis**	**Patient Age (Years)**	**Clinical Clues**
Proximal to the ligament of Treitz	Cameron erosion	20-60	Large hiatal hernia
	NSAID ulcerations	>20	Medication review
	Dieulafoy lesion	>40	Intermittent large-volume bleeding
	Crohn disease	20-60	Family history, extraintestinal manifestations; may also occur in small bowel and colon
	Gastric antral vascular ectasia	20-60	Female, autoimmune disease
Small bowel	Angiodysplasia	>60	Intermittent, usually occult bleeding; may also occur in colon
	Peutz-Jeghers syndrome	<20	Perioral pigmentation, obstructive symptoms
	Meckel diverticulum	20-60	Possible abdominal pain
	Hemangioma	<20	Possible cutaneous hemangiomas
	Malignancy	>50	Weight loss, abdominal pain
	Hereditary hemorrhagic telangiectasia	>50	Mucocutaneous telangiectasias
Colon	Diverticulosis	>50	Intermittent, painless bleeding
	Malignancy	>50	Weight loss, family history

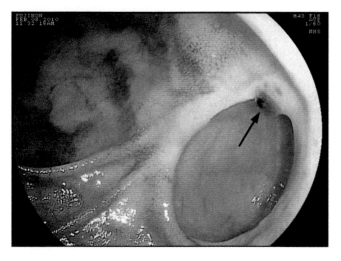

FIGURE 34. Meckel diverticulum diagnosed on balloon-assisted enteroscopy. A diverticulum is seen in the small bowel. At the top of the diverticulum is a visible vessel, which is the raised black spot at the top (*arrow*).

radiation enteropathy, Dieulafoy lesion, hemosuccus pancreaticus, and small-bowel varices. Sources found by repeat conventional upper endoscopy and colonoscopy include Cameron ulcerations in a hiatal hernia, bleeding colonic diverticula, and vascular lesions.

KEY POINT

- Angiodysplasia is the most common cause of obscure gastrointestinal bleeding.

Evaluation

A comprehensive history and clinical examination can be useful to narrow the differential diagnosis of OGIB. Patients 50 years of age or younger are more likely to have tumors (leiomyoma, carcinoid, adenocarcinoma, or lymphoma), Dieulafoy lesion, or Crohn disease. However, older patients are more likely to have vascular lesions, such as angiodysplasia. Patients should be asked about NSAID use (NSAIDs induce small-bowel ulcers), aortic aneurysm repair (raises concern for an aortoenteric fistula), necrotizing pancreatitis (causes hemosuccus pancreaticus), or liver damage (trauma, tumor, or recent biopsy causing hemobilia). Physical examination of the skin may identify lesions associated with hereditary hemorrhagic telangiectasia (also known as Osler-Weber-Rendu syndrome) or celiac disease (associated with dermatitis herpetiformis).

Patients thought to have OGIB should be considered for repeat upper endoscopy and/or colonoscopy; studies have shown that lesions can be missed during initial examinations. Up to 50% of lesions can be identified using this strategy.

For patients with obscure active GIB, initial imaging studies may include nuclear studies followed by angiography to localize the bleeding. The next steps in patients with active bleeding are push enteroscopy, balloon-assisted enteroscopy (deep enteroscopy), or surgery and intraoperative enteroscopy as a last diagnostic option.

For patients with occult GIB, a small-bowel evaluation is indicated after endoscopy and colonoscopy are both negative. The next most appropriate test is capsule endoscopy. Other options include push or deep enteroscopy. If these tests are negative, the next step in a patient with continued bleeding is repeated endoscopic examinations (upper endoscopy, colonoscopy, capsule endoscopy, or deep enteroscopy). If the patient is stable, observation with iron replacement is a reasonable approach.

KEY POINT

- Patients thought to have obscure gastrointestinal bleeding should be considered for repeat upper endoscopy and/or colonoscopy; studies have shown that lesions can be missed during initial examinations.

Technetium-Labeled Nuclear Scan

Technetium 99m-labeled red blood cell or sulfur colloid nuclear scans may be useful in evaluating overt OGIB. They are able to detect bleeding rates between 0.1 and 0.4 mL/min, with accuracy varying from 24% to 91%. Nuclear scans can identify only a general area where bleeding is occurring; they cannot offer accuracy or intervention. Follow-up studies after a positive scan can include repeat endoscopy or angiography; both can offer more accurate localization and therapy. Nuclear scans are often done before angiography.

Angiography

Angiography can identify bleeding in overt OGIB if the bleeding rate is greater than 0.5 mL/min. It is more effective at localizing bleeding but is technically less sensitive than a nuclear bleeding scan. The diagnostic yield ranges from 27% to 77% in OGIB. Angiography allows for intervention such as selective mesenteric embolization. Complications include acute kidney injury, organ necrosis, embolism, hematoma, and vascular dissection or aneurysm.

Wireless Capsule Endoscopy

Capsule endoscopy is a wireless capsule camera (**Figure 35**) that is swallowed by the patient to take images of the small

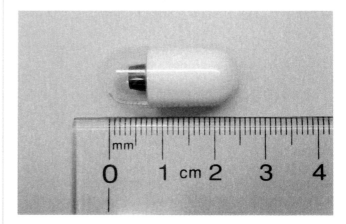

FIGURE 35. Image of an endoscopy capsule.

Courtesy of Dr. Elizabeth Rajan, Mayo Clinic.

CONT.

bowel. These images are transmitted to a radiofrequency receiver worn by the patient. Capsule endoscopy allows visualization of the entire small bowel in up to 90% of patients and has a diagnostic yield of 83%. Limitations of capsule endoscopy include inability to perform therapeutic interventions and difficulty localizing lesions. Complications may include capsule retention in the setting of obstruction or strictures. Capsule endoscopy has become the first-line test in evaluating the small bowel after a negative endoscopy and colonoscopy in patients with OGIB.

> **KEY POINT**
>
> - Capsule endoscopy has become the first-line test in evaluating the small bowel after a negative endoscopy and colonoscopy in patients with obscure gastrointestinal bleeding.

Push Enteroscopy

Push enteroscopy is performed with advancement of the endoscope beyond the ligament of Treitz into the jejunum. Depth of insertion is operator dependent but is also limited owing to looping of the scope in the stomach. The diagnostic yield is between 24% and 56%. Push enteroscopy allows for diagnostic intervention with biopsy and therapeutic intervention with cautery. The most common lesions found are angiodysplasia, which are treated with thermal cautery. This test is done after a negative upper endoscopy and colonoscopy or after a positive capsule endoscopy.

Spiral Enteroscopy

Spiral enteroscopy is performed with deep enteroscopy beyond the ligament of Treitz; it uses a spiral-shaped tube that fits over the endoscope and allows it to be advanced progressively into the small bowel. The technique involves rotary clockwise and counterclockwise maneuvers, similar to the motion of a corkscrew. Depth of insertion has been reported to be up to 260 cm beyond the ligament of Treitz. This modality allows for diagnostic intervention with tissue biopsy and therapeutic intervention (with hemostasis, polypectomy, and foreign body retrieval). The major complication of spiral enteroscopy is perforation of the small bowel, which occurs at a low rate (0.27%). This procedure is used to find a lesion seen on capsule endoscopy, such as an angiodysplasia. It can also be used to reach a lesion or abnormal area seen on a radiologic imaging study.

Single- and Double-Balloon Enteroscopy

Balloon-assisted enteroscopy allows for deep insertion of the enteroscope by using an inflatable balloon fixed on an overtube. It allows for pleating of the small intestine on the enteroscope to go deep into the small bowel beyond the reach of traditional push enteroscopy. Balloon-assisted enteroscopy can be performed with an oral or rectal approach. The diagnostic yield of balloon-assisted enteroscopy for OGIB is as high as 80%, which is superior to that of push enteroscopy.

Diagnostic and therapeutic interventions similar to those of spiral enteroscopy can be performed. The complication rate of balloon-assisted enteroscopy is low; the most commonly reported complications are perforation, ileus, and pancreatitis.

Small-Bowel Radiography

The yield of radiographic imaging with small-bowel follow-through for diagnosing OGIB is very low (0%-5%). Enteroclysis (a double-contrast radiographic study of the small bowel using barium and methylcellulose) highlights the small bowel in more detail to identify inflammatory bowel disease or tumors. Either imaging modality is unable to identify angiodysplasia. Small-bowel radiography is not considered a first-line tool for OGIB because of its low diagnostic yield. Furthermore, better diagnostic tools have since been developed, such as capsule endoscopy, which allow for a better examination of the small-bowel mucosa.

Intraoperative Endoscopy

Intraoperative endoscopy should be reserved for patients with OGIB in whom all other modalities have failed to identify or control a bleeding source. It can be performed during laparotomy or laparoscopy to identify the bleeding source. The diagnostic yield has been reported to be in the range of 58% to 80%. The emergence of balloon-assisted enteroscopy has decreased the use of this technique.

Management

Therapy for OGIB is guided by the underlying source of bleeding. Angiodysplasia should be treated with electrocautery, argon plasma coagulation, injection therapy, mechanical hemostasis (hemoclips or banding), or a combination of these techniques. If endoscopic therapy has failed, medical therapy for angiodysplasia may include octreotide, hormonal therapy, or thalidomide. Patients with angiodysplasia in the setting of aortic stenosis (Heyde syndrome) may benefit from valve replacement surgery. Tumors or masses require surgical intervention. In the presence of massive bleeding, interventional radiology may temporize bleeding with localized embolization. Iron supplementation (oral or intravenous) along with blood transfusion may be needed in some patients. If a causative agent such as an NSAID is identified, it should be stopped.

> **KEY POINT**
>
> - Therapy for obscure gastrointestinal bleeding is guided by the underlying source of bleeding.

Bibliography

Disorders of the Esophagus

Dellon ES, Gonsalves N, Hirano I, Furuta GT, Liacouras CA, Katzka DA; American College of Gastroenterology. ACG clinical guideline: Evidenced based approach to the diagnosis and management of esophageal eosinophilia and eosinophilic esophagitis (EoE). Am J Gastroenterol. 2013 May;108(5):679-92. [PMID: 23567357]

Katz PO, Gerson LB, Vela MF. Guidelines for the diagnosis and management of gastroesophageal reflux disease. Am J Gastroenterol. 2013 Mar;108(3):308-28. [PMID: 23419381]

Pandolfino JE, Kahrilas PJ; American Gastroenterological Association. AGA technical review on the clinical use of esophageal manometry. Gastroenterology. 2005 Jan;128(1):209-24. [PMID: 15633138]

Spechler SJ, Sharma P, Souza RF, Inadomi JM, Shaheen NJ; American Gastroenterological Association. American Gastroenterological Association technical review on the management of Barrett's esophagus. Gastroenterology. 2011 Mar;140(3):e18-52. [PMID: 21376939]

Vaezi MF, Pandolfino JE, Vela MF. ACG clinical guideline: diagnosis and management of achalasia. Am J Gastroenterol. 2013 Aug;108(8):1238-49. [PMID: 23877351]

Wang KK, Sampliner RE; Practice Parameters Committee of the American College of Gastroenterology. Updated guidelines 2008 for the diagnosis, surveillance and therapy of Barrett's esophagus. Am J Gastroenterol. 2008 Mar;103(3):788-97. [PMID: 18341497]

Disorders of the Stomach and Duodenum

Bhatt DL, Scheiman J, Abraham NS, et al; American College of Cardiology Foundation Task Force on Clinical Expert Consensus Documents. ACCF/ACG/AHA 2008 expert consensus document on reducing the gastrointestinal risks of antiplatelet therapy and NSAID use: a report of the American College of Cardiology Foundation Task Force on Clinical Expert Consensus Documents. J Am Coll Cardiol. 2008 Oct 28;52(18):1502-17. [PMID: 19017521]

Camilleri M, Parkman HP, Shafi MA, Abell TL, Gerson L; American College of Gastroenterology. Clinical guideline: management of gastroparesis. Am J Gastroenterol. 2013 Jan;108(1):18-37; quiz 38. [PMID: 23147521]

Chey WD, Wong BC; Practice Parameters Committee of the American College of Gastroenterology. American College of Gastroenterology guideline on the management of Helicobacter pylori infection. Am J Gastroenterol. 2007 Aug;102(8):1808-25. [PMID: 17608775]

Goddard AF, Badreldin R, Pritchard DM, Walker MM, Warren B; British Society of Gastroenterology. The management of gastric polyps. Gut. 2010 Sep;59(9):1270-6. [PMID: 20675692]

Guggenheim DE, Shah MA. Gastric cancer epidemiology and risk factors. J Surg Oncol. 2013 Mar;107(3):230-6. [PMID: 23129495]

Hammer HF. Medical complications of bariatric surgery: focus on malabsorption and dumping syndrome. Dig Dis. 2012;30(2):182-6. [PMID: 22722436]

Heber D, Greenway FL, Kaplan LM, Livingston E, Salvador J, Still C; Endocrine Society. Endocrine and nutritional management of the post-bariatric surgery patient: an Endocrine Society Clinical Practice Guideline. J Clin Endocrinol Metab. 2010 Nov;95(11):4823-43. [PMID: 21051578]

Hirota WK, Zuckerman MJ, Adler DG, et al; Standards of Practice Committee, American Society for Gastrointestinal Endoscopy. ASGE guideline: the role of endoscopy in the surveillance of premalignant conditions of the upper GI tract. Gastrointest Endosc. 2006 Apr;63(4):570-80. [PMID: 16564854]

Hwang JH, Rulyak SD, Kimmey MB; American Gastroenterological Association Institute. American Gastroenterological Association Institute technical review on the management of gastric subepithelial masses. Gastroenterology. 2006 Jun;130(7):2217-28. [PMID: 16762644]

Lacy BE, Talley NJ, Locke GR 3rd, et al. Review article: current treatment options and management of functional dyspepsia. Aliment Pharmacol Ther. 2012 Jul;36(1):3-15. [PMID: 22591037]

Landi B, Palazzo L. The role of endosonography in submucosal tumours. Best Pract Res Clin Gastroenterol. 2009;23(5):679-701. [PMID: 19744633]

Lanza FL, Chan FK, Quigley EM; Practice Parameters Committee of the American College of Gastroenterology. Guidelines for prevention of NSAID-related ulcer complications. Am J Gastroenterol. 2009 Mar;104(3):728-38. [PMID: 19240698]

Longitudinal Assessment of Bariatric Surgery (LABS) Consortium, Flum DR, Belle SH, King WC, et al. Perioperative safety in the longitudinal assessment of bariatric surgery. N Engl J Med. 2009 Jul 30;361(5):445-54. [PMID: 19641201]

Tack J, Talley NJ, Camilleri M, et al. Functional gastroduodenal disorders. Gastroenterology. 2006 Apr;130(5):1466-79. Erratum in: Gastroenterology. 2006 Jul;131(1):336. [PMID: 16678560]

Disorders of the Pancreas

Askew J, Connor S. Review of the investigation and surgical management of resectable ampullary adenocarcinoma. HPB (Oxford). 2013 Nov;15(11):829-838 [PMID: 23458317]

Banks PA, Bollen TL, Dervenis C, et al; Acute Pancreatitis Classification Working Group. Classification of acute pancreatitis–2012: revision of the Atlanta classification and definitions by international consensus. Gut. 2013 Jan;62(1):102-11. [PMID: 23100216]

Burns WR, Edil BH. Neuroendocrine pancreatic tumors: guidelines for management and update. Curr Treat Options Oncol. 2012 Mar;13(1):24-34. [PMID: 22198808]

Canto MI, Harinck F, Hruban RH, et al; International Cancer of Pancreas Screening (CAPS) Consortium. International Cancer of the Pancreas Screening (CAPS) Consortium summit on the management of patients with increased risk for familial pancreatic cancer. Gut. 2013 Mar;62(3):339-47. [PMID: 23135763]

Forsmark CE. Management of chronic pancreatitis. Gastroenterology. 2013 Jun;144(6):1282-91. [PMID: 23622138]

Hart PA, Kamisawa T, Brugge WR, et al. Long-term outcomes of autoimmune pancreatitis: a multicentre, international analysis. Gut. 2013 Dec;62(12):1771-6. [PMID: 23232048]

Mounzer R, Langmead CJ, Wu BU, et al. Comparison of existing clinical scoring systems to predict persistent organ failure in patients with acute pancreatitis. Gastroenterology. 2012 Jun;142(7):1476-82; quiz e15-6. [PMID: 22425589]

Tanaka M, Fernández-del Castillo C, Adsay V, et al; International Association of Pancreatology. International consensus guidelines 2012 for the management of IPMN and MCN of the pancreas. Pancreatology. 2012 May-Jun;12(3):183-97. [PMID: 22687371]

Tenner S, Baillie J, Dewitt J, Vege SS. American college of gastroenterology guideline: management of acute pancreatitis. Am J Gastroenterol. 2013 Sep;108(9):1400-15. [PMID: 23896955]

Vege SS, Ziring B, Jain R, Moayyedi P; Clinical Guidelines Committee. American gastroenterological association institute guideline on the diagnosis and management of asymptomatic neoplastic pancreatic cysts. Gastroenterology. 2015 Apr;148(4):819-22. [PMID: 25805375]

Disorders of the Small and Large Bowel

American College of Gastroenterology Task Force on Irritable Bowel Syndrome, Brandt LJ, Chey WD, Foxx-Orenstein AE, et al. An evidence-based position statement on the management of irritable bowel syndrome. Am J Gastroenterol. 2009 Jan;104 Suppl 1:S1-35. [PMID: 19521341]

Bharucha AE, Pemberton JH, Locke GR 3rd. American Gastroenterological Association technical review on constipation. Gastroenterology. 2013 Jan;144(1):218-38. [PMID: 23261065]

Biondo S, Lopez Borao J, Millan M, Kreisler E, Jaurrieta E. Current status of the treatment of acute colonic diverticulitis: a systematic review. Colorectal Dis. 2012 Jan;14(1):e1-e11. [PMID: 21848896]

Costilla VC, Foxx-Orenstein AE, Mayer AP, Crowell MD. Office-based management of fecal incontinence. Gastroenterol Hepatol (N Y). 2013 Jul;9(7):423-33. [PMID: 23935551]

Kornbluth A, Sachar DB; Practice Parameters Committee of the American College of Gastroenterology. Ulcerative colitis practice guidelines in adults: American College Of Gastroenterology, Practice Parameters Committee. Am J Gastroenterol. 2010 Mar;105(3):501-23. Erratum in: Am J Gastroenterol. 2010 Mar;105(3):500. [PMID: 20068560]

Lakatos PL, Lakatos L, Kiss LS, Peyrin-Biroulet L, Schoepfer A, Vavricka S. Treatment of extraintestinal manifestations in inflammatory bowel disease. Digestion. 2012;86 Suppl 1:28-35. [PMID: 23051724]

Lichtenstein GR, Hanauer SB, Sandborn WJ; Practice Parameters Committee of American College of Gastroenterology. Management of Crohn's disease in adults. Am J Gastroenterol. 2009 Feb;104(2):465-83. [PMID: 19174807]

Longstreth GF, Thompson WG, Chey WD, Houghton LA, Mearin F, Spiller RC. Functional bowel disorders. Gastroenterology. 2006 Apr;130(5):1480-91. Erratum in: Gastroenterology. 2006 Aug;131(2):688. [PMID: 16678561]

Murray JA, Rubio-Tapia A. Diarrhoea due to small bowel diseases. Best Pract Res Clin Gastroenterol. 2012 Oct;26(5):581-600. [PMID: 23384804]

Pardi DS, Kelly CP. Microscopic colitis. Gastroenterology. 2011 Apr;140(4):1155-65. [PMID: 21303675]

Pecoraro F, Rancic Z, Lachat M, et al. Chronic mesenteric ischemia: critical review and guidelines for management. Ann Vasc Surg. 2013 Jan;27(1):113-22. [PMID: 23088809]

Perry WB, Dykes SL, Buie WD, Rafferty JF; Standards Practice Task Force of the American Society of Colon and Rectal Surgeons. Practice parameters for the management of anal fissures (3rd revision). Dis Colon Rectum. 2010 Aug;53(8):1110-5. [PMID: 20628272]

Rivadeneira DE, Steele SR, Ternent C, Chalasani S, Buie WD, Rafferty JL; Standards Practice Task Force of The American Society of Colon and Rectal Surgeons. Practice parameters for the management of hemorrhoids (revised 2010). Dis Colon Rectum. 2011 Sep;54(9):1059-64. [PMID: 21825884]

Schiller LR, Pardi DS, Spiller R, et al. Gastro 2013 APDW/WCOG Shanghai working party report: chronic diarrhea: definition, classification, diagnosis. J Gastroenterol Hepatol. 2014 Jan;29(1):6-25. [PMID: 24117999]

Sinclair JA, Wasan SK, Farraye FA. Health maintenance in the inflammatory bowel disease patient. Gastroenterol Clin North Am. 2012 Jun;41(2):325-37. [PMID: 22500521]

Singh S, Rao SS. Pharmacologic management of chronic constipation. Gastroenterol Clin North Am. 2010 Sep;39(3):509-27. [PMID: 20951915]

Steele SR, Varma MG, Melton GB, Ross HM, Rafferty JF, Buie WD; Standards Practice Task Force of the American Society of Colon and Rectal Surgeons. Practice parameters for anal squamous neoplasms. Dis Colon Rectum. 2012 Jul;55(7):735-49. [PMID: 22706125]

Rubio-Tapia A, Hill ID, Kelly CP, Calderwood AH, Murray JA; American College of Gastroenterology. ACG clinical guidelines: diagnosis and management of celiac disease. Am J Gastroenterol. 2013 May;108(5):656-76; quiz 677. [PMID: 23609613]

Terdiman JP, Gruss CB, Heidelbaugh JJ, Sultan S, Falck-Ytter YT; AGA Institute Clinical Practice and Quality Management Committee. American Gastroenterological Association Institute guideline on the use of thiopurines, methotrexate, and anti-TNF-α biologic drugs for the induction and maintenance of remission in inflammatory Crohn's disease. Gastroenterology. 2013 Dec;145(6):1459-63. [PMID: 24267474]

Wyers MC. Acute mesenteric ischemia: diagnostic approach and surgical treatment. Semin Vasc Surg. 2010 Mar;23(1):9-20. [PMID: 20298945]

Colorectal Neoplasia

Atkin WS, Edwards R, Kralj-Hans I, et al; UK Flexible Sigmoidoscopy Trial Investigators. Once-only flexible sigmoidoscopy screening in prevention of colorectal cancer: a multicentre randomised controlled trial. Lancet. 2010 May 8;375(9726):1624-33. [PMID: 20430429]

Giardiello FM, Allen JI, Axilbund JE, et al. Guidelines on Genetic Evaluation and Management of Lynch Syndrome: A Consensus Statement by the US Multi-Society Task Force on Colorectal Cancer. Gastroenterology. 2014 Aug;147(2):502-26. [PMID: 25043945]

Hetzel JT, Huang CS, Coukos JA, et al. Variation in the detection of serrated polyps in an average risk colorectal cancer screening cohort. Am J Gastroenterol. 2010 Dec;105(12):2656-64. [PMID: 20717107]

Kaminski MF, Regula J, Kraszewska E, et al. Quality indicators for colonoscopy and the risk of interval cancer. N Engl J Med. 2010 May 13;362(19):1795-803. [PMID: 20463339]

Lieberman DA, Rex DK, Winawer SJ, Giardiello FM, Johnson DA, Levin TR; United States Multi-Society Task Force on Colorectal Cancer. Guidelines for colonoscopy surveillance after screening and polypectomy: a consensus update by the US Multi-Society Task Force on Colorectal Cancer. Gastroenterology. 2012 Sep;143(3):844-57. [PMID: 22763141]

NCCN Clinical Guidelines in Oncology. Genetic/Familial High-Risk Assessment: Colorectal. Version 2.2014. NCCN.org. www.nccn.org/professionals/physician_gls/pdf/genetics_colon.pdf. Accessed February 13, 2015.

Rex DK, Ahnen DJ, Baron JA, et al. Serrated lesions of the colorectum: review and recommendations from an expert panel. Am J Gastroenterol. 2012 Sep;107(9):1315-29; quiz 1314, 1330. [PMID: 22710576]

Rex DK, Johnson DA, Anderson JC, Schoenfeld PS, Burke CA, Inadomi JM; American College of Gastroenterology. American College of Gastroenterology guidelines for colorectal cancer screening 2009 [corrected]. Am J Gastroenterol. 2009 Mar;104(3):739-50. Erratum in: Am J Gastroenterol. 2009 Jun;104(6):1613. [PMID: 19240699]

Schoen RE, Pinsky PF, Weissfeld JL, et al; PLCO Project Team. Colorectal-cancer incidence and mortality with screening flexible sigmoidoscopy. N Engl J Med. 2012 Jun 21;366(25):2345-57. [PMID: 22612596]

Siegel R, Naishadham D, Jemal A. Cancer statistics, 2013. CA Cancer J Clin. 2013 Jan;63(1):11-30. [PMID: 23335087]

St John DJ, McDermott FT, Hopper JL, Debney EA, Johnson WR, Hughes ES. Cancer risk in relatives of patients with common colorectal cancer. Ann Intern Med. 1993 May 15;118(10):785-90. [PMID: 8470852]

U.S. Preventive Services Task Force. Screening for colorectal cancer: U.S. Preventive Services Task Force recommendation statement. Ann Intern Med. 2008 Nov 4;149(9):627-37. [PMID: 18838716]

Zauber AG, Winawer SJ, O'Brien MJ, et al. Colonoscopic polypectomy and long-term prevention of colorectal-cancer deaths. N Engl J Med. 2012 Feb 23;366(8):687-96. [PMID: 22356322]

Disorders of the Liver

Bacon BR, Adams PC, Kowdley KV, Powell LW, Tavill AS; American Association for the Study of Liver Diseases. Diagnosis and management of hemochromatosis: 2011 practice guideline by the American Association for the Study of Liver Diseases. Hepatology. 2011 Jul;54(1):328-43. [PMID: 21452290]

Bass NM, Mullen KD, Sanyal A, et al. Rifaximin treatment in hepatic encephalopathy. N Engl J Med. 2010 Mar 25;362(12):1071-81. [PMID: 20335583]

Bruix J, Sherman M; American Association for the Study of Liver Diseases. Management of hepatocellular carcinoma: an update. Hepatology. 2011 Mar;53(3):1020-2. [PMID: 21374666]

Centers for Disease Control and Prevention (CDC). Testing for HCV infection: an update of guidance for clinicians and laboratorians. MMWR Morb Mortal Wkly Rep. 2013 May 10;62(18):362-5. [PMID: 23657112]

Chalasani N, Younossi Z, Lavine JE, et al. The diagnosis and management of non-alcoholic fatty liver disease: practice Guideline by the American Association for the Study of Liver Diseases, American College of Gastroenterology, and the American Gastroenterological Association. Hepatology. 2012 Jun;55(6):2005-23. [PMID: 22488764]

DeLeve LD, Valla DC, Garcia-Tsao G; American Association for the Study Liver Diseases. Vascular disorders of the liver. Hepatology. 2009 May;49(5):1729-64. [PMID: 19399912]

Eaton JE, Talwalkar JA, Lazaridis KN, Gores GJ, Lindor KD. Pathogenesis of primary sclerosing cholangitis and advances in diagnosis and management. Gastroenterology. 2013 Sep;145(3):521-36. [PMID: 23827861]

El-Serag HB. Hepatocellular carcinoma. N Engl J Med. 2011 Sep 22;365(12):1118-27. [PMID: 21992124]

Garcia-Tsao G, Bosch J. Management of varices and variceal hemorrhage in cirrhosis. N Engl J Med. 2010 Mar 4;362(9):823-32. Erratum in: N Engl J Med. 2011 Feb 3;364(5):490. [PMID: 20200386]

Ginès P, Schrier RW. Renal failure in cirrhosis. N Engl J Med. 2009 Sep 24;361(13):1279-90. Erratum in: N Engl J Med. 2011 Jan 27;364(4):389. [PMID: 19776409]

Hay JE. Liver disease in pregnancy. Hepatology. 2008 Mar;47(3):1067-76. [PMID: 18265410]

Kansagara D, Papak J, Pasha AS, et al. Screening for hepatocellular carcinoma in chronic liver disease: a systematic review. Ann Intern Med. 2014 Aug 19;161(4):261-9. [PMID: 24934699]

Liang TJ, Ghany MG. Current and future therapies for hepatitis C virus infection. N Engl J Med. 2013 May 16;368(20):1907 17. [PMID: 23675659]

Lok AS, Ward JW, Perrillo RP, McMahon BJ, Liang TJ. Reactivation of hepatitis B during immunosuppressive therapy: potentially fatal yet preventable. Ann Intern Med. 2012 May 15;156(10):743-5. [PMID: 22586011]

Manns MP, Czaja AJ, Gorham JD, et al; American Association for the Study of Liver Diseases. Diagnosis and management of autoimmune hepatitis. Hepatology. 2010 Jun;51(6):2193-213. [PMID: 20513004]

Nault JC, Bioulac-Sage P, Zucman-Rossi J. Hepatocellular benign tumors-from molecular classification to personalized clinical care. Gastroenterology. 2013 May;144(5):888-902. [PMID: 23485860]

O'Shea RS, Dasarathy S, McCullough AJ; Practice Guideline Committee of the American Association for the Study of Liver Diseases; Practice Parameters Committee of the American College of Gastroenterology. Alcoholic liver disease. Hepatology. 2010 Jan;51(1):307-28. [PMID: 20034030]

Rosen HR. Clinical practice. Chronic hepatitis C infection. N Engl J Med. 2011 Jun 23;364(25):2429-38. [PMID: 21696309]

Runyon BA; AASLD Practice Guidelines Committee. Management of adult patients with ascites due to cirrhosis: an update. Hepatology. 2009 Jun;49(6):2087-107. [PMID: 19475696]

Verma S, Kaplowitz N. Diagnosis, management and prevention of drug-induced liver injury. Gut. 2009 Nov;58(11):1555-64. [PMID: 19834119]

Disorders of the Gallbladder and Bile Ducts

Razumilava N, Gores GJ. Classification, diagnosis, and management of cholangiocarcinoma. Clin Gastroenterol Hepatol. 2013 Jan;11(1):13-21.e1; quiz e3-4. [PMID: 22982100]

Thistle JL, Longstreth GF, Romero Y, et al. Factors that predict relief from upper abdominal pain after cholecystectomy. Clin Gastroenterol Hepatol. 2011 Oct;9(10):891-6. [PMID: 21699805]

Gastrointestinal Bleeding

ASGE Standards of Practice Committee, Fisher L, Lee Krinsky M, Anderson MA, et al. The role of endoscopy in the management of obscure GI bleeding. Gastrointest Endosc. 2010 Sep;72(3):471-9. [PMID: 20801285]

Barkun AN, Bardou M, Kuipers EJ, et al; International Consensus Upper Gastrointestinal Bleeding Conference Group. International consensus recommendations on the management of patients with nonvariceal upper gastrointestinal bleeding. Ann Intern Med. 2010 Jan 19;152(2):101-13. [PMID: 20083829]

Chan FK, Ching JY, Suen BY, Tse YK, Wu JC, Sung JJ. Effects of Helicobacter pylori infection on long-term risk of peptic ulcer bleeding in low-dose aspirin users. Gastroenterology. 2013 Mar;144(3):528-35. [PMID: 23333655]

García-Iglesias P, Villoria A, Suarez D, et al. Meta-analysis: predictors of rebleeding after endoscopic treatment for bleeding peptic ulcer. Aliment Pharmacol Ther. 2011 Oct;34(8):888-900. [PMID: 21899582]

Ghassemi KA, Jensen DM. Lower GI bleeding: epidemiology and management. Curr Gastroenterol Rep. 2013 Jul;15(7):333. [PMID: 23737154]

Hwang JH, Fisher DA, Ben-Menachem T, et al; Standards of Practice Committee of the American Society for Gastrointestinal Endoscopy. The role of endoscopy in the management of acute non-variceal upper GI bleeding. Gastrointest Endosc. 2012 Jun;75(6):1132-8. [PMID: 22624808]

Laine L, Jensen DM. Management of patients with ulcer bleeding. Am J Gastroenterol. 2012 Mar;107(3):345-60; quiz 361. [PMID: 22310222]

Lau JY, Barkun A, Fan DM, Kuipers EJ, Yang YS, Chan FK. Challenges in the management of acute peptic ulcer bleeding. Lancet. 2013 Jun 8;381(9882):2033-43. [PMID: 23746903]

Leighton JA. The role of endoscopic imaging of the small bowel in clinical practice. Am J Gastroenterol. 2011 Jan;106(1):27-36; quiz 37. [PMID: 20978483]

Qureshi W, Mittal C, Patsias I, et al. Restarting anticoagulation and outcomes after major gastrointestinal bleeding in atrial fibrillation. Am J Cardiol. 2014 Feb 15;113(4):662-8. [PMID: 24355310]

Srygley FD, Gerardo CJ, Tran T, Fisher DA. Does this patient have a severe upper gastrointestinal bleed? JAMA. 2012 Mar 14;307(10):1072-9. [PMID: 22416103]

Villanueva C, Colomo A, Bosch A, et al. Transfusion strategies for acute upper gastrointestinal bleeding. N Engl J Med. 2013 Jan 3;368(1):11-21. Erratum in: N Engl J Med. 2013 Jun 13;368(24):2341. [PMID: 23281973]

Gastroenterology and Hepatology Self-Assessment Test

This self-assessment test contains one-best-answer multiple-choice questions. Please read these directions carefully before answering the questions. Answers, critiques, and bibliographies immediately follow these multiple-choice questions. The American College of Physicians is accredited by the Accreditation Council for Continuing Medical Education (ACCME) to provide continuing medical education for physicians.

The American College of Physicians designates MKSAP 17 **Gastroenterology and Hepatology** for a maximum of **16** *AMA PRA Category 1 Credits*™. Physicians should claim only the credit commensurate with the extent of their participation in the activity.

Earn "Instantaneous" CME Credits Online

Print subscribers can enter their answers online to earn Continuing Medical Education (CME) credits instantaneously. You can submit your answers using online answer sheets that are provided at mksap.acponline.org, where a record of your MKSAP 17 credits will be available. To earn CME credits, you need to answer all of the questions in a test and earn a score of at least 50% correct (number of correct answers divided by the total number of questions). Take any of the following approaches:

> ➤ Use the printed answer sheet at the back of this book to record your answers. Go to mksap.acponline.org, access the appropriate online answer sheet, transcribe your answers, and submit your test for instantaneous CME credits. There is no additional fee for this service.

> ➤ Go to mksap.acponline.org, access the appropriate online answer sheet, directly enter your answers, and submit your test for instantaneous CME credits. There is no additional fee for this service.

> ➤ Pay a $15 processing fee per answer sheet and submit the printed answer sheet at the back of this book by mail or fax, as instructed on the answer sheet. Make sure you calculate your score and fax the answer sheet to 215-351-2799 or mail the answer sheet to Member and Customer Service, American College of Physicians, 190 N. Independence Mall West, Philadelphia, PA 19106-1572, using the courtesy envelope provided in your MKSAP 17 slipcase. You will need your 10-digit order number and 8-digit ACP ID number, which are printed on your packing slip. Please allow 4 to 6 weeks for your score report to be emailed back to you. Be sure to include your email address for a response.

If you do not have a 10-digit order number and 8-digit ACP ID number or if you need help creating a user name and password to access the MKSAP 17 online answer sheets, go to mksap.acponline.org or email custserv@acponline.org.

CME credit is available from the publication date of July 31, 2015, until July 31, 2018. You may submit your answer sheets at any time during this period.

*Each of the numbered items is followed by lettered answers. Select the **ONE** lettered answer that is **BEST** in each case.*

Item 1

A 55-year-old man is evaluated during a routine examination. He feels well other than mild knee pain. He drinks six to eight cans of beer per night. He has no personal history of liver disease, but his older brother was recently diagnosed with hereditary hemochromatosis.

On physical examination, vital signs are normal; BMI is 24. He is tanned on sun-exposed body surfaces. Cardiac examination is normal. Abdominal examination reveals hepatomegaly. Bilateral bony hypertrophy of the knees is noted.

Laboratory studies:

Alanine aminotransferase	70 U/L
Aspartate aminotransferase	160 U/L
Ferritin	592 ng/mL (592 µg/L)
Transferrin saturation	40%

Genetic testing for hemochromatosis reveals heterozygosity for *C282Y*. Abdominal ultrasound reveals a change in liver echotexture consistent with fatty changes.

Which of the following is the most appropriate treatment?

(A) Administer deferoxamine
(B) Perform phlebotomy
(C) Repeat serum iron tests now
(D) Stop alcohol intake

Item 2

A 40-year-old man is evaluated for a 6-month history of intermittent episodes of two to four loose stools per day. When he has diarrhea, he also notices crampy abdominal pain and bloating. He has not had nausea, vomiting, anorexia, fever, melena, hematochezia, recent travel, or any new medications, including antibiotics. He is overweight but has been exercising and watching his diet for the past 6 months, and he has intentionally lost 6.8 kg (15.0 lb). The main change in his diet has been switching to diet soda and using sugar-free sweeteners. He takes no medications.

On physical examination, vital signs are normal. The abdomen is obese but soft with normal bowel sounds and no distention or tenderness.

Which of the following is the most appropriate management?

(A) Abdominal CT scan
(B) Colonoscopy with biopsies
(C) Discontinuation of sugar-free sweeteners
(D) Gluten-free diet
(E) Tissue transglutaminase IgA antibody testing

Item 3

A 68-year-old man is evaluated for new-onset ascites with lower-extremity edema. Symptoms have increased gradually over the past 4 weeks. He has consumed three alcoholic beverages per day for many years. His medical history is notable for coronary artery bypass graft surgery 8 months ago and dyslipidemia. His medications are low-dose aspirin, atorvastatin, and metoprolol.

On physical examination, temperature is 36.8 °C (98.2 °F), blood pressure is 122/84 mm Hg, pulse rate is 64/min, and respiration rate is 16/min; BMI is 28. Cardiac examination reveals an elevated jugular venous pressure, a normal S_1 and S_2, and no murmurs. Pulmonary examination findings are normal. Abdominal examination reveals hepatomegaly, distention, dullness to percussion over the flanks, and a positive fluid wave. There is 2+ pitting edema of the lower extremities.

Laboratory studies reveal a serum albumin level of 3.5 g/dL (35 g/L). Other studies, including serum alanine aminotransferase and aspartate aminotransferase levels, are normal.

Paracentesis reveals a total nucleated cell count of 120/µL with 30% polymorphonucleocytes. Ascitic fluid albumin level is 2.3 g/dL (23 g/L) and total protein is 3.5 g/dL (35 g/L).

Which of the following is the most likely cause of this patient's ascites?

(A) Alcoholic cirrhosis
(B) Constrictive pericarditis
(C) Nonalcoholic cirrhosis
(D) Tuberculous peritonitis

Item 4

A 48-year-old woman is evaluated at an urgent care center for a 2-day history of severe retrosternal chest pain. She has not had heartburn or dysphagia. She is finishing a course of treatment for Lyme disease, but she has no other medical problems and otherwise feels well. Her only medication is doxycycline.

Physical examination is unremarkable, and laboratory studies are normal.

Which of the following is the most likely diagnosis?

(A) Barrett esophagus
(B) *Candida* esophagitis
(C) Eosinophilic esophagitis
(D) Pill-induced esophagitis

Item 5

A 56-year-old woman is hospitalized for new-onset confusion. She has a history of decompensated hepatitis B cirrhosis with chronic ascites. Her medications are spironolactone, furosemide, lactulose, and entecavir.

On physical examination, temperature is 36.8 °C (98.2 °F), blood pressure is 118/62 mm Hg, pulse rate is 88/min, and respiration rate is 20/min; BMI is 23. She is disoriented to time and date. Asterixis is noted. The abdomen is moderately distended with ascites.

Laboratory studies reveal a serum bilirubin level of 2.9 mg/dL (49.6 µmol/L), a serum creatinine level of 1.3 mg/dL

H CONT.

(114.9 µmol/L), and a blood urea nitrogen level of 34 mg/dL (12.1 mmol/L).

Diagnostic paracentesis reveals a nucleated cell count of 820/µL with 70% polymorphonuclear leukocytes. Gram stain and culture results are pending.

Which of the following is the most appropriate treatment?

(A) Cefotaxime and albumin
(B) Cefotaxime and normal saline
(C) Norfloxacin
(D) Rifaximin

Item 6

A 58-year-old man is evaluated for a 6-month history of episodic epigastric abdominal pain. In addition, his wife was recently diagnosed with *Helicobacter pylori* infection, and she is concerned that he may be infected as well. His epigastric pain occurs on most days and may occur several times during the day. He characterizes it as a vague discomfort that does not affect most activities. The discomfort is not closely related to eating, but he has been eating less. The discomfort typically resolves spontaneously within 30 to 60 minutes, but it has been occurring more frequently. He has also noted occasional nausea without vomiting. His weight is 2.3 kg (5.0 lb) lower than it was 1 year ago at his last appointment. Family history is negative for gastrointestinal malignancy.

On physical examination, blood pressure is 138/79 mm Hg, and pulse rate is 80/min. Other vital signs are normal. BMI is 35. Abdominal examination reveals generalized tenderness to deep palpation but no palpable mass.

Laboratory studies reveal a hemoglobin level of 12.5 g/dL (125 g/L) and a mean corpuscular volume of 94 fL.

Which of the following is the most appropriate management?

(A) Empiric treatment of *H. pylori*
(B) Empiric trial of omeprazole
(C) *H. pylori* serologic testing
(D) Upper endoscopy

Item 7

A 28-year-old man is evaluated in follow-up for elevated liver chemistry test results, which were performed to assess a 3-month history of fatigue. He has no history of liver disease and has not had abdominal pain or fever. His medical history is significant for a 3-year history of diarrhea.

On physical examination, vital signs are normal; BMI is 24. Spider angiomata and jaundice are absent. Abdominal examination reveals hepatomegaly but no splenomegaly or ascites.

Laboratory studies:

Alanine aminotransferase	75 U/L
Aspartate aminotransferase	87 U/L
Alkaline phosphatase	456 U/L
Total bilirubin	1.2 mg/dL (20.5 µmol/L)
Direct bilirubin	0.4 mg/dL (6.8 µmol/L)

Abdominal CT shows a thickened extrahepatic bile duct but no intrahepatic biliary dilatation and no hepatic or pancreatic mass. Magnetic resonance cholangiopancreatography reveals changes consistent with primary sclerosing cholangitis.

Which of the following is the most appropriate next step in management?

(A) Colonoscopy
(B) Endoscopic retrograde cholangiopancreatography
(C) Liver biopsy
(D) Serum IgG4 measurement

Item 8

H

A 25-year-old woman is evaluated in the emergency department for a 3-day history of nausea with nonradiating epigastric burning. She also has had a 24-hour history of frequent black stools, fatigue, and lightheadedness. For the past 5 days she has been taking ibuprofen for migraine. She takes no other medications. There is no history of gastrointestinal bleeding, alcoholism, chronic liver disease, or bleeding disorders.

On physical examination, temperature is 37.0 °C (98.6 °F), blood pressure is 110/65 mm Hg supine and 92/53 mm Hg standing, pulse rate is 85/min supine and 115/min standing, and respiration rate is 14/min. Abdominal examination reveals epigastric tenderness without guarding or rebound. Rectal examination is positive for melena. Laboratory studies reveal a hemoglobin level of 9.2 g/dL (92 g/L) and a blood urea nitrogen level of 28 mg/dL (10 mmol/L); all other tests are normal.

After intravenous fluid resuscitation, upper endoscopy is performed and reveals a 1.5-cm duodenal bulb ulcer with a central, nonbleeding visible vessel.

Which of the following is the most appropriate management?

(A) Endoscopic therapy
(B) Immediate surgical intervention
(C) Octreotide infusion
(D) Observation

Item 9

H

A 49-year-old woman is hospitalized for altered mental status. She has alcoholic cirrhosis complicated by ascites. She has not had fever, focal infection symptoms, hematemesis, hematochezia, or melena. She takes lactulose, but she is now having four to five loose stools per day. She also takes furosemide and spironolactone.

On physical examination, temperature is 36.4 °C (97.5 °F), blood pressure is 102/74 mm Hg, pulse rate is 78/min, and respiration rate is 16/min; BMI is 24. She is disoriented to time and date. Scleral icterus, spider angiomata, and asterixis are noted. The mucous membranes are dry. Ascites is present.

Laboratory studies:

INR	1.3 (normal range, 0.8-1.2)
Albumin	2.6 g/dL (26 g/L)
Total bilirubin	3.5 mg/dL (59.9 µmol/L)
Blood urea nitrogen	38 mg/dL (13.6 mmol/L)
Creatinine	2.5 mg/dL (221 µmol/L)
Urinalysis	Normal

CONT.

Blood culture results are pending. Her diuretics and lactulose are discontinued.

Which of the following is the most appropriate treatment for acute kidney injury in this patient?

(A) Midodrine
(B) Midodrine and octreotide
(C) Norepinephrine
(D) 25% albumin

Item 10

A 73-year-old woman was admitted to the hospital 12 hours ago with fever, epigastric abdominal pain, and jaundice. She was hypotensive on admission to the emergency department but improved after receiving intravenous antibiotics and fluids. One hour ago the epigastric pain recurred and she again became febrile and hypotensive. She is transferred to the ICU, and her blood pressure improves with administration of fluids. She has no history of liver or biliary disease. Her only medication is piperacillin-tazobactam.

On physical examination, temperature is 39.3 °C (102.7 °F), blood pressure is 106/60 mm Hg, pulse rate is 102/min, and respiration rate is 22/min. Oxygen saturation is 96% breathing ambient air. Jaundice is noted. Abdominal examination reveals right upper quadrant tenderness but no hepatomegaly, ascites, abdominal guarding, or tenderness to percussion.

Laboratory studies:

Hemoglobin	13 g/dL (130 g/L)
Leukocyte count	19,000/µL (19 × 10⁹/L), with 80% segmented neutrophils and 15% band forms
Alanine aminotransferase	453 U/L
Total bilirubin	8.3 mg/dL (141.9 µmol/L)

Ultrasound of the right upper quadrant reveals dilated intrahepatic and extrahepatic bile ducts, gallstones, a normal gallbladder wall, and no pericholecystic fluid. The pancreas is not well visualized.

Which of the following is the most appropriate management?

(A) Abdominal CT
(B) Cholecystectomy
(C) Endoscopic retrograde cholangiopancreatography
(D) Percutaneous cholecystostomy

Item 11

A 67-year-old woman is evaluated during a routine examination. She has a history of hip and knee pain related to degenerative joint disease. The joint pain is now well controlled with diclofenac, which was started 3 months ago. A previous trial of high-dose acetaminophen was not effective. She does not have any gastrointestinal symptoms, and she takes the diclofenac with food most of the time. Her medical history is otherwise notable for type 2 diabetes mellitus, hyperlipidemia, and hypertension. Her parents both had coronary artery disease. Her medications are low-dose aspirin, metformin, chlorthalidone, simvastatin, and diclofenac.

On physical examination, vital signs are normal. Abdominal examination is unremarkable.

Which of the following is the most appropriate management?

(A) Change to enteric-coated aspirin
(B) Continue the current medication regimen
(C) Initiate omeprazole, 20 mg once daily
(D) Initiate omeprazole, 40 mg once daily

Item 12

A 66-year-old man is evaluated for a several-year history of one to three bulky, semisolid, foul-smelling bowel movements daily that are associated with excess flatulence. Associated symptoms are episodic epigastric pain, a ravenous appetite, and a 9.0-kg (19.8-lb) weight loss over the last year. Medical history is notable for alcoholism; he has not consumed alcohol since his last attack of pancreatitis 15 years ago. He has an 80-pack-year history of smoking but currently does not smoke. He takes no medications.

On physical examination, temperature is 37.0 °C (98.6 °F), blood pressure is 133/72 mm Hg, pulse rate is 77/min, and respiration rate is 14/min; BMI is 21. He is thin with temporal wasting and poor dentition. Abdominal examination reveals mild epigastric tenderness with no masses. The liver and spleen are not enlarged. Borborygmi is audible without a stethoscope. There is no abdominal distention. No jaundice is present.

Laboratory studies reveal a serum albumin level of 3.3 g/dL (33 g/L), a serum lipase level of 46 U/L, and tissue transglutaminase serology is negative.

Abdominal ultrasound shows pancreatic calcification but no masses. Fecal fat testing reveals a stool fat of 40 g/d.

Which of the following is the most appropriate treatment?

(A) Fiber
(B) Gluten-free diet
(C) Loperamide
(D) Pancreatic enzymes

Item 13

A 23-year-old man is evaluated for chronic diarrhea. He has had intermittent loose stools over the past 2 to 3 years; however, over the past 6 months, diarrhea has become more severe (five to six bowel movements per day) and constant. Stools are described as mushy and malodorous and are accompanied by crampy abdominal pain and bloating. He has lost 2.3 kg (5.0 lb) over the past 6 months despite consuming more calories. He has not had fever or gastrointestinal bleeding and has no history of foreign travel. He has type 1 diabetes mellitus that is well controlled with insulin. He does not smoke cigarettes or drink alcohol.

On physical examination, vital signs are normal. He has evidence of muscle wasting and pedal edema. The abdomen is scaphoid but soft with increased bowel sounds. No distention or tenderness is noted.

Laboratory studies reveal a hemoglobin level of 10.4 g/dL (104 g/L) and a mean corpuscular volume of 100 fL.

Which of the following is the most appropriate diagnostic test to perform next?

(A) Anti-*Saccharomyces cerevisiae* antibodies
(B) Flexible sigmoidoscopy
(C) Tissue transglutaminase antibody testing
(D) Upper endoscopy with small-bowel biopsies
(E) Video capsule endoscopy

Item 14

A 25-year-old woman is evaluated for a 6-month history of constipation characterized by straining and infrequent bowel movements (once every 3 days). She has also had frequent passage of mucus, generalized abdominal discomfort, and bloating. She has not had weight loss. Symptoms began gradually and have slowly progressed. Her symptoms are severe enough to affect her appetite; she deliberately avoids some meals because eating often worsens her symptoms. Bran supplementation made her symptoms worse. There is no family history of colon cancer. Her medications are a multivitamin and an oral contraceptive agent.

On physical examination, vital signs are normal. Abdominal examination reveals generalized tenderness to light palpation but no masses. Rectal examination findings are normal.

Laboratory studies reveal a hemoglobin level of 13 g/dL (130 g/L).

In addition to starting polyethylene glycol, which of the following is the most appropriate initial management?

(A) Obtain a comprehensive metabolic panel
(B) Obtain colonoscopy
(C) Obtain tissue transglutaminase testing
(D) Reassurance and patient education

Item 15

A 35-year-old man is evaluated for a 2-month history of upper abdominal discomfort after eating. He has recently returned from working in a rural area of a developing country. He takes no medications. There is no family history of esophageal or gastric cancer.

On physical examination, vital signs are normal. BMI is 40. Centripetal obesity is noted, but abdominal examination findings are otherwise normal.

Laboratory studies reveal a hemoglobin level of 15 g/dL (150 g/L).

Which of the following is the most appropriate management?

(A) Barium esophagogram
(B) Empiric *Helicobacter pylori* eradication therapy
(C) *H. pylori* testing
(D) Upper endoscopy

Item 16

An 18-year-old woman is hospitalized for a 1-day history of confusion, which was preceded by a 1-week history of fatigue and a 2-day history of jaundice. She has not had fever or abdominal pain. She has not had liver disease previously, and she has never used injection drugs. No one else in her family is ill.

On physical examination, temperature is 37.1 °C (98.8 °F), blood pressure is 88/58 mm Hg, pulse rate is 110/min, and respiration rate is 22/min; BMI is 24. She is oriented to person but disoriented to time and place. Jaundice and asterixis are noted. The spleen is palpable below the left costal margin, and there is no ascites.

Laboratory studies:

Hemoglobin	9 g/dL (90 g/L)
Reticulocyte count	9% of erythrocytes
INR	1.7 (normal range, 0.8-1.2)
Alanine aminotransferase	239 U/L
Aspartate aminotransferase	243 U/L
Alkaline phosphatase	34 U/L
Total bilirubin	8.4 mg/dL (143.6 µmol/L)
Direct bilirubin	2.6 mg/dL (44.5 µmol/L)

A drug screen is positive for acetaminophen. Bedside abdominal ultrasound reveals a small liver, splenomegaly, and no ascites.

Which of the following is the most likely diagnosis?

(A) Acetaminophen hepatotoxicity
(B) Budd-Chiari syndrome
(C) Herpes hepatitis
(D) Wilson disease

Item 17

A 53-year-old woman is evaluated in follow-up after a recent hospitalization for right flank pain. Ultrasound performed in the hospital showed a dilated right renal collecting system and a 12-mm gallbladder polyp. Two hours after admission, she passed a stone in the urine and the right flank pain resolved. Since her hospitalization, she has had no other episodes of pain and otherwise feels well.

On physical examination, vital signs are normal; BMI is 34. Abdominal examination reveals a normal liver and spleen, no tenderness, and a negative Murphy sign.

Laboratory studies, including a complete blood count, alkaline phosphatase, alanine aminotransferase, and bilirubin, are normal.

Which of the following is the most appropriate management?

(A) Abdominal CT
(B) Cholecystectomy
(C) Endoscopic retrograde cholangiopancreatography
(D) Magnetic resonance cholangiopancreatography
(E) Ultrasound in 1 year

Item 18

A 55-year-old man is evaluated in the emergency department for a 6-hour history of severe epigastric

H
CONT.
abdominal pain, nausea, and vomiting. In the previous 6 weeks he had two episodes of postprandial right upper quadrant pain. He is otherwise healthy and takes no medications.

On physical examination, temperature is 36.8 °C (98.2 °F), blood pressure is 130/75 mm Hg, pulse rate is 89/min, and respiration rate is 17/min; BMI is 29. Scleral icterus is present. Abdominal examination reveals epigastric abdominal tenderness without guarding or rebound. Bowel sounds are present but hypoactive, and there is abdominal distention.

He is admitted to the hospital, and fluid resuscitation is started.

Laboratory studies:

Test	On presentation	After 12 hours of fluid resuscitation
Leukocyte count	14,000/µL (14×10^9/L)	12,000/µL (12×10^9/L)
Alanine amino-transferase	350 U/L	98 U/L
Aspartate ami-notransferase	310 U/L	86 U/L
Total bilirubin	4.5 mg/dL (77 µmol/L)	1.6 mg/dL (27 µmol/L)
Lipase	3250 U/L	1220 U/L

Abdominal ultrasound shows cholelithiasis with no gallbladder wall thickening or pericholecystic fluid. The common bile duct is not dilated. There is no choledocholithiasis.

Which of the following is the most appropriate management?

(A) Cholecystectomy prior to hospital discharge
(B) Cholecystokinin hepatobiliary (CCK-HIDA) scintigraphy
(C) Endoscopic retrograde cholangiopancreatography with biliary sphincterotomy
(D) Intravenous imipenem

Item 19

A 22-year-old woman is evaluated for a flare of Crohn disease. A colonoscopy performed 6 months ago showed moderate, patchy, left-sided colitis extending from the descending colon to the splenic flexure. She responded to therapy with prednisone but declined maintenance therapy in advance of conceiving. She is now 12 weeks pregnant and for the past 2 weeks has experienced bloody diarrhea and left-sided abdominal pain.

On physical examination, temperature is 37.2 °C (99.0 °F), blood pressure is 110/66 mm Hg, and pulse rate is 76/min. Abdominal examination reveals left-sided abdominal tenderness without guarding or rebound.

Flexible sigmoidoscopy shows recurrent left-sided patchy colitis, and stool studies are negative for *Clostridium difficile* infection.

Which of the following is the most appropriate treatment?

(A) Certolizumab
(B) Ciprofloxacin and metronidazole

(C) Controlled ileal-release budesonide
(D) Mesalamine
(E) Methotrexate

Item 20

A 25-year-old woman is evaluated for an 8-month history of epigastric abdominal pain. The pain is episodic, but it is present more often than not. There do not seem to be any factors that clearly exacerbate or alleviate the pain. She notes occasional nausea and poor appetite but has not had weight loss. Her medical history is notable for gastroesophageal reflux disease. There is no family history of gastrointestinal malignancy. Her only medication is omeprazole, 20 mg/d.

On physical examination, vital signs are normal. Abdominal examination reveals generalized abdominal tenderness to light palpation but is otherwise normal.

Testing for *Helicobacter pylori* is negative. Owing to ongoing symptoms despite antisecretory therapy, upper endoscopy with gastric and small-bowel biopsies is performed; results are normal.

Which of the following is the most appropriate treatment?

(A) Increase omeprazole to twice daily
(B) Initiate hydrocodone/acetaminophen as needed
(C) Initiate metoclopramide
(D) Initiate nortriptyline
(E) Switch omeprazole to ranitidine

Item 21

A 64-year-old man is evaluated in follow-up after recent abnormal findings on intraoperative liver biopsy. Two days ago he underwent right colon resection for a large villous adenoma with high-grade dysplasia. At the time of surgery, an abnormal-appearing liver was noted and biopsy was performed. His medical history is notable for type 2 diabetes mellitus, hypertension, and obesity. Medications are metformin and lisinopril. He drinks two cans of beer daily but does not use tobacco.

On physical examination, vital signs are normal; BMI is 38. No jaundice or spider angiomata are noted. Abdominal examination reveals healing laparoscopic scars and hepatomegaly. The spleen is not palpable, and there is no ascites. No peripheral edema is seen.

Laboratory studies:

Complete blood count	Normal
INR	Normal
Alanine aminotransferase	79 U/L
Aspartate aminotransferase	68 U/L
Albumin	Normal
Alkaline phosphatase	126 U/L
Total bilirubin	Normal
Ferritin	389 ng/mL (389 µg/L)
Iron	Normal
Total iron-binding capacity	Normal
Iron saturation	Normal

Liver biopsy demonstrates a mildly active steatohepatitis without fibrosis. An iron stain is negative.

Which of the following is the most appropriate management?

(A) Bariatric surgery
(B) Phlebotomy
(C) Surveillance for hepatocellular carcinoma
(D) Weight loss

Item 22

A 29-year-old man is evaluated during a routine examination. His medical history is significant for ulcerative colitis involving the entire colon, which was diagnosed 4 years ago. His symptoms responded to therapy with mesalamine and have remained in remission on this medication. His family history is significant for a maternal uncle who died of colon cancer at the age of 50 years.

Physical examination is unremarkable.

Serum alkaline phosphatase, alanine aminotransferase, and aspartate aminotransferase levels are normal.

Which of the following is the most appropriate interval at which to perform colonoscopy with biopsies in this patient?

(A) Begin now and repeat annually
(B) Begin in 4 years and repeat every 1 to 2 years
(C) Begin in 4 years and repeat every 10 years
(D) Begin at age 40 years and repeat every 5 years

Item 23

A 58-year-old woman is evaluated in the emergency department for a 2-day history of left lower abdominal discomfort. The pain began insidiously and has gradually progressed. She has felt warm but has not had shaking chills, urinary symptoms such as dysuria or urgency, change in bowel habits, or apparent blood in her stool. She is able to eat and drink normally; however, her appetite is decreased. She has never had symptoms like this before. Her medical history is unremarkable.

On physical examination, temperature is 36.6 °C (97.9 °F), blood pressure is 135/68 mm Hg, pulse rate is 94/min, and respiration rate is 18/min. She appears mildly uncomfortable. Mild left lower quadrant abdominal tenderness is noted, with no fullness or mass, guarding, or rebound tenderness.

Laboratory studies are significant for a hemoglobin level of 11.8 g/dL (118 g/L) and a leukocyte count of 10,800/µL (10.8×10^9/L). Serum electrolyte levels and kidney function studies are normal.

Abdominal CT scan shows inflammation of the sigmoid colon and mesentery consistent with acute diverticulitis; no bowel obstruction or abscess is noted.

In addition to antibiotic therapy, which of the following is the most appropriate management?

(A) Discharge home with close follow-up
(B) Laparoscopic sigmoid resection
(C) Percutaneous drainage
(D) Urgent colonoscopy

Item 24

A 57-year-old woman is evaluated after a recent screening colonoscopy. The colonoscopy disclosed a 12-mm polyp in the ascending colon, which was removed. No other lesions were noted. On pathology, the lesion was found to be a sessile serrated polyp.

Physical examination findings are unremarkable.

Which of the following is the most appropriate time to repeat colonoscopy?

(A) 1 year
(B) 3 years
(C) 5 years
(D) 10 years

Item 25

A 41-year-old woman is evaluated in follow-up after presenting to the emergency department 1 week ago for burning epigastric and chest pain. In the emergency department, a complete blood count and liver chemistry studies were normal, but a radiograph of the chest and upper abdomen demonstrated calcified gallstones. The pain resolved with administration of a liquid antacid, and omeprazole was started. The pain had been present intermittently for approximately 6 months prior to the emergency department visit. It occurred nearly every day, usually after meals and when recumbent, and had been typically burning in nature at night. The pain has not recurred since she started omeprazole. She has not had dysphagia and has a good appetite and stable weight. Her medical history is notable for obesity.

On physical examination, vital signs are normal; BMI is 36. There is no abdominal tenderness, and the liver and spleen are of normal size. Murphy sign is negative.

Which of the following is the most appropriate management for this patient's gallstones?

(A) Annual ultrasonography
(B) Laparoscopic cholecystectomy
(C) Ursodiol
(D) Clinical observation

Item 26

A 24-year-old woman is evaluated for a 1-month history of increasing pain and bleeding from a skin ulcer next to her stoma. The skin symptoms get worse each time she changes her appliance. She underwent proctocolectomy 4 years ago for medically refractory colonic Crohn disease. She has not had small-bowel involvement, and her ostomy output has been stable since surgery.

On physical examination, vital signs are normal. The skin findings are shown (see top of next page). The remainder of the skin examination is normal. The abdomen is soft with normal bowel sounds. There is no distention, tenderness, masses, or organomegaly.

Which of the following is the most likely cause of this patient's skin findings?

(A) Acrodermatitis enteropathica
(B) Erythema nodosum

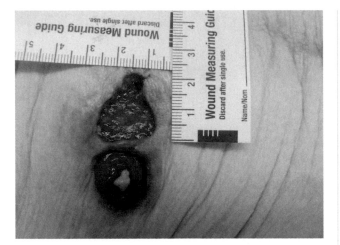

(C) Pyoderma gangrenosum

(D) Squamous cell carcinoma

Item 27

A 30-year-old woman is evaluated for a 2-month history of diarrhea with three to five loose stools per day. She has mild abdominal cramps, bloating, intermittent nausea, and mild anorexia that has resulted in the loss of 2.3 kg (5.0 lb). She has had no fever or blood in the stool. She works in a day care center and has not traveled recently or had exposure to antibiotics. She is otherwise healthy and takes no medications.

On physical examination, temperature is 37.0 °C (98.6 °F), blood pressure is 112/74 mm Hg, and pulse rate is 70/min. The abdomen is soft with normal bowel sounds and mild distention but no tenderness.

Which of the following is the most appropriate management?

(A) Colonoscopy

(B) Stool cultures

(C) Stool testing for ova and parasites

(D) No further testing

Item 28

A 63-year-old man is evaluated for a 1-month history of painless jaundice. He has not had pancreatitis, weight loss, oily stools, or diabetes mellitus. He has never smoked cigarettes and has consumed alcohol only minimally and rarely. His medical and family history is unremarkable, and he takes no medications.

On physical examination, temperature is 37.0 °C (98.6 °F), blood pressure is 136/78 mm Hg, pulse rate is 73/min, and respiration rate is 14/min; BMI is 27. Jaundice is noted. Abdominal examination reveals epigastric tenderness without guarding or rebound.

Laboratory studies:

Alanine aminotransferase	132 U/L
Aspartate aminotransferase	121 U/L
Alkaline phosphatase	353 U/L
Total bilirubin	4.2 mg/dL (71.8 µmol/L)
Serum IgG4	Elevated

Magnetic resonance cholangiopancreatography shows features of sclerosing cholangitis, focal enlargement of the head of the pancreas with a featureless border, and a nondilated pancreatic duct.

Which of the following is the most appropriate management?

(A) Antioxidants

(B) Biliary metal stent

(C) Prednisone

(D) Surgery

Item 29

An 80-year-old man is evaluated for gastrointestinal bleeding. His medical history is notable for a 3-month history of intermittent melena that resulted in a hospitalization 2 days ago, during which he has required fluid resuscitation and erythrocyte transfusions. Upper endoscopy and colonoscopy were normal.

On physical examination, temperature is 37.0 °C (98.6 °F), blood pressure is 135/80 mm Hg, pulse rate is 80/min, and respiration rate is 18/min. Abdominal examination findings are normal.

Laboratory studies show a hemoglobin level of 8.2 g/dL (82 g/L). Capsule endoscopy shows fresh blood in the proximal jejunum and several angiodysplasias.

Which of the following is the most appropriate test to perform next?

(A) Intraoperative endoscopy

(B) Push enteroscopy

(C) Repeat upper endoscopy

(D) Technetium-labeled nuclear scan

Item 30

A 40-year-old man is evaluated in follow-up for irritable bowel syndrome with constipation (IBS-C), which was diagnosed 3 months ago. His IBS symptoms did not respond to a trial of psyllium, which was discontinued owing to bloating. A trial of polyethylene glycol had similar results. He has no other medical problems and takes no other medications.

On physical examination, vital signs are normal. Abdominal examination reveals generalized abdominal tenderness but is otherwise normal.

Which of the following is the most appropriate treatment?

(A) Start a bran-based dietary supplement

(B) Start bisacodyl

(C) Start linaclotide

(D) Start rifaximin

Item 31

A 55-year-old woman is evaluated during a routine examination. She underwent biliopancreatic diversion with duodenal switch 8 years ago for treatment of obesity-related complications and lost 68.0 kg (150.0 lb) in the first year following surgery. Her weight has been relatively stable for the last year. She has had chronic nonbloody diarrhea since her bariatric surgery. She also has had generalized fatigue, dry skin, dry and itchy eyes, and increased difficulty seeing road signs at night while driving. Her other medical problems are type 2 diabetes mellitus and hypertension. Her prescription medications are metformin and lisinopril, and she also takes an over-the-counter multivitamin with iron. Her last colonoscopy, performed 5 years ago, was normal.

On physical examination, blood pressure is 140/79 mm Hg and pulse rate is 63/min. BMI is 25. The examination is otherwise unremarkable.

Laboratory studies reveal a hemoglobin level of 10.5 g/dL (105 g/L) and a mean corpuscular volume of 95 fL.

Which of the following deficiencies best explains this patient's current findings?

(A) Copper
(B) Iron
(C) Vitamin A
(D) Vitamin B$_{12}$

Item 32

A 68-year-old woman is evaluated for a 3-month history of gradually progressive abdominal distention. Her medical history is notable for a 20-year history of obesity, type 2 diabetes mellitus, hyperlipidemia, and hypertension. She also has had a 10-year history of elevation of serum aminotransferase levels, which was attributed to nonalcoholic fatty liver disease. She does not consume alcohol. Her medications are metformin, lisinopril, low-dose aspirin, and simvastatin.

On physical examination, vital signs are normal; BMI is 38. Spider angiomata are present. Abdominal examination is limited by obesity, but there is mild abdominal distention consistent with ascites. There is no obvious hepatomegaly or splenomegaly.

Laboratory studies:

Platelet count	68,000/μL (68 × 10^9/L)
Alanine aminotransferase	54 U/L
Aspartate aminotransferase	64 U/L
Albumin	3.2 g/dL (32 g/L)
Total bilirubin	2 mg/dL (34.2 μmol/L)
Direct bilirubin	1.4 mg/dL (24 μmol/L)
Urinalysis	1+ protein

Which of the following is the most appropriate next step in management?

(A) Echocardiogram
(B) Liver biopsy
(C) Stop simvastatin
(D) Ultrasound of the liver and spleen

Item 33

A 70-year-old man is evaluated in follow-up for heartburn of 7 years' duration. He has frequent nocturnal reflux but has not had odynophagia or dysphagia, and his weight has been stable. He was recently started on once-daily omeprazole

with good control of his symptoms. He has a 30-pack-year history of cigarette smoking and continues to smoke.

On physical examination, vital signs are normal; BMI is 29. The remainder of the physical examination is normal.

He is concerned about his long-term heartburn symptoms and expresses an interest in further evaluation to assess his risk of cancer because of his prolonged symptoms. Based on his risk factors and after discussing with the patient the benefits and harms of screening endoscopy for Barrett esophagus, upper endoscopy is performed. An area of salmon-colored mucosa is seen in the esophagus, and biopsies confirm Barrett esophagus without dysplasia.

Which of the following is the most appropriate next step in management?

(A) Endoscopic ablation
(B) Esophagectomy
(C) Fundoplication
(D) Repeat upper endoscopy in 3 to 5 years

Item 34

A 58-year-old woman is evaluated for a 6-month history of gradually progressive fatigue and a 1-month history of generalized pruritus without rash. She also has dry eyes and dry mouth. She has not had fever, jaundice, or weight loss. She has a 3-year history of hypercholesterolemia for which she takes simvastatin. She has no other medical problems.

On physical examination, vital signs are normal; BMI is 24. Other than excoriations on her arms, legs, and upper back, the physical examination is normal.

Laboratory studies:

Alanine aminotransferase	75 U/L
Aspartate aminotransferase	54 U/L
Alkaline phosphatase	328 U/L
Total bilirubin	1.2 mg/dL (20.5 μmol/L)
Direct bilirubin	0.6 mg/dL (10.3 μmol/L)
Antimitochondrial antibody	1:640

Ultrasound of the right upper quadrant is normal.

Which of the following is the most likely diagnosis?

(A) Autoimmune hepatitis
(B) Cholangiocarcinoma
(C) Primary biliary cirrhosis
(D) Primary sclerosing cholangitis

Item 35

A 67-year-old man is re-evaluated for a 3-month history of iron deficiency anemia due to obscure gastrointestinal bleeding. At the time of diagnosis he was evaluated with two upper endoscopies and a colonoscopy that failed to reveal the source of gastrointestinal bleeding. He has remained hemodynamically stable but requires oral iron therapy. His medical history is notable for chronic atrial fibrillation, for which he takes diltiazem and warfarin.

On physical examination, temperature is 37.0 °C (98.6 °F), blood pressure is 130/78 mm Hg, pulse rate is 80/min, and respiration rate is 18/min. Abdominal examination findings are normal.

Laboratory studies show a hemoglobin level of 9.2 g/dL (92 g/L) and an INR of 2.5 (normal range, 0.8-1.2). A guaiac fecal occult blood test is positive.

Which of the following is the most appropriate diagnostic test to perform next?

(A) Angiography
(B) Capsule endoscopy
(C) Intraoperative endoscopy
(D) Technetium-labeled nuclear scan

Item 36

A 35-year-old man is evaluated in the emergency department for a 6-hour history of epigastric abdominal pain that radiates to the back. He also has nausea and occasional bilious vomiting. He has consumed between six and twelve beers daily for 10 to 15 years.

On physical examination, temperature is 37.2 °C (99.0 °F), blood pressure is 110/65 mm Hg, pulse rate is 105/min, and respiration rate is 22/min. Abdominal examination discloses epigastric tenderness without guarding or rebound. Bowel sounds are present but hypoactive, and there is mild abdominal distention. No jaundice is noted.

Laboratory studies reveal a leukocyte count of 14,000/µL (14 × 10^9/L), a blood urea nitrogen level of 25 mg/dL (8.9 mmol/L), and a serum lipase level of 952 U/L.

Abdominal ultrasound shows a normal-appearing gallbladder and no biliary dilation. The patient is admitted to the hospital. Over the next 48 hours, he has ongoing abdominal pain, nausea, and poor appetite despite supportive therapy consisting of pain medication and aggressive intravenous fluid replacement. Subsequent contrast-enhanced CT of the abdomen shows nonenhancing areas of the head and body of the pancreas (consistent with necrosis) and several peripancreatic fluid collections.

Which of the following is the most appropriate management?

(A) Drainage of the fluid collections
(B) Endoscopic retrograde cholangiopancreatography
(C) Enteral nutrition by nasojejunal tube
(D) Total parenteral nutrition

Item 37

A 30-year-old woman is evaluated in an urgent care facility for a 1-day history of rectal bleeding and anal pain associated with a bowel movement. She has a lifelong history of constipation. She is otherwise well and her only medication is a daily laxative.

On physical examination, vital signs are normal; BMI is 27. Upon separating the buttocks, a midline posterior anal fissure is observed. There is no evidence of fresh blood or clots. Topical treatment is provided.

Which of the following is the most appropriate management?

(A) Admission to the hospital for observation
(B) Colonoscopy
(C) Outpatient follow-up
(D) Surgery

Item 38

A 42-year-old woman is evaluated after an incidental liver lesion was found during a recent CT urogram, which was performed for evaluation of kidney stones. Follow-up CT of the lesion demonstrates a well-circumscribed 6-cm lesion with peripheral enhancement on the early arterial phase, centripetal flow on the portal phase, and isodensity on the late phase. Biopsy of the lesion confirms a hepatocellular adenoma, and β-catenin activation mutation is positive. Her only medication is an estrogen and progesterone oral contraceptive.

On physical examination, vital signs are normal; BMI is 28. Abdominal examination findings are normal.

Which of the following is the most appropriate treatment?

(A) Discontinuation of the oral contraceptive
(B) Resection
(C) Surveillance CT imaging every 6 months
(D) Transarterial chemoembolization

Item 39

A 60-year-old woman is evaluated for a 5-day history of painful swallowing with both liquids and solids. The pain is worse when swallowing solid foods. She otherwise feels well. She underwent liver transplantation 4 months ago. Her only medication is mycophenolate mofetil, and she recently stopped taking prednisone.

On physical examination, vital signs are normal. The oral pharynx appears normal, and abdominal examination reveals no tenderness.

Upper endoscopy findings are shown.

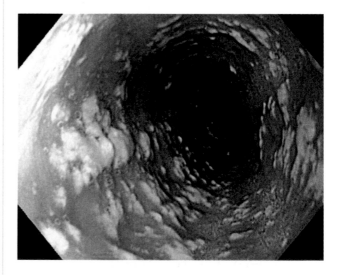

Which of the following is the most appropriate treatment?

(A) Acyclovir
(B) Fluconazole
(C) Ganciclovir
(D) Swallowed aerosolized fluticasone
(E) Swallowed nystatin

Item 40

A 36-year-old woman is evaluated for a 12-year history of refractory constipation. Her symptoms began after a difficult childbirth. She has constipation marked by straining, bloating, and a constant sensation of incomplete emptying. She sometimes has 4 or more days between bowel movements. When she does have a bowel movement, the stool is soft-formed. Trials of several fiber supplements, lactulose, milk of magnesia, docusate, bisacodyl, polyethylene glycol, and lubiprostone have provided only transient relief for no more than 4 weeks before the gradual return of symptoms. There is no family history of gastrointestinal malignancies or inflammatory bowel disease. Medications are polyethylene glycol, psyllium, and bisacodyl.

On physical examination, vital signs are normal. BMI is 17. Tenderness to palpation is noted in the lower abdomen. No masses are noted. Rectal examination reveals normal resting tone, an increase in external anal sphincter tone, and poor relaxation of the pelvic floor when bearing down. Soft stool is noted in the rectal vault.

Anorectal manometry confirms paradoxical muscle contraction during the Valsalva maneuver consistent with pelvic floor dyssynergia.

Which of the following is the most appropriate management?

(A) Increase polyethylene glycol
(B) Increase psyllium
(C) Start biofeedback therapy
(D) Start enema therapy

Item 41

A 54-year-old man is evaluated for a 4-month history of intermittent, nonprogressive solid-food dysphagia. He has a long-standing history of heartburn that has been well controlled with once-daily proton pump inhibitor (PPI) therapy for the past 5 years. Results of a screening colonoscopy 4 years ago were normal. There is no family history of colorectal cancer.

Physical examination findings are unremarkable.

Upper endoscopy reveals a 3-cm hiatal hernia, an esophageal (Schatzki) ring, and approximately six polyps smaller than 4 mm in the fundus and upper body of the stomach. The duodenum is normal. The esophageal ring is dilated, and biopsy of random gastric polyps confirms fundic gland polyps without dysplasia.

Which of the following is the most appropriate next step in management?

(A) Perform *APC* gene testing
(B) Perform excision of all fundic gland polyps
(C) Repeat colonoscopy
(D) Stop PPI therapy
(E) Reassurance

Item 42

A 50-year-old man is evaluated in follow-up after hospitalization 6 months ago for a large bleeding gastric ulcer. Tests performed for *Helicobacter pylori* infection at that time were negative. However, for the 3 months before hospitalization he had been taking ibuprofen for chronic back pain. He was discharged from the hospital on omeprazole, and his ibuprofen was discontinued. Owing to the large size of the ulcer and increased suspicion for underlying malignancy, follow-up upper endoscopy was performed 3 months later and showed complete ulcer healing; the omeprazole was stopped. He has not found any other treatment as effective as ibuprofen for his back pain, and he wishes to restart the ibuprofen. He does not have cardiovascular disease and is at low risk for developing cardiovascular disease.

Physical examination is unremarkable.

Which of the following is the most appropriate management?

(A) Celecoxib
(B) Celecoxib and omeprazole
(C) Ibuprofen
(D) Ibuprofen and sucralfate

Item 43

A 28-year-old woman is evaluated for an 8-week history of increasing lower abdominal crampy pain and diarrhea. She now has 6 to 10 bowel movements per day with one or two nocturnal stools. Stools are loose to watery with intermittent blood streaking. The pain is in the lower abdomen and has increased to 6 to 8 out of 10 in severity over the past week. She has anorexia and nausea but no vomiting or fever. She takes no medications, including NSAIDs.

On physical examination, temperature is 37.8 °C (100.0 °F), blood pressure is 100/54 mm Hg, and pulse rate is 96/min. She appears thin, pale, and in moderate distress. The abdomen is distended with diffuse tenderness that is most prominent in the lower quadrants. There is no rigidity, guarding, rebound tenderness, masses, or organomegaly.

Representative colonoscopy findings seen in a patchy distribution throughout the ascending, transverse, and descending colon are shown. The terminal ileum and rectum show no inflammation.

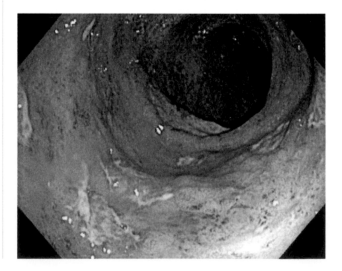

Which of the following is the most likely diagnosis?

(A) Collagenous colitis

(B) Crohn colitis

(C) Ischemic colitis

(D) Ulcerative colitis

Item 44

A 48-year-old woman is evaluated for a 3-month history of anorexia associated with a 9.1-kg (20.0-lb) weight loss. Six months ago she began having nausea, vomiting, meal-related abdominal pain and bloating, and diarrhea. Other medical problems include dyslipidemia and hypertension treated with simvastatin, chlorthalidone, and lisinopril. She has a 25-pack-year history of smoking.

On physical examination, blood pressure is 140/85 mm Hg and pulse rate is 88/min; BMI is 17. A bruit is audible in the upper abdomen and over both femoral arteries. Dorsalis pedis and posterior tibial pulses are diminished bilaterally.

Upper endoscopy findings are normal. CT scan of the abdomen and pelvis demonstrates a dilated and debris-filled stomach and diffuse dilation of the small bowel.

Which of the following diagnostic tests should be done next?

(A) Abdominal ultrasonography

(B) Capsule endoscopy

(C) CT angiography

(D) Splanchnic angiography

Item 45

A 38-year-old woman is evaluated in follow-up after recent surgery for endometrial cancer. Her family history is significant for colon cancer in her sister (diagnosed at age 45 years) and her mother (diagnosed at age 65 years). Her maternal grandfather was diagnosed with rectal cancer at age 47 years. The patient has never had colon cancer screening with colonoscopy.

Which of the following is the most appropriate time to start colon cancer screening with colonoscopy?

(A) Now

(B) Age 40 years

(C) Age 47 years

(D) Age 50 years

Item 46

A 45-year-old man is evaluated in follow-up after a recent diagnosis of hepatitis B infection, which was discovered after a blood donation. His medical history is notable for illicit parenteral drug use 10 years ago. He has no family history of hepatitis B infection. He is otherwise well and takes no medications.

On physical examination, vital signs are normal, and he appears well. No spider angiomata are noted. The liver span is normal, and the spleen is not palpable. No ascites or edema is present.

Laboratory studies:

Alanine aminotransferase	Normal
Hepatitis B serologic studies:	
Hepatitis B surface antigen	Positive
IgM antibody to hepatitis B core antigen	Negative
IgG antibody to hepatitis B core antigen	Positive
Hepatitis B e antigen	Negative
Antibody to hepatitis B e antigen	Positive
Hepatitis B virus DNA	<20 IU/mL

Which of the following is the most appropriate management?

(A) Entecavir

(B) Lamivudine

(C) Pegylated interferon

(D) No treatment at this time

Item 47

A 23-year-old woman is evaluated for an 8-month history of alternating diarrhea and constipation, generalized abdominal discomfort, bloating, increased flatulence, nausea, and occasional passage of mucus following bowel movements. She has up to five loose, nonbloody bowel movements daily, described as oatmeal in consistency, alternating with periods of constipation. Abdominal discomfort is described as a generalized ache coming in waves and sometimes improves after a bowel movement. She has not had any improvement in her symptoms with the avoidance of milk or a short course of probiotics. Her medical history is unremarkable. There is no family history of gastrointestinal malignancies or inflammatory bowel disease. Her medications are ibuprofen and loperamide.

On physical examination, blood pressure is 130/80 mm Hg, and pulse rate is 62/min. Abdominal examination reveals generalized abdominal tenderness but is otherwise normal. Rectal examination findings are normal.

Which of the following is the most appropriate diagnostic test to perform next?

(A) Colonoscopy

(B) Flexible sigmoidoscopy

(C) Lactose hydrogen breath test

(D) Thyroid-stimulating hormone level

(E) Tissue transglutaminase serology

Item 48

A 72-year-old woman is re-evaluated for iron deficiency anemia and intermittent dark-colored stools. Since the incidental discovery of iron deficiency anemia 3 months ago, she has been evaluated with upper endoscopy that showed a large hiatal hernia and specks of old blood in the stomach but no clear bleeding source. Colonoscopy was normal. Her only medication is iron sulfate.

On physical examination, temperature is 37.0 °C (98.6 °F), blood pressure is 122/78 mm Hg, pulse rate is 72/min, and respiration rate is 18/min. Abdominal examination findings are normal.

Laboratory studies show a hemoglobin level of 11.5 g/dL (115 g/L) and a mean corpuscular volume of 77 fL. A guaiac fecal occult blood test is positive.

Which of the following is the most appropriate diagnostic test to perform next?

(A) Balloon enteroscopy
(B) Intraoperative endoscopy
(C) Push enteroscopy
(D) Repeat colonoscopy
(E) Repeat upper endoscopy

Item 49

A 60-year-old woman is evaluated for a 3-week history of substernal chest pain. The pain is dull, nonradiating, and unrelated to activities. Sometimes the pain is worse after eating spicy foods and can be occasionally triggered by emotional stress. She has not had shortness of breath or weakness. She is moderately active, walking a mile each day. She generally eats a "healthy heart" diet but has never had her lipid levels evaluated. She has never smoked cigarettes. There is no family history of heart disease. Other than the current problem, she is well and takes no medications.

On physical examination, blood pressure is 135/75 mm Hg, pulse rate is 70/min, and respiration rate is 12/min. The remainder of the examination is normal.

An electrocardiogram is normal.

Which of the following is the most appropriate next step in management?

(A) Ambulatory pH testing
(B) Esophageal manometry
(C) Exercise stress test
(D) Upper endoscopy

Item 50

A 34-year-old woman is evaluated in follow-up after a recent diagnosis of hepatitis C virus (HCV) infection, which was discovered after a blood donation. Her medical history is notable for injection drug use 12 years ago. Her only medication is an oral contraceptive.

Vital signs and general physical examination are normal.

Laboratory studies:

Alanine aminotransferase (ALT)	Normal
Antibody to HCV	Positive
HCV RNA	1.2 million IU/mL
Hepatitis B surface antibody	Positive
Hepatitis B surface antigen	Negative
IgG antibody to hepatitis A virus	Positive
Antibody to HIV	Negative

HCV genotyping reveals that she has HCV genotype 2. Liver biopsy demonstrates moderate portal inflammation (grade 2 of 4) and periportal fibrosis with rare portal-portal septa (stage 2 of 4).

Which of the following is the most appropriate management?

(A) Hepatitis A vaccination
(B) Hepatitis B vaccination
(C) Serial monitoring of ALT levels
(D) Testing for IgM antibody to hepatitis A virus
(E) Treatment for hepatitis C virus infection

Item 51

A 55-year-old man is evaluated in follow-up for acid reflux. He has an 8-year history of heartburn, which was previously well controlled with once-daily pantoprazole. His dosage was increased to twice daily 10 weeks ago because he was having nocturnal heartburn. Despite the increase in medication, he has had minimal improvement in symptoms. The patient verified that he is taking the medication 30 minutes before meals. He takes no other medications.

Physical examination is unremarkable.

Upper endoscopy findings are normal.

Which of the following is the most appropriate next step in management?

(A) Ambulatory pH impedance monitoring
(B) Barium esophagogram
(C) Esophageal manometry
(D) Fundoplication

Item 52

A 59-year-old woman is evaluated for a 3-month history of watery diarrhea. She has six to eight nonbloody bowel movements per day with one or two nocturnal stools. She has crampy abdominal pain that improves after a bowel movement. She has significant fecal urgency and has had three episodes of fecal incontinence. She has not had nausea or weight loss and otherwise feels well. Her only other medical problem is frequent tension-type headaches that are treated with daily over-the-counter ibuprofen.

On physical examination, vital signs are normal. Abdominal examination is unremarkable.

Colonoscopy reveals sigmoid diverticulosis but no inflammatory changes. Random colon biopsies show expansion of the lamina propria with acute and chronic inflammatory cells, increased intraepithelial lymphocytes, and no subepithelial collagen thickening.

Which of the following is the most likely diagnosis?

(A) *Clostridium difficile* colitis
(B) Collagenous colitis
(C) Ischemic colitis
(D) Lymphocytic colitis

Item 53

A 41-year-old woman is evaluated in the ICU 7 days after induction chemotherapy for acute myeloid leukemia. Twenty-four hours ago she developed fever of 39.4 °C

(102.9 °F) and severe hypotension and was begun on intravenous fluids, broad-spectrum antibiotics, antifungal therapy, norepinephrine, and vasopressin. Last night she developed diarrhea and a 1 g/dL (10 g/L) drop in hemoglobin.

On physical examination today, temperature is 38.1 °C (100.6 °F), blood pressure is 89/47 mm Hg, pulse rate is 100/min, and respiration rate is 22/min. Oxygen saturation is 94% on a 50% rebreather mask. Palpation of the abdomen elicits left lower abdominal pain without rebound tenderness. Liquid brown stool is present.

A review of the patient's cardiac monitor recordings for the past 24 hours documents only sinus tachycardia.

Laboratory studies reveal a hemoglobin level of 8 g/dL (80 g/L), a leukocyte count of 150/µL (0.15 × 10^9/L), and a platelet count of 10,000/µL (10 × 10^9/L).

CT of the abdomen and pelvis reveals mild proximal jejunal wall thickening and dilation, mild mesenteric edema, and a trace amount of free pelvic fluid.

Which of the following is the most likely diagnosis for this patient's gastrointestinal findings?

(A) Hemorrhage into the bowel wall
(B) Ischemic colitis
(C) Nonocclusive mesenteric ischemia
(D) Superior mesenteric artery embolism

Item 54

A 58-year-old man is evaluated in follow-up for hepatitis C–related cirrhosis that is complicated by nonbleeding small esophageal varices and ascites. His ascites has recently worsened and has required large-volume paracentesis three times per month. He has been on a low-salt diet, spironolactone, and furosemide.

On physical examination, temperature is 36.8 °C (98.2 °F), blood pressure is 98/60 mm Hg, pulse rate is 65/min, and respiration rate is 16/min; BMI is 26. He appears chronically ill. Scleral icterus, jaundice, and spider angiomata are noted. The abdomen is distended with ascites. The spleen tip is palpable.

Laboratory studies reveal a serum creatinine level of 2.2 mg/dL (194.5 µmol/L).

The Model for End-Stage Liver Disease (MELD) score is 21.

Which of the following is the most appropriate next step in management?

(A) Continuation of current medical therapy
(B) Evaluation for liver transplantation
(C) Surgical portosystemic shunt
(D) Transjugular intrahepatic portosystemic shunt

Item 55

A 28-year-old woman was hospitalized 2 days ago for gallstone pancreatitis. She is in the sixteenth week of pregnancy. She now feels well and is tolerating oral intake. Approximately 2 weeks ago she had an episode of severe right upper quadrant and shoulder pain associated with nausea that lasted 2 hours and then resolved. Her medical history is otherwise unremarkable, and her only medication is a prenatal vitamin.

On physical examination, vital signs are normal. Abdominal examination reveals an enlarged uterus consistent with pregnancy, and no hepatomegaly or abdominal tenderness is noted.

Laboratory studies, including a complete blood count, serum amylase, and serum total bilirubin, are normal.

Ultrasound of the right upper quadrant reveals gallbladder stones, no bile duct dilatation, and a normal pancreas.

Which of the following is the most appropriate management?

(A) Bile acid dissolution therapy
(B) Cholecystectomy after delivery
(C) Cholecystectomy prior to hospital discharge
(D) Endoscopic retrograde cholangiopancreatography with sphincterotomy
(E) Extracorporeal shock-wave lithotripsy

Item 56

A 45-year-old man is evaluated in the emergency department for two episodes of hematemesis and lightheadedness. He has no history of gastrointestinal bleeding, bleeding disorders, alcoholism, chronic liver disease, cardiovascular disease, or cancer. He takes no medications.

On physical examination, temperature is 37.0 °C (98.6 °F), blood pressure is 103/62 mm Hg supine and 78/50 mm Hg standing, pulse rate is 101/min supine and 125/min standing, and respiration rate is 14/min. There is no jaundice, spider angiomata, or palmar erythema. Abdominal examination reveals no tenderness, guarding, or rebound. Rectal examination identifies melena.

Laboratory studies:

Hemoglobin	10 g/dL (100 g/L)
Platelet count	200,000/µL (200 × 10^9/L)
Prothrombin time	11 s
Alanine aminotransferase	28 U/L
Aspartate aminotransferase	22 U/L
Blood urea nitrogen	34 mg/dL (12.1 mmol/L)
Creatinine	0.9 mg/dL (79.6 µmol/L)

Which of the following is the most likely cause of this patient's gastrointestinal bleeding?

(A) Duodenal angiodysplasia
(B) Erosive gastritis
(C) Esophageal varices
(D) Peptic ulcer disease
(E) Portal gastropathy

Item 57

A 65-year-old man is evaluated after a recent colonoscopy, which disclosed a 2.5-cm pedunculated polyp in the sigmoid colon. The polyp was removed in its entirety in a single piece. Biopsy results showed a well-differentiated adeno-carcinoma confined to the submucosa without evidence of lymphovascular involvement and a 1-mm margin. There is no family history of colorectal cancer.

Physical examination findings are unremarkable.

Which of the following is the most appropriate management?

(A) Colon resection
(B) CT scan of the abdomen and pelvis
(C) Radiation therapy
(D) Repeat colonoscopy in 3 months

Item 58

A 42-year-old man is evaluated in the emergency department for a 2-day history of bright red blood per rectum. He reports feeling lightheaded, which started this morning and prompted him to come to the emergency department. His medical history is otherwise unremarkable.

On physical examination, temperature is 37.0 °C (98.6 °F), blood pressure is 95/60 mm Hg, pulse rate is 110/min, and respiration rate is 20/min. He is clammy. Abdominal examination findings are normal. Rectal examination shows fresh blood.

He is admitted to the hospital and is stabilized with fluid resuscitation and erythrocyte transfusions.

Laboratory studies show a hemoglobin level of 8.5 g/dL (85 g/L). Upper endoscopy results are normal. Colonoscopy shows fresh blood throughout the colon and terminal ileum.

He stabilizes overnight, but the next morning he has several large bowel movements of fresh blood. He is hemodynamically unstable, and fluid resuscitation is initiated.

Which of the following is the most appropriate test to perform next?

(A) Angiography
(B) Balloon enteroscopy
(C) Repeat colonoscopy
(D) Technetium-labeled nuclear scan

Item 59

A 73-year-old man is evaluated in the hospital for a 2-day history of fever and abdominal pain. He has been on mechanical ventilation for 3 weeks owing to an exacerbation of COPD related to pneumonia. His medical history is also notable for coronary artery disease and ischemic cardiomyopathy with a left ventricular ejection fraction of 35%. His medications are piperacillin-tazobactam, albuterol, lisinopril, metoprolol, and diltiazem.

On physical examination, temperature is 38.9 °C (102.0 °F), blood pressure is 92/60 mm Hg, pulse rate is 110/min, and respiration rate is 18/min on the ventilator. BMI is 32. He is ventilated and sedated. Cardiopulmonary examination reveals a grade 3/6 holosystolic murmur at the apex and coarse breath sounds. Abdominal examination reveals right upper quadrant tenderness. No ascites or hepatosplenomegaly is noted.

Laboratory studies:

Hemoglobin	11 g/dL (110 g/L)
Leukocyte count	17,000/µL (17 × 10⁹/L), with 92% segmented neutrophils and 5% band forms
Creatinine	1.6 mg/dL (141.4 µmol/L)
Alanine aminotransferase	Normal
Alkaline phosphatase	Normal
Bilirubin	Normal

Ultrasound of the right upper quadrant reveals an enlarged gallbladder, a thickened gallbladder wall, pericholecystic fluid, no bile duct dilatation, no gallstones, and no hydronephrosis.

Which of the following is the most appropriate management?

(A) Abdominal CT with intravenous contrast
(B) Endoscopic retrograde cholangiopancreatography with biliary sphincterotomy
(C) Laparoscopic cholecystectomy
(D) Magnetic resonance cholangiopancreatography
(E) Percutaneous cholecystostomy

Item 60

A 55-year-old man is evaluated in the emergency department for a 2-day history of mild nausea and dyspepsia that is worse with fasting and improved with eating. He has also had a 24-hour history of frequent black stools and fatigue. He has no history of gastrointestinal bleeding, alcoholism, chronic liver disease, bleeding disorders, cardiovascular disease, or cancer.

On physical examination, temperature is 37.0 °C (98.6 °F), blood pressure is 114/66 mm Hg, pulse rate is 85/min, and respiration rate is 14/min; BMI is 27. Abdominal examination reveals epigastric tenderness without guarding or rebound. Rectal examination identifies melena. Laboratory studies are normal except for a hemoglobin level of 7.9 g/dL (79 g/L). He is admitted to the hospital and is given intravenous fluid resuscitation and intravenous proton pump inhibitor (PPI) therapy.

Upper endoscopy identifies a 1-cm clean-based gastric ulcer.

Which of the following is the most appropriate next step in management?

(A) Blood transfusion
(B) Endoscopic treatment
(C) Octreotide
(D) Substitute oral for intravenous PPI

Item 61

A 57-year-old man is evaluated during a routine examination. His medical history is notable for chronic hepatitis C infection with cirrhosis, which was diagnosed 3 years ago. He undergoes surveillance ultrasound for hepatocellular carcinoma every 6 months.

On physical examination, temperature is 36.8 °C (98.2 °F), blood pressure is 110/82 mm Hg, pulse rate is

65/min, and respiration rate is 18/min; BMI is 22. Muscle wasting and scleral icterus are noted. There is no flank dullness and no asterixis.

Ultrasound demonstrates three new liver masses. A four-phase CT demonstrates three lesions (1.8 cm, 2.5 cm, and 2.9 cm in size) that show arterial enhancement with venous washout. Splenomegaly and esophageal varices are also noted.

Which of the following is the most appropriate next step in management?

(A) Liver biopsy
(B) Liver transplantation evaluation
(C) Sorafenib
(D) Surgical resection
(E) Transarterial chemoembolization

Item 62

A 55-year-old man is evaluated in follow-up after a recent routine screening for antibody to hepatitis C virus (HCV) was positive. His medical history is unremarkable; he has not used illicit drugs or had any history of blood transfusions. He currently feels well and takes no medications.

Vital signs and physical examination are normal.

Laboratory studies reveal a positive HCV antibody test, but HCV RNA testing is negative. The serum alanine aminotransferase level is normal.

Which of the following is the most appropriate diagnostic test to perform next?

(A) Perform liver ultrasound
(B) Perform serial alanine aminotransferase monitoring
(C) Repeat HCV antibody testing
(D) Repeat HCV RNA testing
(E) No further testing

Item 63

A 46-year-old man is evaluated for intermittent rectal bleeding of 3 months' duration. He is otherwise well and takes no medications. His father had a few polyps removed from the colon when he was 71 years old, but no other details are known about his father's medical history. The patient and his wife have three children aged 8, 12, and 18 years.

On physical examination, vital signs and the remainder of the examination are normal.

Colonoscopy reveals 12 polyps ranging in size from 2 to 7 mm, all of which are removed from the colon. He undergoes genetic testing, which reveals biallelic mutations in the *MYH* gene and confirms a diagnosis of *MYH*-associated polyposis (MAP).

Genetic testing of which of the following persons will provide the most cost-effective approach to determining if the patient's children have inherited MAP?

(A) The patient's father
(B) The patient's mother
(C) The patient's 18-year-old child
(D) The patient's wife

Item 64

A 47-year-old woman is evaluated in the emergency department after vomiting bright-red blood. She has alcoholic cirrhosis with ascites, which has been well controlled with diuretics. She has had jaundice and intermittent confusion for the past month. She has not consumed alcohol in the past 11 months. Her medications are spironolactone and furosemide, and octreotide was begun in the emergency department.

On physical examination, temperature is 36.8 °C (98.2 °F), blood pressure is 72/54 mm Hg, pulse rate is 112/min, and respiration rate is 20/min; BMI is 26. She is confused. Scleral icterus, jaundice, and spider angiomata over the chest are noted. The left lobe of the liver is firm and is palpated 3 cm below the costal margin. There is no abdominal pain or flank dullness.

Laboratory studies reveal a hemoglobin level of 8.7 g/dL (87 g/L).

Ultrasound shows a coarsened liver echotexture, left lobe hypertrophy, and splenomegaly but no ascites.

Intravenous fluid resuscitation is initiated.

Which of the following is the most appropriate next step in management?

(A) Antibiotics
(B) Nonselective β-blocker
(C) Transjugular intrahepatic portosystemic shunt placement
(D) Upper endoscopy

Item 65

A 38-year-old man is evaluated for a 6-month history of fatigue. He was recently discovered to have anemia and elevated liver chemistry test results. He has had a long history of loose and occasionally malodorous stools. He has a good appetite but has unintentionally lost 2.3 kg (5.0 lb) over the past 6 weeks. He has not had blood in the stool, melena, or other obvious source of blood loss. He drinks approximately five alcoholic beverages per week and never more than two per occasion.

On physical examination, temperature is 36.8 °C (98.2 °F), blood pressure is 108/54 mm Hg, pulse rate is 82/min, and respiration rate is 16/min; BMI is 18. He appears thin, and muscle wasting is noted. He is not in acute distress. Abdominal examination reveals a normal liver and spleen.

Laboratory studies:

Hemoglobin	11 g/dL (110 g/L)
Mean corpuscular volume	78 fL
Ferritin	8 ng/mL (8 µg/L)
Alanine aminotransferase	82 U/L
Aspartate aminotransferase	78 U/L
Alkaline phosphatase	135 U/L
Total bilirubin	Normal

Stool is negative for occult blood.

Which of the following is the most likely diagnosis?

(A) Alcohol-induced liver disease
(B) Celiac disease
(C) Chronic viral hepatitis
(D) Primary biliary cirrhosis

Item 66

A 43-year-old woman is evaluated in the emergency department for a 4-day history of abdominal pain. She underwent laparoscopic cholecystectomy 1 week ago for symptomatic gallbladder stones. The surgery had no complications, and she left the hospital the same day. Three days after surgery she began to have episodes of epigastric pain and nausea that last 30 minutes to 2 hours. She has not had vomiting, fever, abdominal distention, jaundice, or bleeding. She is currently pain free.

On physical examination, temperature is 36.8 °C (98.2 °F), blood pressure is 106/60 mm Hg, pulse rate is 82/min, and respiration rate is 16/min. Abdominal examination reveals well-healed laparoscopic surgery port sites. No hepatomegaly, ascites, abdominal guarding, or abdominal tenderness is noted.

Initial laboratory studies show a serum alanine aminotransferase level of 84 U/L and a serum aspartate aminotransferase level of 62 U/L. Other laboratory studies, including a complete blood count and serum alkaline phosphatase and amylase levels, are normal. Ultrasound of the right upper quadrant reveals no abdominal fluid collections; the intrahepatic and extrahepatic bile ducts are dilated, and the pancreas is not well visualized. Laboratory studies checked 24 hours later are normal.

Which of the following is the most likely diagnosis?

(A) Acute pancreatitis
(B) Bile leak
(C) Cholangitis
(D) Choledocholithiasis
(E) Sphincter of Oddi dysfunction

Item 67

A 60-year-old woman is evaluated during a routine follow-up appointment. She has gastroparesis associated with long-standing type 2 diabetes mellitus. Improved blood sugar control and efforts to eat small, frequent meals did not result in symptom improvement. In addition to these interventions, metoclopramide was started 6 months ago, after which her nausea and periodic vomiting resolved. However, she has had some restlessness at night with the urge to repeatedly cross and uncross her legs. Several weeks ago she developed a tremor in her right hand. In addition to metoclopramide, her medications are glyburide and metformin.

On physical examination, blood pressure is 125/65 mm Hg and pulse rate is 75/min. Other vital signs are normal. Tremor is noted in the lower lip and resting tremor is seen in the right hand.

In addition to dietary modification and blood glucose control, which of the following is the most appropriate management?

(A) Decrease in the metoclopramide dosage
(B) Discontinue metoclopramide and begin promethazine
(C) Gastric pacemaker placement
(D) Pyloric botulinum toxin injection

Item 68

A 38-year-old woman is hospitalized for new-onset confusion and jaundice. She noticed a yellowish discoloration of the eyes 4 days before admission. Six weeks ago she developed sinus infection symptoms that were treated with amoxicillin-clavulanate. She has no history of liver disease. She does not drink alcohol or use illicit drugs or herbal supplements. She is now taking no medications.

On physical examination, temperature is 37.2 °C (99.0 °F), blood pressure is 118/82 mm Hg, pulse rate is 72/min, and respiration rate is 20/min; BMI is 27. She appears ill and is disoriented to time and date. Asterixis, scleral icterus, and jaundice are noted. Examination is negative for spider angiomata, palmar erythema, muscle wasting, and rash. The liver edge is palpable 2 cm below the costal margin. The spleen is not palpable.

Laboratory studies:

INR	1.9 (normal range 0.8-1.2)
Prothrombin time	28 s
Alanine aminotransferase	199 U/L
Aspartate aminotransferase	398 U/L
Total bilirubin	9.5 mg/dL (162.5 μmol/L)
Creatinine	1.2 mg/dL (106.1 μmol/L)

Serologic studies for hepatitis A IgM, hepatitis B surface antigen, hepatitis B core IgM, Epstein-Barr virus, cytomegalovirus IgM, antinuclear antibody, anti-smooth muscle antibody, and ceruloplasmin are all negative. The serum acetaminophen level is 0 μg/mL. A pregnancy test is negative.

In addition to evaluation for liver transplantation, which of the following is the most appropriate treatment?

(A) Intravenous acyclovir
(B) Intravenous glucocorticoids
(C) Intravenous *N*-acetylcysteine
(D) Oral pentoxifylline

Item 69

A 28-year-old man is evaluated in the emergency department for a piece of food stuck in his esophagus. He notes that this has happened in the past, but he was previously able to induce vomiting to relieve the blockage. He has no symptoms of gastroesophageal reflux disease, and he takes no medications.

Physical examination findings are unremarkable.

Upper endoscopy reveals a food bolus in the mid-esophagus, and gentle pressure with the endoscope passes the food bolus into the stomach. Upper endoscopy findings are shown (see top of next page).

Which of the following is the most likely diagnosis?

(A) Achalasia
(B) Barrett esophagus
(C) Diffuse esophageal spasm
(D) Eosinophilic esophagitis

Item 70

A 27-year-old woman is evaluated during a routine examination. She has a personal and family history of familial

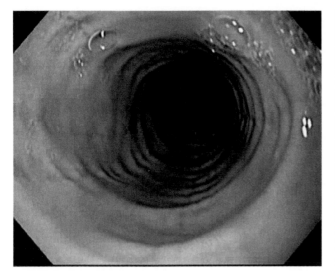

ITEM 69

adenomatous polyposis (FAP) and has undergone a total colectomy and ileorectal anastomosis.

On physical examination, vital signs are normal. The physical examination is remarkable only for a well-healed surgical scar on the abdomen.

In addition to annual sigmoidoscopy to assess for postoperative rectal polyp burden, which of the following should be recommended for FAP-related surveillance?

(A) CT of the abdomen and pelvis
(B) Ophthalmology consultation
(C) Small-bowel capsule endoscopy
(D) Upper endoscopy

Item 71

A 21-year-old man is evaluated for a 2-week history of fatigue and a 1-week history of right upper quadrant discomfort and dark urine. He drinks three alcoholic beverages per day and uses injection drugs. There is no personal or family history of liver disease or hepatocellular carcinoma.

On physical examination, temperature is 38.0 °C (100.4 °F), blood pressure is 120/68 mm Hg, pulse rate is 112/min, and respiration rate is 20/min. He is alert and oriented. Needle marks are noted on the arms. There is no asterixis. Scleral icterus is present. There is right upper quadrant tenderness, and the liver is enlarged, soft, and tender. There is no ascites and no splenomegaly.

Laboratory studies:

INR	1.2 (normal range, 0.8-1.2)
Alanine aminotransferase	1843 U/L
Aspartate aminotransferase	1598 U/L
Total bilirubin	4.8 mg/dL (82.1 µmol/L)
Anti–hepatitis A virus IgG antibodies	Positive
Anti–hepatitis A virus IgM antibodies	Negative
Hepatitis B surface antigen	Positive
IgM antibody to hepatitis B core antigen	Positive

Hepatitis B e antigen	Positive
IgG antibody to hepatitis B core antigen	Negative
Hepatitis B surface antibody	Negative
Antibody to hepatitis B e antigen	Negative
Hepatitis B virus DNA	69,000 IU/mL

Ultrasound of the right upper quadrant reveals an enlarged liver with no masses. The spleen is normal, and there is no ascites.

Which of the following is the most appropriate management?

(A) CT of the abdomen with contrast
(B) Lamivudine
(C) Pegylated interferon
(D) Serial monitoring of liver enzymes
(E) Tenofovir

Item 72

A 31-year-old woman is evaluated for a 9-year history of episodic attacks of idiopathic pancreatitis. She previously had no pain between attacks; however, over the last 6 months, epigastric pain has become more constant and has increased in severity. The pain has not responded well to enzyme replacement, ibuprofen, and acetaminophen. She was recently started on tramadol with modest but not sufficient relief of her symptoms. Current medications are enteric-coated pancreatic enzyme replacement, ibuprofen, and tramadol.

On physical examination, vital signs are normal; BMI is 24. Abdominal examination reveals epigastric and left upper abdominal tenderness with no guarding or rebound.

Contrast-enhanced multidetector CT shows evidence of chronic pancreatitis. There is no pancreatic cyst, mass, enlargement, or pancreatic ductal dilation and no bile duct dilation or gallstones. Endoscopic ultrasonography confirms findings of chronic pancreatitis.

Which of the following is the most appropriate additional treatment?

(A) Celiac plexus blockade
(B) Extracorporeal shock wave lithotripsy
(C) Pancreaticoduodenectomy
(D) Pregabalin

Item 73

A 44-year-old man is evaluated in follow-up for symptoms of gastroesophageal reflux disease. Eight weeks ago he was evaluated for heartburn and a sour taste in his mouth and was started on once-daily pantoprazole. Despite improvement in his heartburn symptoms, he continues to wake up with an acid taste in the middle of the night. He has not had difficulty swallowing and has no reflux symptoms during the day. He confirms that he takes the medication 30 minutes before a meal.

Physical examination is unremarkable.

Which of the following is the most appropriate next step in management?

(A) Add metoclopramide

(B) Increase pantoprazole to twice daily

(C) Perform upper endoscopy

(D) Switch to omeprazole

Item 74

A 38-year-old man is evaluated in follow-up after a diagnosis of ulcerative colitis. Ten days ago he was started on prednisone, 60 mg/d, but his symptoms have not improved. He has six to nine bloody bowel movements per day and moderate abdominal pain. He has decreased his oral intake because eating exacerbates his pain and diarrhea.

On physical examination, temperature is 37.0 °C (98.6 °F), blood pressure is 110/56 mm Hg, and pulse rate is 96/min. He is pale but in no distress. The abdomen is diffusely tender without distention, guarding, or rebound.

Laboratory studies reveal a hemoglobin level of 9.7 g/dL (97 g/L) and a leukocyte count of 6300/μL (6.3×10^9/L).

Stool culture and *Clostridium difficile* assay are negative.

Which of the following is the most appropriate treatment?

(A) Increase prednisone to 80 mg/d

(B) Initiate adalimumab

(C) Initiate ciprofloxacin and metronidazole

(D) Initiate mesalamine

(E) Initiate sulfasalazine

Item 75

A 60-year-old man is evaluated in the emergency department for a 24-hour history of frequent black stools and fatigue without abdominal pain. His medical history is notable for a myocardial infarction 1 year ago and hypertension. He has no history of gastrointestinal bleeding, alcoholism, chronic liver disease, bleeding disorders, or cancer. His medications are aspirin, metoprolol, lisinopril, and atorvastatin.

On physical examination, temperature is 37.0 °C (98.6 °F), blood pressure is 122/69 mm Hg, pulse rate is 87/min, and respiration rate is 14/min; BMI is 29. Abdominal examination is normal. Rectal examination identifies melena. Laboratory studies are normal except for a hemoglobin level of 10.2 g/dL (102 g/L).

He is admitted to the hospital. Aspirin is discontinued, and he is given intravenous fluid resuscitation and intravenous proton pump inhibitor (PPI) therapy (bolus followed by continuous intravenous infusion). Upper endoscopy identifies a 1-cm clean-based duodenal ulcer. Intravenous PPI is switched to an oral PPI. *Helicobacter pylori* testing is negative. He tolerates refeeding without problems and is now ready for discharge.

Which of the following adjustments should be made to this patient's medication on discharge?

(A) Change aspirin to clopidogrel

(B) Discontinue aspirin

(C) Resume aspirin before discharge

(D) Resume aspirin 4 weeks after discharge

Item 76

A 63-year-old woman is evaluated in follow-up after a colonoscopy performed last month demonstrated a 12-mm sessile serrated polyp in the transverse colon. A screening colonoscopy performed when she was 50 years old disclosed a 15-mm hyperplastic polyp in the ascending colon and two hyperplastic polyps measuring 4 and 6 mm in the transverse colon; all polyps were removed. Follow-up colonoscopy at age 55 years revealed a 5-mm sessile serrated polyp in the transverse colon and a 4-mm hyperplastic polyp in the descending colon. There is no family history of colon cancer or family members with colonic polyps.

Physical examination findings are unremarkable.

Which of the following is the most likely diagnosis?

(A) Familial adenomatous polyposis

(B) Lynch syndrome

(C) Peutz-Jeghers syndrome

(D) Serrated polyposis syndrome

Item 77

A 42-year-old man is evaluated for a 2-month history of two to four loose stools per day and abdominal cramps. He was diagnosed 1 year ago with celiac disease. Until recently, his symptoms responded to a strict gluten-free diet, with resolution of weight loss, diarrhea, abdominal pain, and iron deficiency anemia. He has not had fever, melena, or hematochezia. He has not taken any new medications.

On physical examination, vital signs are normal. The abdomen is soft with normal bowel sounds. There is no distention, tenderness, masses, or organomegaly.

Which of the following is the most appropriate management?

(A) Abdominal CT scan

(B) Careful dietary review

(C) Colonoscopy with biopsies

(D) Upper endoscopy with small-bowel biopsy

Item 78

A 45-year-old woman is evaluated in follow-up after being treated for a *Helicobacter pylori*–related duodenal ulcer 1 month ago. Despite completing a 10-day course of clarithromycin, amoxicillin, and omeprazole, urea breath testing is positive. She has no antibiotic allergies.

Physical examination is unremarkable.

Which of the following is the most appropriate treatment?

(A) Initiate a 7-day course of levofloxacin, amoxicillin, and omeprazole

(B) Initiate a 10-day course of clarithromycin, metronidazole, and omeprazole

(C) Initiate a 10-day course of levofloxacin, amoxicillin, and omeprazole

(D) Initiate a 14-day course of clarithromycin, amoxicillin, and omeprazole

(E) Repeat the 10-day course of clarithromycin, amoxicillin, and omeprazole

Item 79

A 25-year-old man is evaluated for scleral icterus. He is a graduate student in physical chemistry; a professor noticed that he had "yellow eyes" and suggested that this finding be evaluated. The patient has no symptoms, no history of previous medical problems, and takes no medications.

On physical examination, vital signs are normal. Scleral icterus is present. The abdomen is soft and nontender. The liver and spleen are not enlarged.

Laboratory studies:

Hemoglobin	14 g/dL (140 g/L)
Reticulocyte count	1.5% of erythrocytes
Alanine aminotransferase	25 U/L
Aspartate aminotransferase	28 U/L
Alkaline phosphatase	75 U/L
Total bilirubin	2.9 mg/dL (49.6 µmol/L)
Direct bilirubin	0.2 mg/dL (3.4 µmol/L)

A blood smear is normal.

Which of the following is the most appropriate management?

(A) Direct antiglobulin (Coombs) test

(B) Hepatitis B and C serology

(C) Magnetic resonance cholangiopancreatography

(D) No further tests

Item 80

A 72-year-old man is evaluated during a routine examination. He underwent a sigmoid colectomy and adjuvant chemotherapy 4 years ago for stage III adenocarcinoma of the colon. Results of colonoscopies performed 1 year postoperatively and last year were normal.

On physical examination, he appears healthy and has no evidence of recurrent disease.

Which of the following is the most appropriate time to repeat colonoscopy?

(A) 1 year

(B) 3 years

(C) 5 years

(D) 10 years

Item 81

A 48-year-old man is evaluated for a 4-week history of heartburn that awakens him at night. The symptoms occur about three times per week. He has been taking over-the-counter antacids with incomplete relief. Food triggers include coffee and spicy foods. He has not had unintentional weight loss or difficulty swallowing.

Physical examination and laboratory studies are normal.

Which of the following is the most appropriate next step in management?

(A) Ambulatory esophageal pH monitoring

(B) Esophageal manometry

(C) Trial of a proton pump inhibitor

(D) Upper endoscopy

Item 82

A 58-year-old woman is evaluated in the emergency department for a 1-day history of nausea and pain in the left lower abdomen, which was followed by the onset of several episodes of dark-red rectal bleeding. Her bowel habits were previously normal, and she has not had tenesmus, fecal urgency, constipation, diarrhea, weight change, or previous abdominal pain. She has no history of gastrointestinal bleeding, alcoholism, chronic liver disease, bleeding disorders, or cancer. Other medical problems are hypertension, hyperlipidemia, and peripheral vascular disease. Her medications are chlorthalidone, ramipril, and simvastatin. She continues to smoke 1 pack of cigarettes daily.

On physical examination, temperature is 37.0 °C (98.6 °F), blood pressure is 125/68 mm Hg, pulse rate is 87/min, and respiration rate is 14/min; BMI is 27. Abdominal examination reveals pain in the left lower abdomen with no guarding or rebound. No abdominal masses are noted, and the liver and spleen are not enlarged. Bowel sounds are diminished in frequency, and abdominal distention is noted. Rectal examination identifies a small amount of fresh blood and clots; no external hemorrhoids or anal fissure are noted. Femoral, popliteal, and dorsalis pedis pulses are diminished bilaterally.

Laboratory studies reveal a hemoglobin level of 10 g/dL (100 g/L), a leukocyte count of 14,000/µL (14 × 10⁹/L), and a platelet count of 215,000/µL (215 × 10⁹/L).

Which of the following is the most likely diagnosis?

(A) Angiodysplasia

(B) Colon cancer

(C) Diverticular bleeding

(D) Ischemic colitis

(E) Ulcerative colitis

Item 83

A 62-year-old man is evaluated after a recent screening colonoscopy. The colonoscopy disclosed a 3-mm sigmoid polyp and an 8-mm hepatic flexure polyp, both of which were removed. On pathology, the sigmoid polyp is noted to be a hyperplastic polyp, and the hepatic flexure polyp is found to be a tubulovillous adenoma with high-grade dysplasia.

Physical examination findings are unremarkable.

Which of the following is the most appropriate time to repeat colonoscopy?

(A) 3 to 6 months

(B) 1 year

(C) 3 years

(D) 5 years

Item 84

A 72-year-old man is evaluated for a 3-month history of difficulty swallowing solid foods. He has lost 4.5 kg (10.0 lb) over the last 2 months. He has a 10-year history of heartburn, which is controlled with omeprazole once daily. His other medical problems include obesity and a 35-pack-year history of cigarette smoking. His BMI before the onset of his symptoms was 30.

On physical examination, vital signs are normal; BMI is 29. The remainder of the physical examination is unremarkable.

Laboratory studies are normal.

Which of the following is the most appropriate next step in management?

(A) CT of the chest
(B) Esophageal manometry
(C) pH study
(D) Upper endoscopy

Item 85

A 68-year-old woman undergoes upper endoscopy for evaluation of dyspepsia. She has a history of pernicious anemia. She has no other medical problems and her only medication is oral vitamin B_{12}.

On physical examination, vital signs are normal, as is the remainder of the physical examination.

Upper endoscopy discloses a 6-mm polyp in the body of the stomach, which is removed by polypectomy. Other endoscopic findings, including biopsy of the duodenum to evaluate for celiac disease, are normal. Pathologic examination of the polyp confirms a well-differentiated neuroendocrine tumor.

The fasting serum gastrin level is 1025 pg/mL (1025 ng/L).

Which of the following is the most appropriate management?

(A) CT of the abdomen and pelvis
(B) Partial gastrectomy
(C) Radiolabeled somatostatin receptor scintigraphy
(D) Observation

Item 86

A 58-year-old man is evaluated for a 10-year history of intermittent difficulty swallowing both solids and liquids. Over the last 6 months the symptoms have worsened and now include regurgitation and weight loss of 4.5 kg (10.0 lb). He has tried antacids but has had no improvements in his symptoms.

Physical examination is unremarkable.

Laboratory studies are normal. A barium radiograph is shown (see top of next column). Upper endoscopy reveals no luminal mass. Esophageal manometry demonstrates aperistalsis and incomplete lower esophageal sphincter relaxation.

Which of the following is the most likely diagnosis?

(A) Achalasia
(B) Diffuse esophageal spasm

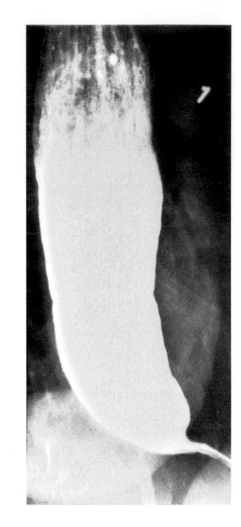

(C) Esophageal hypomotility
(D) Nutcracker esophagus

Item 87

A 38-year-old woman is evaluated for a 6-month history of generalized abdominal pain, nonbloody diarrhea, increased flatulence, and bloating following meals. She underwent Roux-en-Y gastric bypass with cholecystectomy 2 years ago for morbid obesity. She has no history of gastrointestinal malignancies or inflammatory bowel disease. Her medications are dicyclomine, loperamide, a multivitamin, and calcium with vitamin D.

On physical examination, vital signs are normal. BMI is 29. Abdominal examination reveals a well-healed midline incision but is otherwise normal.

Laboratory studies, including liver chemistry studies and hemoglobin level, are normal.

Which of the following is the most appropriate management?

(A) Colonoscopy
(B) Empiric treatment with antibiotics
(C) Omeprazole
(D) Right upper quadrant ultrasound
(E) Stool cultures

Item 88

A 25-year-old woman is evaluated for a 3-day history of diarrhea with four or five loose to watery stools per day. She has had mild to moderate abdominal cramps, intermittent nausea, and muscle aches but no fever, blood in the stool, or vomiting. She has had no recent travel outside her home town and has not recently been exposed to antibiotics. She is otherwise healthy and takes no medications.

On physical examination, temperature is 37.6 °C (99.7 °F), blood pressure is 110/70 mm Hg, and pulse rate is 85/min. She appears mildly ill. The abdomen is soft, non-tender, and nondistended.

Which of the following is the most appropriate management?

(A) Colonoscopy

(B) Stool cultures

(C) Stool testing for ova and parasites

(D) Supportive care

Item 89

A 24-year-old woman is evaluated for a 2-month history of painless bright red blood per rectum that is usually associated with defecation. She has noted a protrusion of tissue from the rectum during these episodes. Her medical history is otherwise unremarkable. There is no family history of inflammatory bowel disease, colorectal polyps, or colorectal cancer.

Anoscopy discloses a rectal polyp.

Colonoscopy reveals a 14-mm pedunculated polyp in the rectum, which is removed. Colonoscopy findings are otherwise normal. Biopsy confirmed the polyp to be a juvenile polyp. Upper endoscopy is performed and is normal.

Which of the following is the most appropriate management?

(A) Genetic counseling

(B) Repeat colonoscopy in 2 years

(C) Repeat upper endoscopy in 2 years

(D) Repeat both colonoscopy and upper endoscopy in 2 years

(E) Reassurance

Item 90

A 78-year-old man is evaluated for symptoms of dysphagia that began 2 weeks ago. When he eats, he starts coughing after the first bite of food and occasionally has nasal regurgitation.

On physical examination, blood pressure is 135/90 mm Hg, pulse rate is 78/min, and respiration rate is 12/min. Left-sided weakness is noted in both extremities, upper greater than lower.

Which of the following is the most appropriate diagnostic test to evaluate this patient's dysphagia?

(A) Barium swallow

(B) Esophageal manometry

(C) Upper endoscopy

(D) Videofluoroscopy

Item 91

A 38-year-old man is evaluated in follow-up after starting therapy for ulcerative colitis. A colonoscopy performed 3 months ago showed moderate colitis extending from the rectum to the proximal transverse colon. He was initially treated with mesalamine without any improvement in his symptoms. On prednisone, 40 mg/d, his symptoms have steadily improved, with cessation of bleeding and a decrease in diarrhea. The dose of prednisone has been tapered to 20 mg/d, and he is now having one to two mostly formed stools per day.

On physical examination, vital signs are normal. Abdominal examination is unremarkable.

Laboratory studies reveal a normal complete blood count, and the serum thiopurine methyltransferase level is undetectable.

Which of the following is the most appropriate maintenance therapy?

(A) Azathioprine

(B) Infliximab

(C) 6-Mercaptopurine

(D) Methotrexate

(E) Prednisone

Item 92

A 25-year-old man is evaluated in follow-up after recently testing positive for hepatitis B surface antigen. He underwent testing as part of the immigration process from Somalia. Two other siblings also have hepatitis B virus (HBV) infection.

On physical examination, he is a young, healthy-appearing man. Vital signs are normal. No jaundice is noted, and the abdominal examination is unremarkable.

Laboratory studies:

Alanine aminotransferase	Normal
Aspartate aminotransferase	Normal
α-Fetoprotein	Normal
Hepatitis B surface antigen	Positive
Hepatitis B e antibody	Positive
Hepatitis B e antigen	Negative
HBV DNA	896 IU/mL

Ultrasound of the upper abdomen is normal.

Which of the following is the most appropriate management?

(A) Administration of hepatitis B vaccine

(B) Administration of pegylated interferon

(C) Administration of tenofovir

(D) α-Fetoprotein measurement every 12 months

(E) Ultrasound imaging of the liver every 6 months

Item 93

A 55-year-old man is hospitalized for a 3-day history of melena and a 2-week history of epigastric abdominal pain.

His medical history is notable for degenerative arthritis of the knee, for which he takes an NSAID.

On physical examination, blood pressure is 139/65 mm Hg and pulse rate is 75/min. Other vital signs are normal. Abdominal examination reveals epigastric tenderness to light palpation.

Initial laboratory studies reveal a hemoglobin level of 12 g/dL (120 g/L). An intravenous proton pump inhibitor (PPI) and intravenous hydration are initiated.

Upper endoscopy reveals three cratered, clean-based gastric ulcers smaller than 1 cm. The esophagus, stomach, and small bowel are well visualized, and no other source of gastrointestinal bleeding is identified. Gastric biopsies are taken to test for *Helicobacter pylori*.

The patient is examined 24 hours after admission. Vital signs are stable and the abdominal examination reveals diminished tenderness to palpation. Laboratory studies reveal a hemoglobin level of 11.5 g/dL (115 g/L).

In addition to discontinuing the NSAID, which of the following is the most appropriate management?

(A) Begin oral feeding, switch to an oral PPI, and observe for 24 hours
(B) Continue intravenous PPI therapy for another 24 hours
(C) Discharge and switch to oral PPI therapy
(D) Perform repeat upper endoscopy before discharge

Item 94

A 65-year old man is evaluated for a 4-week history of worsening reflux and heartburn. He has a 10-year history of heartburn that was previously well controlled with omeprazole. Recently he noticed that the medication is less effective, and he is experiencing heartburn in the afternoon. He has no dysphagia, nausea, vomiting, or weight loss. He takes no other medications.

On physical examination, vital signs are normal. The remainder of the examination, including abdominal examination, is unremarkable.

Upper endoscopy shows a small hiatal hernia and salmon-colored mucosa in the distal esophagus. Pathology results reveal a diagnosis of Barrett esophagus with high-grade dysplasia.

Which of the following is the most appropriate next step in management?

(A) Endoscopic ablation
(B) Esophagectomy
(C) Fundoplication
(D) Repeat upper endoscopy in 1 year

Item 95

A 51-year-old woman is evaluated in the emergency department after running her car into a stop sign several hours ago. Emergency personnel reported that she had confusion, tremulousness, and a low blood glucose level, all of which resolved after ingestion of glucose tablets. Her medical history is significant for a 1.5-year history of episodic confusion. She has no history of diabetes mellitus and has not used insulin or oral hypoglycemic agents. She has not had upper abdominal pain, pancreatitis, or weight loss. She takes no medications.

In the emergency department, vital signs and physical examination are normal.

To further investigate the hypoglycemia, she is admitted to the hospital for a 72-hour fast. Confusion is observed after 10 hours of fasting, but the neurologic examination is otherwise nonfocal. Blood samples are immediately drawn and the symptoms resolve with administration of glucose.

Laboratory studies show an elevated C-peptide level, a plasma glucose level of 45 mg/dL (2.5 mmol/L), and an elevated fasting insulin level.

Contrast-enhanced multidetector CT shows a normal-appearing pancreas.

Which of the following is the most appropriate diagnostic test to perform next?

(A) Endoscopic retrograde cholangiopancreatography
(B) Endoscopic ultrasound
(C) Octreotide scan
(D) Transabdominal ultrasound

Item 96

A 63-year-old woman is evaluated in follow-up after a recent diagnosis of collagenous colitis. She initially presented with a 3-month history of watery diarrhea that included 7 to 10 nonbloody bowel movements per day and one or two nocturnal stools. She continues to have crampy abdominal pain and urgency but no fecal incontinence. She has been treated with loperamide, diphenoxylate, and then bismuth subsalicylate for 6 months without any improvement in her symptoms. She takes no other medications.

On physical examination, vital signs are normal. Abdominal examination is unremarkable.

Which of the following is the most appropriate treatment?

(A) Budesonide
(B) Ciprofloxacin
(C) Infliximab
(D) Mesalamine

Answers and Critiques

Item 1   Answer: D

Educational Objective: Treat alcohol-induced liver disease with alcohol cessation.

This patient has alcohol-induced liver disease, and the most appropriate treatment is to stop alcohol intake. In alcohol-induced liver disease, serum aspartate aminotransferase (AST) and alanine aminotransferase (ALT) levels are typically elevated two to six times the upper limit of normal but AST levels above 500 U/L and ALT levels above 200 U/L are uncommon. An AST/ALT ratio above 2 to 3 is typical for alcoholic liver disease.

Hereditary hemochromatosis is an autosomal recessive disease, and homozygosity for *C282Y* is generally required to cause iron overload. The initial step in evaluating patients with suspected hemochromatosis is a serum transferrin saturation measurement, which is the most sensitive test in diagnosing this condition. Elevated serum transferrin saturations suggest hemochromatosis, and further assessment is advised, usually with serum ferritin measurement and hemochromatosis gene testing. Serum ferritin, although not usually used as an initial diagnostic study for suspected hemochromatosis, is a surrogate measure of iron stores; values greater than 1000 ng/mL (1000 µg/L) in the absence of an inflammatory state or another cause for liver disease suggest hemochromatosis. Serum ferritin measurement is therefore used as a follow-up study for elevated transferrin saturation levels. A liver biopsy specimen stained for iron confirms tissue iron overload. This patient is heterozygous for *C282Y* and has a slightly elevated serum ferritin level but a normal transferrin saturation; these findings do not support the diagnosis of hemochromatosis. Isolated elevations of serum ferritin, as seen in this patient, can be due to inflammatory states such as liver injury from another cause, including alcohol-induced liver disease. Phlebotomy (the treatment of choice for hemochromatosis) and iron chelation with deferoxamine (the typical treatment for secondary iron overload conditions) are not necessary at this time.

Repeating serum iron tests now will not add much useful information at this time; however, repeat testing should be performed later after the patient decreases his alcohol intake, as iron overload may result in some patients despite an absence of homozygosity for *C282Y*.

KEY POINT

- Isolated elevations of serum ferritin levels can be due to inflammatory states such as liver injury from another cause, including alcohol-induced liver disease.

Bibliography

Adams PC. Evaluation of cirrhosis with an elevated ferritin. Clin Gastroenterol Hepatol. 2012 Apr;10(4):368-70. [PMID: 22037432]

Item 2   Answer: C

Educational Objective: Manage chronic diarrhea caused by malabsorption of sugar-free sweeteners.

The most appropriate management is discontinuation of sugar-free sweeteners. The appearance of this patient's diarrhea coincided with healthy lifestyle changes that include the ingestion of artificial sweeteners. The temporal association between the onset of this patient's diarrhea and his dietary changes makes it highly likely that the exposure to nonabsorbable sugar alcohols ("sugar-free sweeteners") is the cause of his symptoms. The presence of bloating is also characteristic of diarrhea due to non-absorbed carbohydrates. In this patient, further testing is not necessary before recommending the discontinuation of sugar-free sweeteners. However, if the likely diagnosis was less clear, assessment of his stool electrolytes would be helpful. In diarrhea caused by malabsorbed carbohydrates, an elevation in the osmotic gap would be expected. The osmotic gap is calculated using the following equation:

$$290 - 2 \times [\text{stool sodium} + \text{stool potassium}]$$

A gap greater than 100 mOsm/kg (100 mmol/kg) indicates an osmotic diarrhea. If the gap is less than 50 mOsm/kg (50 mmol/kg), the diarrhea is not osmotic. A gap between 50 and 100 mOsm/kg (50 and 100 mmol/kg) is equivocal. Sugar-free sweeteners are metabolized by gut bacteria, liberating gas and osmotically active substances that cause diarrhea and account for the osmotic gap.

Pancreatic cancer could present with diarrhea and weight loss, but this patient's age, absence of abdominal pain, and correlation of symptoms with dietary changes make this diagnosis less likely. Therefore, a CT scan should be deferred until a dietary cause of his symptoms is excluded.

Patients with microscopic colitis lack signs of systemic inflammation and present with painless watery diarrhea without bleeding. Diagnosis can only be made when biopsies of the colon show a predominance of intraepithelial lymphocytes in the colonic mucosa (lymphocytic colitis) or the addition of a thickened subepithelial collagen band (collagenous colitis). Colonoscopy with biopsies would be useful to exclude microscopic colitis, but this diagnosis is uncommon in younger males and would not cause an osmotic diarrhea.

Celiac disease is thought to affect nearly 0.5% to 1% of individuals in the United States. The typical features of celiac disease are diarrhea, bloating, and weight loss. Tissue transglutaminase (tTG) IgA antibody measurement would be useful to evaluate for celiac disease, but this patient's symptoms began after a dietary change, making celiac disease unlikely. In addition, the empiric use of a gluten-free diet is not recommended in the absence of a confirmed diagnosis of celiac disease.

> **KEY POINT**
>
> - Artificial sweeteners have little or no absorption in the small intestine and, when taken in excess, can cause symptoms of carbohydrate malabsorption.

Bibliography

Schiller LR. Definitions, pathophysiology, and evaluation of chronic diarrhoea. Best Pract Res Clin Gastroenterol. 2012 Oct;26(5):551-62. [PMID: 23384801]

Item 3   Answer: B

Educational Objective: Diagnose constrictive pericarditis as a cause of ascites.

The most likely diagnosis is constrictive pericarditis. This patient has undergone previous cardiac surgery, which is a risk factor for constrictive pericarditis. Ascitic fluid analysis should include measurement of albumin and total protein; cell count and bacterial cultures should be checked when infection is suspected. The serum-ascites albumin gradient (SAAG) should be calculated by subtracting the ascitic fluid albumin level from the serum albumin level. The main factors that distinguish a cardiac source for ascites from other sources are a SAAG of 1.1 g/dL (11 g/L) or greater and an ascitic fluid total protein level of 2.5 g/dL (25 g/L) or greater. This patient meets these criteria, making a cardiac cause for his ascites likely. In addition, over 90% of patients with constrictive pericarditis have evidence of jugular venous distention and clear lungs on auscultation. Other less commonly observed findings include Kussmaul sign (rise in jugular pressure on inspiration), paradoxical pulse, and a pericardial knock on cardiac auscultation.

Patients with cirrhosis, portal hypertension, and resultant ascites will also have a SAAG greater than 1.1 g/dL (11 g/L), but the ascitic fluid total protein level will be less than 2.5 g/dL (25 g/L). Therefore, alcoholic and nonalcoholic cirrhosis are not the likely cause of this patient's ascites.

Tuberculous peritonitis is very uncommon and is associated with a SAAG less than 1.1 g/dL (11 g/L), an ascitic fluid total protein level greater than 3 g/dL (30 g/L), and a lymphocytic predominance in the cell count with differential. Although this patient has a high ascitic fluid total protein level, the SAAG is greater than 1.1 g/dL (11 g/L) and he does not have a predominance of lymphocytes on the ascitic fluid cell count.

> **KEY POINT**
>
> - A serum-ascites albumin gradient (SAAG) of 1.1 g/dL (11 g/L) or greater with an ascitic fluid total protein level of 2.5 g/dL (25 g/L) or greater indicates a cardiac cause of ascites.

Bibliography

Gordon FD. Ascites. Clin Liver Dis. 2012 May;16(2):285-99. [PMID: 22541699]

Item 4   Answer: D

Educational Objective: Diagnose pill-induced esophagitis.

The most likely diagnosis is pill-induced esophagitis. This patient has retrosternal chest pain after taking doxycycline for Lyme disease. Pill-induced esophagitis has been observed with alendronate, quinidine, tetracycline, doxycycline, potassium chloride, ferrous sulfate, and mexiletine. Pills typically cause local injury at sites of anatomic narrowing of the esophagus, such as the aortic arch, gastroesophageal junction, or the esophageal indentation caused by an enlarged left atrium. Clinical symptoms include chest pain, dysphagia, and odynophagia. Symptoms may begin hours to days after starting therapy, and stopping the medication will often lead to symptom relief. Preventive strategies to decrease pill-induced esophagitis are to drink plenty of water with the medication and avoid lying down for 30 minutes after ingestion.

Barrett esophagus (BE) is present when columnar epithelium replaces the normal squamous epithelium in the distal esophagus. BE is a consequence of gastroesophageal reflux disease (GERD) and by itself is often asymptomatic. There is nothing in this patient's clinical picture to suggest BE or GERD.

Patients with infectious esophagitis may be asymptomatic or may have odynophagia or dysphagia. Infectious esophagitis is typically caused by *Candida albicans*, herpes simplex virus, and cytomegalovirus. These infections typically occur in patients who are immunosuppressed owing to medications (such as glucocorticoids, azathioprine, or tumor necrosis factor-α inhibitors) or congenital or acquired immunodeficiencies. Use of swallowed aerosolized glucocorticoids may put an immunocompetent patient at risk for some of these infections. *Candida* infection is characterized by small, white, raised plaques on upper endoscopy, and esophageal brushings confirm the diagnosis. Pill-induced esophagitis is a much more likely diagnosis for this immunocompetent patient taking doxycycline than is *Candida* esophagitis.

Eosinophilic esophagitis (EoE) is defined as esophageal squamous mucosal inflammation caused by eosinophilic infiltration. EoE is usually seen in young men who present with dysphagia and a food-bolus obstruction. This patient does not have symptoms characteristic of EoE.

> **KEY POINT**
>
> - Pill-induced esophagitis is characterized by chest pain, dysphagia, and odynophagia and has been associated with alendronate, quinidine, tetracycline, doxycycline, potassium chloride, ferrous sulfate, and mexiletine.

Bibliography

Geagea A, Cellier C. Scope of drug-induced, infectious and allergic esophageal injury. Curr Opin Gastroenterol. 2008 Jul;24(4):496-501. [PMID: 18622166]

Item 5   Answer: A

Educational Objective: Treat spontaneous bacterial peritonitis.

The most appropriate treatment is cefotaxime and albumin. This patient has been hospitalized with overt hepatic encephalopathy, which in many instances may be the sole presenting feature of spontaneous bacterial peritonitis (SBP). It is important to perform a diagnostic paracentesis in patients with ascites who are admitted to the hospital, especially those with overt hepatic encephalopathy. This patient's ascitic fluid analysis demonstrates a polymorphonuclear cell count of 820/μL, which exceeds the diagnostic threshold for SBP of 250/μL. The most important therapeutic intervention at this time is treatment of SBP, which precipitated this patient's hepatic encephalopathy. Appropriate treatment of SBP consists of a systemic antibiotic and intravenous albumin. For patients without nosocomial SBP or recent exposure to β-lactams, intravenous cefotaxime is the drug of choice. Patients with a serum creatinine level greater than 1 mg/dL (88.4 μmol/L), a serum bilirubin level greater than 4 mg/dL (68.4 μmol/L), or a blood urea nitrogen level greater than 30 mg/dL (10.7 mmol/L) should receive 1.5 g/kg of intravenous albumin (25%) on the day of diagnosis and 1 g/kg of albumin on day 3; this practice has demonstrated a survival benefit.

Cefotaxime and normal saline are not appropriate because this patient's survival will be improved with the use of intravenous albumin, whereas use of normal saline may result in worsening ascites.

Norfloxacin (or ciprofloxacin) is effective for secondary prevention of SBP and should be given to this patient indefinitely after completion of intravenous cefotaxime. However, norfloxacin is a poorly absorbed second-generation fluoroquinolone that is not appropriate for treatment of newly diagnosed SBP.

Treatment of overt hepatic encephalopathy is aimed at treating the underlying precipitant, in this case SBP. In these cases treatment consists of administering lactulose to achieve two to three, soft, formed bowel movements per day. Rifaximin is FDA approved for maintenance of remission in patients with previous episodes of overt hepatic encephalopathy, but it is not approved for initial treatment of overt hepatic encephalopathy or as treatment for SBP.

KEY POINT

- Appropriate treatment of spontaneous bacterial peritonitis consists of a third-generation cephalosporin and, in many patients, intravenous albumin.

Bibliography

Runyon BA; AASLD. Introduction to the revised American Association for the Study of Liver Diseases Practice Guideline management of adult patients with ascites due to cirrhosis 2012. Hepatology. 2013 Apr;57(4):1651-3. [PMID: 23463403]

Item 6   Answer: D

Educational Objective: Evaluate dyspepsia with alarm features.

The most appropriate management is further investigation with upper endoscopy. Guidelines recommend upper endoscopy for patients with dyspepsia and alarm features. Alarm features include onset after age 50 years; anemia; dysphagia; odynophagia; vomiting; weight loss; family history of upper gastrointestinal malignancy; personal history of peptic ulcer disease, gastric surgery, or gastrointestinal malignancy; and abdominal mass or lymphadenopathy on examination. For patients younger than 50 years without alarm features, a test-and-treat approach for *Helicobacter pylori* is reasonable and cost effective when the patient is from an area where the prevalence of *H. pylori* is high (such as developing countries). However, a proton pump inhibitor is the most appropriate first-line strategy if the patient is from an area where the prevalence of *H. pylori* is low. Endoscopic evaluation should be reserved for those who do not respond to therapy. Cost-effective tests for *H. pylori* include urea breath testing and fecal antigen testing. This patient with uninvestigated dyspepsia has multiple alarm features, including age, progressive symptoms of recent onset, nausea, change in eating habits, weight loss, and anemia. These alarm features warrant prompt structural evaluation.

Although *H. pylori* gastritis is a possibility in this patient, empiric treatment of *H. pylori* infection is not an appropriate management strategy in patients with uninvestigated dyspepsia with alarm features.

An empiric trial of omeprazole would not be appropriate because it may mask a gastric ulcer or cancer. Given this patient's alarm features, a structural evaluation of the upper gastrointestinal tract should be performed before a trial of PPI therapy.

The serologic antibody test for *H. pylori* does not accurately identify active infection. Furthermore, treatment for a positive antibody may mask a more serious upper gastrointestinal condition such as an ulcer or gastric cancer.

KEY POINT

- Upper endoscopy is recommended for the exclusion of upper gastrointestinal structural causes of dyspepsia; it should be performed in patients who have alarm features.

Bibliography

Graham DY, Rugge M. Clinical practice: diagnosis and evaluation of dyspepsia. J Clin Gastroenterol. 2010 Mar;44(3):167-72. [PMID: 20009950]

Item 7   Answer: A

Educational Objective: Evaluate for ulcerative colitis in a patient with primary sclerosing cholangitis.

The most appropriate next step in management is colonoscopy. Primary sclerosing cholangitis (PSC) is diagnosed by measuring liver enzymes and performing cholangiography.

Serum alkaline phosphatase values are 3 to 10 times the upper limit of normal, and serum alanine aminotransferase and aspartate aminotransferase levels are two to three times the upper limit of normal. Serum total bilirubin levels may be normal in 60% of patients. Serum antinuclear and anti-smooth muscle antibodies are present in 20% to 50% of patients, but antimitochondrial antibodies are rarely found in PSC. The gold standard for diagnosis of PSC is cholangiography. Diagnostic findings consist of segmental bile duct fibrosis with saccular dilatation of normal intervening areas, resulting in the characteristic "beads on a string" appearance. Magnetic resonance cholangiopancreatography (MRCP) has been increasingly used and has an overall diagnostic accuracy rate of 90%. This patient's clinical presentation and cholangiographic findings are consistent with PSC. Eighty percent of patients with PSC have ulcerative colitis. Given this patient's 3-year history of diarrhea, colonoscopy should be performed to evaluate for ulcerative colitis. Patients with PSC and ulcerative colitis are at increased risk for colon cancer and should receive surveillance. There is no effective medical therapy for PSC. Endoscopic dilatation of biliary strictures and removal of stones may be necessary in patients with progressive cholestasis or symptoms of cholangitis. PSC is generally a progressive disease that often requires liver transplantation.

MRCP has already been performed; endoscopic retrograde cholangiopancreatography (ERCP) will not add any additional useful information to the clinical picture. ERCP will be useful in managing choledocholithiasis, occurring in 10% to 25% of symptomatic patients, and dilatation of dominant strictures, occurring in 5% to 10% of patients.

Liver biopsy is usually not necessary for the diagnosis of PSC. Liver biopsy is required for making a diagnosis of small-duct PSC when cholangiography is normal. Periductal fibrosis with inflammation, bile duct proliferation, and ductopenia are the main histologic findings.

IgG4-associated cholangitis may mimic PSC, but patients will usually have abnormalities in the pancreas on cross-sectional imaging. This patient did not have these findings, so serum IgG4 measurement is not required.

KEY POINT

- Eighty percent of patients with primary sclerosing cholangitis have ulcerative colitis.

Bibliography

Chapman R, Fevery J, Kalloo A, et al; American Association for the Study of Liver Diseases. Diagnosis and management of primary sclerosing cholangitis. Hepatology. 2010 Feb;51(2):660-78. [PMID: 20101749]

Item 8 Answer: A

Educational Objective: Manage upper gastrointestinal bleeding caused by a high-risk ulcer.

The most appropriate management is endoscopic therapy. Upper endoscopy should be performed at the time of an upper gastrointestinal bleed after appropriate volume resuscitation to diagnose the cause of bleeding, provide a prognosis, and provide endoscopic therapy if required. An ulcer with a visible vessel has an approximately 50% risk of rebleeding if not treated endoscopically. These ulcers can be effectively treated with injection of sclerosants, thermal coagulation via endoscopic probes, or mechanical modalities such as hemostatic clips. Clean-based ulcers rebleed in less than 5% of cases and do not require endoscopic therapy.

Prospective trials have shown a 5% to 10% rebleeding rate following endoscopic hemostasis. In these patients, endoscopic therapy may be repeated if the patient remains hemodynamically stable and if the endoscopist thinks that the bleeding lesion is amenable to endoscopic therapy. If repeat endoscopy is unsuccessful or the bleeding vessel is inaccessible or too large, surgical consultation should be obtained. However, in this patient, endoscopic intervention is the first management choice for an accessible and small visible vessel.

Octreotide may have a marginal benefit by decreasing the rate of nonvariceal bleeding, but it is inferior to intravenous proton pump inhibitors. Octreotide is most useful in patients with variceal bleeding.

Observation is not appropriate for this patient with a high-risk lesion seen on endoscopy. Without endoscopic therapy, patients with this type of lesion have a 30% to 50% chance of rebleeding.

KEY POINT

- High-risk ulcers are characterized by active arterial spurting or a nonbleeding visible vessel; they should be treated endoscopically with hemostatic clips, thermal therapy, or injection of sclerosants.

Bibliography

Barkun AN, Bardou M, Kuipers EJ, et al; International Consensus Upper Gastrointestinal Bleeding Conference Group. International consensus recommendations on the management of patients with nonvariceal upper gastrointestinal bleeding. Ann Intern Med. 2010 Jan 19;152(2):101-13. [PMID: 20083829]

Item 9 Answer: D

Educational Objective: Treat acute kidney injury in the context of cirrhosis with a colloid fluid challenge.

The most appropriate treatment for acute kidney injury in this patient is 25% albumin. This patient has acute kidney injury (AKI) and hepatic encephalopathy, most likely precipitated by dehydration from lactulose-induced diarrhea. AKI is common and occurs in approximately 20% of hospitalized patients with cirrhosis. In approximately 70% of patients with cirrhosis and AKI, the precipitant is prerenal, from sources such as infection, gastrointestinal bleeding, excessive diuresis, or diarrhea. This patient has dry mucous membranes, diarrhea, and no obvious signs of infection or bleeding and has been treated with diuretics. Approximately two thirds of patients with prerenal AKI are fluid responsive. After stopping diuretics and lactulose, the best initial treatment is intravenous colloid administration, usually in the form of 25% albumin, administered at 1 g/kg body weight per day in divided doses.

The other third of patients who are not fluid responsive generally have type 1 or type 2 hepatorenal syndrome (HRS). HRS diagnostic criteria consist of (1) an increase in the serum creatinine level to greater than 1.5 g/dL (132.6 µmol/L) over days to weeks, (2) lack of response to an albumin challenge of 1 g/kg/d for 2 days, and (3) the absence of shock, nephrotoxic drugs, active urine sediment, proteinuria greater than 500 mg/d, and ultrasound evidence of parenchymal kidney disease or obstruction. Although this patient could have evolving HRS, this cannot be diagnosed until fluid responsiveness has been evaluated. If she is not fluid responsive and does not have evidence of acute tubular necrosis on urinalysis, then treatment for type 1 HRS could begin. Norepinephrine with albumin infusion is effective for patients with type 1 HRS who are in the ICU. Midodrine, octreotide, and albumin are the appropriate treatments for type 1 HRS in patients outside of the ICU. Terlipressin is effective for type 1 HRS but is not available in the United States.

KEY POINT

- Acute kidney injury occurs in approximately 20% of hospitalized patients with cirrhosis; such patients should receive a fluid challenge (usually with 25% albumin) to evaluate fluid responsiveness before hepatorenal syndrome can be diagnosed.

Bibliography

Garcia-Tsao G, Parikh CR, Viola A. Acute kidney injury in cirrhosis. Hepatology. 2008 Dec;48(6):2064-77. [PMID: 19003880]

Item 10   Answer: C

Educational Objective: Manage acute cholangitis.

The most appropriate management is endoscopic retrograde cholangiopancreatography (ERCP). The presence of fever, abdominal pain, and jaundice (Charcot triad) is consistent with acute cholangitis, and ERCP is indicated. Dilation of the extrahepatic and intrahepatic bile ducts on abdominal ultrasound or noncontrast CT scan is consistent with a diagnosis of choledocholithiasis, although dilated bile ducts may not be identified in patients with acute biliary obstruction. Acute cholangitis is usually caused by *Escherichia coli*, *Klebsiella* species, *Pseudomonas* species, and enterococci and can progress to septic shock with or without liver abscess formation. Empiric antibiotics targeting these likely organisms should be administered immediately when cholangitis is suspected. If improvement is not seen rapidly, urgent ERCP should be performed to remove the common bile duct stone. When duct decompression with ERCP is not possible, percutaneous cholangiography with biliary tube placement can be performed.

Abdominal CT is not appropriate because it would delay ERCP, which is needed urgently. In addition, it would not add much useful information to this patient's ultrasound findings.

Cholecystectomy will remove the source of future gallstones, but it will not decompress this patient's obstructed common bile duct or reduce her risk of dying from sepsis. Cholecystectomy will eventually be recommended for this patient; however, it must be delayed until the cholangitis is resolved.

Percutaneous cholecystostomy could be considered if this patient had acute cholecystitis, but her clinical history suggests common bile duct obstruction rather than simple cystic duct obstruction. The pain of acute cholecystitis typically lasts longer than 3 hours and shifts to the right upper quadrant, causing localized tenderness. The pain is due to gallbladder distention, ongoing gallbladder contraction against the obstructed outlet, and occasionally bacterial infection, leading to inflammation of the gallbladder wall. Fever, nausea, and vomiting are frequent findings, but jaundice is unusual. Findings of gallbladder inflammation may include thickening of the gallbladder wall (>2 mm), intramural gas, and pericholecystic fluid. These findings are not present in this patient.

KEY POINT

- Patients with cholangitis should receive immediate broad-spectrum antimicrobial therapy; if rapid improvement is not seen, urgent endoscopic stone removal should be performed.

Bibliography

Khashab MA, Tariq A, Tariq U, et al. Delayed and unsuccessful endoscopic retrograde cholangiopancreatography are associated with worse outcomes in patients with acute cholangitis. Clin Gastroenterol Hepatol. 2012 Oct;10(10):1157-61. [PMID: 22507875]

Item 11   Answer: C

Educational Objective: Provide the appropriate prevention strategy for NSAID-induced injury.

The most appropriate management is to start standard-dose omeprazole (20 mg/d). The chronic use of NSAIDs is associated with significant gastrointestinal risk. Nearly one in four chronic NSAID users will develop ulcer disease and as many as 4% will have bleeding or perforation complications. Risk factors for NSAID-related gastrointestinal complications include a history of peptic ulcer disease or other gastrointestinal bleeding event; *Helicobacter pylori* infection; age 65 years or older; concomitant use of aspirin (of any dose), anticoagulants, other NSAIDs, or glucocorticoids; high-dose NSAID use; and chronic comorbid illness. Although this patient is currently tolerating her daily NSAID well, she has several risk factors that put her at increased risk for NSAID-associated gastric injury (age older than 65 years and daily low-dose aspirin for cardiovascular risk reduction). Therefore, the most appropriate strategy for gastric protection is omeprazole, 20 mg/d. Standard-dose daily proton pump inhibitor (PPI) therapy has consistently demonstrated superiority to placebo in significantly reducing the risk of NSAID-induced gastric injury. Higher PPI doses have not demonstrated superiority to standard-dose therapy. If PPI therapy cannot be used, misoprostol, 200 µg four times daily, is an alternative; however, side effects such as abdominal cramps and diarrhea may be limiting.

Changing this patient's aspirin to an enteric-coated formulation will not reduce the risk of NSAID-induced gastrointestinal injury.

Answers and Critiques

Given this patient's risk profile, preventive measures should be pursued. Therefore, continued observation alone on the current medication regimen is not appropriate.

> **KEY POINT**
>
> • Standard-dose daily proton pump inhibitor therapy significantly reduces the risk of NSAID-induced gastric injury.

Bibliography

Lanza FL, Chan FK, Quigley EM; Practice Parameters Committee of the American College of Gastroenterology. Guidelines for prevention of NSAID-related ulcer complications. Am J Gastroenterol. 2009 Mar;104(3): 728-38. [PMID: 19240698]

Item 12   Answer: D

Educational Objective: Treat chronic pancreatitis with pancreatic enzymes.

The most appropriate treatment is pancreatic enzymes. This patient has steatorrhea and evidence of malnutrition (temporal wasting, poor dentition, hypoalbuminemia, and weight loss) that is attributable to exocrine pancreatic insufficiency from chronic pancreatitis. This diagnosis is based on established risk factors (past heavy and sustained alcohol use and cigarette smoking), clinical features (previous attacks of pancreatitis, current weight loss), and objective findings (pancreatic calcifications and steatorrhea). Exocrine insufficiency is treated using enteric-coated pancreatic enzymes. Steatorrhea that persists despite enzyme replacement may be treated by increasing the dose to 90,000 units of lipase per meal; confirming the diagnosis of pancreatic insufficiency by performing direct pancreatic function testing (if available); and excluding nonpancreatic causes, including bacterial overgrowth, celiac disease, and terminal ileal disease. Fat-soluble vitamin replacement is also important. Endocrine insufficiency can be difficult to manage because patients with chronic pancreatitis often lose counter-regulatory hormones such as glucagon when their islet cells are destroyed, rendering their plasma glucose levels more labile. If diabetes mellitus occurs, it should be treated with insulin.

Loperamide and fiber are symptomatic therapies for chronic diarrhea. These are not appropriate in this patient because they do not treat the cause of steatorrhea or the associated weight loss and malnutrition.

A gluten-free diet is not appropriate because this patient's serologic testing for celiac disease was negative. Celiac disease is an established risk factor for acute and chronic pancreatitis and a cause of steatorrhea.

> **KEY POINT**
>
> • Common criteria for diagnosis of chronic pancreatitis consist of clinical features (pain, recurrent attacks of pancreatitis, weight loss) with objective findings of steatorrhea and pancreatic calcifications.

Bibliography

Forsmark CE. Management of chronic pancreatitis. Gastroenterology. 2013 Jun;144(6):1282-91.e3. [PMID: 23622138]

Item 13   Answer: C

Educational Objective: Evaluate for celiac disease in a patient with chronic diarrhea.

The most appropriate diagnostic test to perform next is testing for serum tissue transglutaminase antibodies. This patient has chronic diarrhea with clinical evidence of steatorrhea, the differential diagnosis of which includes small-bowel mucosal diseases, pancreatic insufficiency, small intestinal bacterial overgrowth, and lymphatic obstruction. Celiac disease is a chronic inflammatory enteropathy caused by an immune-mediated reaction to gluten and gliadins and is present in 0.5% to 1% of the U.S. population. The chronic diarrhea, abdominal pain, and malabsorption present in this patient suggest this diagnosis, and the initial step is testing for serologic markers for the disease. IgA tissue transglutaminase antibody is the screening test of choice for celiac disease and is both sensitive and specific; initial testing for celiac disease should be done while the patient is consuming gluten.

While anti-*Saccharomyces cerevisiae* antibodies (ASCA) have been proposed as a serologic method for differentiating Crohn disease from ulcerative colitis, they are neither adequately sensitive nor specific and can lead to false-positive results if used as a screening test for gastrointestinal symptoms. There is no role for ASCA in the evaluation of a patient with suspected celiac disease.

Endoscopy (flexible sigmoidoscopy or colonoscopy) can be an important test in evaluating selected patients with chronic diarrhea, but it would not be the most appropriate next study in this patient with diarrhea with a high pretest probability of celiac disease given his history of type 1 diabetes mellitus with clear evidence of malabsorption. Flexible sigmoidoscopy in particular would only visualize the distal aspects of the colon, and because colonic disorders do not cause malabsorption, this test would not be diagnostic in this patient. A positive tissue transglutaminase test and confirmation of celiac disease as the cause of diarrhea in this patient would make colonoscopy unnecessary and avoid the potential risks of the procedure.

Upper endoscopy with small-bowel biopsies is performed in patients with a consistent clinical picture and positive serologic studies to confirm the diagnosis of celiac disease. Characteristic biopsy findings include intraepithelial lymphocytosis, crypt hyperplasia, and villous blunting. However, upper endoscopy with biopsies would not be indicated as an initial study in patients suspected of having celiac disease.

Video capsule endoscopy can visualize the small-bowel mucosa and might show nonspecific changes in a patient with suspected celiac disease; however, it is not indicated as an initial diagnostic study before serologic testing or for confirmation if the patient is a candidate for routine upper endoscopy with biopsy.

> **KEY POINT**
>
> • Serologic testing for tissue transglutaminase antibodies should be performed in patients with suspected celiac disease, which may present with weight loss, steatorrhea, and nutritional deficiencies.

Bibliography

Schiller LR. Definitions, pathophysiology, and evaluation of chronic diarrhoea. Best Pract Res Clin Gastroenterol. 2012 Oct;26(5):551-62. [PMID: 23384801]

Item 14   Answer: D

Educational Objective: Diagnose irritable bowel syndrome.

The most appropriate management is reassurance and patient education that addresses the diagnosis and treatment of irritable bowel syndrome (IBS). The American College of Gastroenterology recommends a simple definition of IBS: abdominal pain or discomfort that occurs in association with altered bowel habits over a period of at least 3 months. The diagnosis of IBS is further subtyped into diarrhea predominant (IBS-D), constipation predominant (IBS-C), or mixed (IBS-M), which alternates between diarrhea and constipation. This young woman has symptoms that fulfill diagnostic criteria for IBS-C in the absence of any alarm features. A recent evidence-based review by the American College of Gastroenterology IBS task force concluded that, in such a setting, no further biochemical or structural testing is indicated given the low yield of testing. The routine pursuit of a complete blood count, serum chemistry studies, thyroid function studies, stool studies for ova and parasites, and abdominal imaging is unnecessary in this setting. An essential initial step in management of IBS is the clear establishment of the diagnosis with explanation of and reassurance regarding the patient's symptoms. In addition to reassurance, over-the-counter remedies addressing constipation or diarrheal symptoms can be recommended, as these agents are safe and potentially effective. In this patient, the osmotic laxative polyethylene glycol is likely to be well tolerated and to improve this patient's constipation symptoms.

This patient has no symptoms of diarrhea or blood in the stool, and there is no family history of colon cancer to justify a colonoscopy. The passage of mucus is commonly reported in IBS, so this symptom alone does not warrant colonoscopy.

The typical features of celiac disease are diarrhea, bloating, and weight loss. A tissue transglutaminase serologic study would be a reasonable screening test for celiac disease in a patient with IBS-D, but it is not necessary in patients with IBS-C.

KEY POINT

- Routine complete blood count, serum chemistry studies, thyroid function studies, stool studies for ova and parasites, and abdominal imaging are unnecessary in establishing the diagnosis of irritable bowel syndrome.

Bibliography

American College of Gastroenterology Task Force on Irritable Bowel Syndrome, Brandt LJ, Chey WD, Foxx-Orenstein AE, et al. An evidence-based position statement on the management of irritable bowel syndrome. Am J Gastroenterol. 2009 Jan;104 Suppl 1:S1-35. [PMID: 19521341]

Item 15   Answer: C

Educational Objective: Diagnose *Helicobacter pylori* infection in a patient at high risk using the appropriate test.

The most appropriate management is noninvasive *Helicobacter pylori* testing, followed by eradication therapy if test results are positive. Noninvasive *H. pylori* testing modalities include serology, the fecal antigen test, or the urea breath test. The recommended and most cost-effective approach for this patient is serologic testing. He is younger than 50 years of age with vague abdominal discomfort without alarm features (anemia; dysphagia; odynophagia; vomiting; weight loss; family history of upper gastrointestinal malignancy; personal history of peptic ulcer disease, gastric surgery, or gastrointestinal malignancy; and abdominal mass or lymphadenopathy on examination), and, most importantly, he has been residing in an area where the prevalence of *H. pylori* is high (a developing country). Serologic testing for *H. pylori* has limitations in that it does not test for active *H. pylori* infection and has poor positive predictive value. Therefore, positive serologic results must be interpreted with caution when performed in populations with a low background prevalence of *H. pylori*, such as those in developed countries. Fecal antigen testing and urea breath testing offer a more accurate means of noninvasive testing for *H. pylori*, as both of these test modalities assess for the presence of active infection. Therefore, these testing modalities should be used to test for *H. pylori* in individuals for whom the background prevalence of *H. pylori* is low. Although these tests are more expensive and logistically more complicated than serology, they offer greater testing accuracy. Fecal antigen and urea breath tests are equivalent in terms of their accuracy. The choice of fecal antigen testing versus urea breath testing will typically depend on test availability and patient preference.

A barium esophagogram would have limited utility in this patient with dyspepsia and no associated symptoms consistent with esophageal disease, such as acid brash, dysphagia, and odynophagia. Even with these symptoms, an empiric trial of a proton pump inhibitor could be considered consider prior to imaging with a barium esophagogram.

Empiric treatment for *H. pylori* is not appropriate because the diagnosis of *H. pylori* should be made before initiating treatment. Empiric therapy for *H. pylori* is expensive and carries the potential harm of medication side effects; therefore, it would not be indicated without first confirming active infection.

Upper endoscopy would be appropriate for patients whose symptoms do not respond to *H. pylori* treatment or PPI therapy. Patients older than 50 years or with alarm features should be evaluated with upper endoscopy. In patients without alarm features, endoscopy as an initial management intervention would be unlikely to find gastritis, peptic ulcer disease, or esophagitis.

KEY POINT

- Before pursuing *Helicobacter pylori* eradication therapy, noninvasive testing for *H. pylori* should be performed to confirm infection.

Answers and Critiques

Bibliography

McColl KE. Clinical practice. Helicobacter pylori infection. N Engl J Med. 2010 Apr 29;362(17):1597-604. [PMID: 20427808]

Item 16   Answer: D

Educational Objective: Diagnose Wilson disease presenting as acute liver failure.

The most likely diagnosis is Wilson disease. Wilson disease is a rare congenital disorder of copper excretion that occurs in approximately 1 in 30,000 live births. Young patients with Wilson disease tend to present with acute liver failure; older patients present with chronic liver disease and/or neurologic manifestations. Wilson disease should be considered in all patients younger than 40 years of age who have unexplained liver disease. When Wilson disease causes acute hepatitis, usually in young patients, the sudden release of copper from liver cells can also induce hemolytic anemia. This patient's low hemoglobin level, increased reticulocyte count, and elevated indirect bilirubin level support the diagnosis of hemolytic anemia. The presence of a low alkaline phosphatase level (copper interferes with the synthesis of alkaline phosphatase enzymes), a moderate elevation of aminotransferase levels despite other evidence of liver dysfunction, and hemolytic anemia make Wilson disease likely. The most common screening test for Wilson disease is serum ceruloplasmin, which is reduced; elevated urine excretion of copper is ascertained to verify the presumptive diagnosis of Wilson disease. In a young patient with elevated liver test results, a low ceruloplasmin level, and elevated urine copper excretion, liver biopsy is typically obtained to confirm the diagnosis of Wilson disease. Liver biopsy demonstrates excessive intrahepatic copper. Kayser-Fleischer rings, noted on ophthalmologic examination, indicate copper deposition in the Descemet membrane of the iris. Patients with acute liver failure due to Wilson disease rarely recover and should be urgently referred for liver transplantation.

Acetaminophen hepatotoxicity and herpes hepatitis present with very high aminotransferase levels, often over 5000 U/L. This patient's aminotransferase levels are not compatible with these conditions.

Budd-Chiari syndrome, characterized by an obstruction of hepatic venous outflow, can occasionally present with acute liver failure but has ascites as a predominant clinical manifestation. This patient does not have ascites, which makes Budd-Chiari syndrome unlikely.

KEY POINT

- Wilson disease should be considered in all patients younger than 40 years of age who have unexplained liver disease.

Bibliography

Eapen CE, Kumar S, Fleming JJ, Ramakrishna B, Abraham L, Ramachandran J. Copper and liver disease. Gut. 2012 Jan;61(1):63. Erratum in: Gut. 2012 May;61(5):773. [PMID: 22139599]

Item 17   Answer: B

Educational Objective: Manage gallbladder polyps.

The most appropriate management is cholecystectomy. The finding of a gallbladder polyp larger than 1 cm is an indication for cholecystectomy, even if the patient is asymptomatic. Gallbladder polyps are found in approximately 5% of ultrasound examinations. Although only a small percentage of gallbladder polyps are neoplastic (adenoma or adenocarcinoma), the risk for neoplasia increases as polyp size increases. In the absence of gallstones, a gallbladder polyp smaller than 1 cm can be followed with serial ultrasound examinations unless the patient is symptomatic or has primary sclerosing cholangitis. For patients with gallstones and any size polyp, cholecystectomy is usually recommended.

Further imaging with abdominal CT, endoscopic retrograde cholangiopancreatography, or magnetic resonance cholangiopancreatography is not necessary in this patient because she has an asymptomatic, incidental gallbladder polyp; however, these tests should be considered if this patient had symptoms or elevated liver chemistry tests suggesting bile duct obstruction or malignancy.

KEY POINT

- The finding of a gallbladder polyp larger than 1 cm is an indication for cholecystectomy, even if the patient is asymptomatic.

Bibliography

Gallahan WC, Conway JD. Diagnosis and management of gallbladder polyps. Gastroenterol Clin North Am. 2010 Jun;39(2):359-67, x. [PMID: 20478491]

Item 18   Answer: A

Educational Objective: Treat acute pancreatitis caused by gallstones.

The most appropriate management is to perform cholecystectomy for gallstone-induced acute pancreatitis prior to hospital discharge. In the United States, 80% of cases of acute pancreatitis are caused by gallstones or alcohol use. The pathophysiology of gallstone-induced pancreatitis is likely related to gallstone obstruction of the common channel (bile-pancreatic duct) or reflux of bile into the pancreatic duct owing to impaction of the stone at the ampulla. Elevation of the alanine aminotransferase concentration is the most clinically useful laboratory test predicting gallstone pancreatitis. In addition, this patient has evidence of gallstones on ultrasonography. Patients with gallstone pancreatitis and no complications should have a cholecystectomy prior to discharge to prevent recurrent attacks. Delaying cholecystectomy is warranted to reduce the risk of sepsis and complications in patients with severe acute pancreatitis, particularly with pancreatic necrosis and acute peripancreatic fluid collections.

Cholecystokinin hepatobiliary (CCK-HIDA) scintigraphy is most commonly used for evaluation of cholecystitis, biliary obstruction, and suspected gallbladder dysfunction.

CONT.

This is not appropriate for this patient because he has no ultrasound evidence of cholecystitis.

Endoscopic retrograde cholangiopancreatography (ERCP) and biliary sphincterotomy are not indicated in the absence of cholangitis or nonresolving biliary obstruction unless the patient is not a surgical candidate for cholecystectomy. Obstruction is typically indicated by a dilated bile duct and persistently elevated liver enzyme levels.

Antibiotics should be reserved for treatment of cholangitis, acute cholecystitis, or other infections, which are absent in this patient. Cholangitis typically presents with fever, jaundice, and pain in the right upper quadrant (Charcot triad). Most patients will have cholelithiasis, elevated aminotransferase levels, and hyperbilirubinemia. Ultrasonography may show a dilated common bile duct. Findings of cholecystitis may include thickening of the gallbladder wall (>2 mm), intramural gas, and pericholecystic fluid. Hepatobiliary scintigraphy is indicated to confirm or exclude the diagnosis of acute cholecystitis when the initial ultrasound is indeterminate.

KEY POINT

- Patients with uncomplicated gallstone-induced acute pancreatitis should undergo cholecystectomy prior to hospital discharge to prevent recurrent attacks.

Bibliography

Tenner S, Baillie J, DeWitt J, Vege SS; American College of Gastroenterology. American College of Gastroenterology guideline: management of acute pancreatitis. Am J Gastroenterol. 2013 Sep;108(9):1400-15; 1416. [PMID: 23896955]

Item 19   Answer: A

Educational Objective: Treat Crohn disease in a pregnant patient.

The most appropriate treatment is certolizumab. The previously used treatment approach for Crohn disease (CD) was to (1) initiate therapy with 5-aminosalicylate drugs such as mesalamine at diagnosis; (2) begin thiopurine therapy with azathioprine or 6-mercaptopurine if a patient requires repeated courses of glucocorticoids; and (3) begin therapy with anti–tumor necrosis factor (anti-TNF) agents if these other therapies are unsuccessful. This paradigm has been challenged by newer studies showing that 5-aminosalicylates have only minimal, if any, efficacy in CD, and the success of treatment is significantly higher when anti-TNF therapy is begun alone or in combination with thiopurines earlier in the disease course. Many experts have abandoned the use of 5-aminosalicylates entirely for CD except perhaps for those with mild Crohn colitis. The decision to use thiopurine or anti-TNF monotherapy versus combination therapy is based on an individual patient's severity of symptoms and risk factors for developing complications of their disease balanced against the potential side effects of these treatments. This patient with new-onset CD is in her first trimester of pregnancy. Treatment with an anti-TNF agent is effective for induction and maintenance of remission in CD and is generally considered to be safe during pregnancy (FDA pregnancy category B). The three anti-TNF agents approved for CD are infliximab, adalimumab, and certolizumab. Because certolizumab is pegylated, it should have very little, if any, placental transfer and therefore is favored by some clinicians in a pregnant patient over the other two agents. Although endoscopic procedures are generally avoided in pregnant patients unless absolutely necessary, flexible sigmoidoscopy is safer than colonoscopy, and in this patient it was useful to confirm that her symptoms are due to active CD before committing her to expensive immunosuppressive medications.

Antibiotics are generally not recommended for induction of remission in CD because no particular class of drug can be endorsed based on available data. Furthermore, ciprofloxacin (pregnancy category C) should be used in pregnancy only if the potential benefits outweigh the risk to the fetus. Metronidazole is a pregnancy category B drug.

Controlled ileal-release budesonide is effective for ileocolonic CD, but it would not be effective in this patient with left-sided colitis. In addition, it is classified as category C for use during pregnancy.

Mesalamine may be used to treat ulcerative colitis, but it is not effective in most patients with CD.

Methotrexate may be effective for inducing and maintaining remission in CD, but it is contraindicated during pregnancy. Methotrexate is a classified as category X for use in pregnancy because it may cause fetal death and/or congenital abnormalities.

KEY POINT

- Treatment with an anti–tumor necrosis factor agent is effective for induction and maintenance of remission in Crohn disease and is generally considered to be safe during pregnancy (FDA pregnancy category B).

Bibliography

Ng SW, Mahadevan U. Management of inflammatory bowel disease in pregnancy. Expert Rev Clin Immunol. 2013 Feb;9(2):161-73; quiz 174. [PMID: 23390947]

Item 20   Answer: D

Educational Objective: Treat functional dyspepsia.

The most appropriate management is to start nortriptyline. This patient has functional dyspepsia (FD), a chronic symptom complex consisting of epigastric pain/discomfort, postprandial fullness, and/or early satiety in the absence of a structural explanation. No universally effective therapy exists, but a variety of treatments are effective in subgroups of FD. Treatment strategies must carefully weigh the therapeutic benefits with the side effects of therapy. Given the low risk of side effects, initial treatment strategies include treatment of *Helicobacter pylori* infection, proton pump inhibitor (PPI) therapy, or H$_2$-blocker therapy. Although generally well tolerated, these treatment strategies frequently fail to adequately alleviate symptoms. In particular, treatment for *H. pylori* is unlikely to be beneficial in this patient with negative test results. Clinical trials have not demonstrated an added benefit of high-dose PPI therapy compared with standard-dose therapy. Therefore, increasing omeprazole to twice daily would not be beneficial for this patient. Additionally, switching from PPI to H_2-blocker therapy is of little benefit given these agents' similar physiologic effect on gastric acid production. Tricyclic antidepressants (TCA) are generally well tolerated, with response rates as high as 70% in small, marginal-quality trials. Despite these limitations, the efficacy and side-effect profile make a trial of a low-dose TCA such as nortriptyline an attractive treatment strategy when symptoms do not respond to PPIs or H_2 blockers. Therefore, nortriptyline is the most appropriate management.

Narcotics such as hydrocodone have no role in the treatment of FD and are likely to promote side effects as well as dependence.

The prokinetic agent metoclopramide has demonstrated limited efficacy. The benefits of its use should be weighed against the substantial risk of potential neurologic side effects, which include akathisia (nervousness, restlessness, anxiety, agitation), parkinsonism (bradykinesia, resting tremor, and rigidity), and tardive dyskinesia (involuntary, repetitive, tic-like movements that involve primarily the facial muscles but also the extremities, digits, hips, or torso).

KEY POINT

- A low-dose tricyclic antidepressant may be effective in the treatment of functional dyspepsia when symptoms do not respond to proton pump inhibitor or H_2-blocker therapy.

Bibliography

Lacy BE, Talley NJ, Locke GR 3rd, et al. Review article: current treatment options and management of functional dyspepsia. Aliment Pharmacol Ther. 2012 Jul;36(1):3-15. [PMID: 22591037]

Item 21   Answer: D

Educational Objective: Manage nonalcoholic fatty liver disease.

The most appropriate management is weight loss. This patient has nonalcoholic fatty liver disease (NAFLD), and weight loss should be recommended. NAFLD is the most common cause of abnormal liver test results in the United States. Approximately 30% of the U.S. population has NAFLD, some of whom have normal liver enzyme levels. Most patients with NAFLD have insulin resistance associated with obesity, hypertriglyceridemia, and/or type 2 diabetes mellitus. Approximately 20% of patients with NAFLD have nonalcoholic steatohepatitis (NASH), which is characterized by hepatic steatosis accompanied by inflammation and often fibrosis. Although NASH requires a liver biopsy for accurate diagnosis, a presumptive diagnosis can be made in a patient with mild abnormalities of aminotransferase levels, risk factors for NAFLD (such as diabetes, obesity, and hyperlipidemia), and imaging features consistent with hepatic steatosis. This patient's liver biopsy is consistent with steato-

hepatitis, and given his risk factors of obesity and diabetes mellitus, NAFLD is the most likely diagnosis.

Patients with NASH who have bariatric surgery and lose weight have improvement in hepatic histology, and bariatric surgery can be considered if conservative attempts at weight loss fail.

Patients with NAFLD may have abnormal iron tests, especially serum ferritin. The absence of iron on this patient's liver biopsy excludes significant iron overload, and therefore phlebotomy is unnecessary.

Patients with NASH and cirrhosis are at significant risk for hepatocellular carcinoma, and surveillance with imaging should be performed every 6 months; however, surveillance is not necessary in the absence of cirrhosis.

KEY POINT

- A presumptive diagnosis of nonalcoholic steatohepatitis can be made in a patient with mild abnormalities of aminotransferase levels, risk factors for nonalcoholic fatty liver disease (such as diabetes mellitus, obesity, and hyperlipidemia), and imaging features consistent with hepatic steatosis.

Bibliography

Chalasani N, Younossi Z, Lavine JE, et al; American Gastroenterological Association; American Association for the Study of Liver Diseases; American College of Gastroenterology. The diagnosis and management of non-alcoholic fatty liver disease: practice guideline by the American Gastroenterological Association, American Association for the Study of Liver Diseases, and American College of Gastroenterology. Gastroenterology. 2012 Jun;142(7):1592-609. Erratum in: Gastroenterology. 2012 Aug;143(2):503. [PMID: 22656328]

Item 22   Answer: B

Educational Objective: Provide colon cancer surveillance in a patient with ulcerative colitis.

The most appropriate colon cancer surveillance strategy is colonoscopy with biopsies beginning in 4 years and repeated every 1 to 2 years. Patients with inflammatory bowel disease have health risks related to their disease or its treatment. Patients with long-standing colitis are at increased risk for colon cancer and should undergo surveillance colonoscopy with biopsies every 1 to 2 years beginning after 8 to 10 years of disease. This recommendation applies to patients with ulcerative colitis involving more than the rectum and those with Crohn colitis involving at least one third of the colon. This patient should begin a surveillance program in approximately 4 years, when his ulcerative colitis has been present for 8 years. He has a single second-degree relative with colon cancer, but this does not affect the surveillance recommendation. Four-quadrant surveillance biopsies should be obtained every 10 cm beginning in the cecum, resulting in approximately 32 to 36 biopsies. In patients with inflammatory bowel disease and concomitant primary sclerosing cholangitis (PSC), the risk of colon cancer is particularly high, and it is recommended that such patients begin yearly surveillance as soon as the diagnosis of PSC is made. However, this patient has normal liver chemistry studies, which makes PSC unlikely.

For patients with Lynch syndrome (hereditary nonpolyposis colorectal cancer), recommended colorectal cancer screening is colonoscopy every 1 to 2 years beginning at age 20 to 25 years, or 2 to 5 years earlier than the youngest age at diagnosis of colorectal cancer if the affected relative was less than 25 years old.

Patients with ulcerative colitis involving the rectum are not at increased risk for colorectal cancer. In these patients, average-risk colorectal cancer screening with colonoscopy is recommended beginning at age 50 years and should be repeated every 10 years.

The 2012 American College of Physicians Guidance Statement on colorectal cancer screening recommends initiation of screening in high-risk patients (a first-degree relative with colon cancer or advanced adenoma diagnosed at age <60 years, or two first-degree relatives diagnosed at any age) at age 40 years, or 10 years younger than the earliest colon cancer diagnosis in the family, whichever is earlier. Colonoscopy is repeated every 5 years.

KEY POINT

- Patients with long-standing colitis associated with inflammatory bowel disease are at increased risk for colon cancer and should undergo surveillance colonoscopy every 1 to 2 years beginning after 8 to 10 years of disease.

Bibliography
Collins PD. Strategies for detecting colon cancer and dysplasia in patients with inflammatory bowel disease. Inflamm Bowel Dis. 2013 Mar-Apr;19(4):860-3. [PMID: 23446340]

Item 23   Answer: A

Educational Objective: Manage diverticulitis.

The most appropriate management for this woman with diverticulitis is treatment with oral antibiotics with home discharge and close clinical follow-up. The therapeutic approach to diverticulitis is dictated by patient-related factors, the severity of clinical features, and the ability to tolerate oral intake. In a healthy, immunocompetent patient with mild symptoms, outpatient therapy is appropriate and should consist of a liquid diet, oral antimicrobial agents that cover colonic organisms and include anaerobic coverage (such as ciprofloxacin and metronidazole), and as-needed analgesia. Close follow-up is warranted to detect any deterioration as soon as possible. For older, frail, sicker patients, and in those with potential complications of diverticulitis (such as peritonitis or fistula formation), hospitalization is recommended for administration of intravenous antimicrobial agents and observation. This patient with diverticulitis has mild symptoms and is otherwise healthy. She is able to maintain oral intake and can therefore be managed as an outpatient with oral antibiotics and close follow-up.

Surgery is pursued acutely only in patients who have free perforation or peritonitis, or in those for whom medical therapy is unsuccessful. If indicated, both laparoscopic and open procedures are options; laparoscopic treatment is associated with a more rapid recovery time. This patient does not have a current indication for surgical intervention.

Percutaneous drainage is typically indicated in patients with diverticulitis with larger abscesses (often considered to be >3 cm) that are procedurally amenable in those without evidence of peritonitis. Smaller abscesses are usually treated with antibiotics alone and close follow-up. This patient does not have evidence of an abscess on imaging; therefore, percutaneous drainage is not indicated.

Colonoscopy is recommended after recovery because diverticulitis may be precipitated by a sigmoid cancer; however, colonoscopy during an attack is contraindicated because it would be very difficult to insert the colonoscope beyond the area of inflammation and obtain adequate mucosal inspection. In addition, it may cause peritonitis.

KEY POINT

- In a healthy, immunocompetent patient with diverticulitis and mild symptoms, outpatient therapy is appropriate and should consist of a liquid diet, oral antimicrobial agents that cover colonic organisms and include anaerobic coverage (such as ciprofloxacin and metronidazole), and as-needed analgesia.

Bibliography
Wilkins T, Embry K, George R. Diagnosis and management of acute diverticulitis. Am Fam Physician. 2013 May 1;87(9):612-20. [PMID: 23668524]

Item 24   Answer: B

Educational Objective: Provide colonoscopy surveillance following a diagnosis of a serrated polyp.

Colonoscopy should be repeated in 3 years. The World Health Organization has classified serrated colorectal polyps into three categories: hyperplastic polyps, sessile serrated polyps, and traditional serrated adenomas. Hyperplastic polyps are believed to have no malignant potential, whereas sessile serrated polyps and traditional serrated adenomas are neoplastic. Sessile serrated polyps are thought to be the precursor of approximately 15% of sporadic colorectal cancers. Recent guidelines have established recommendations for postpolypectomy surveillance colonoscopy intervals in patients with serrated polyps; the rationale for postpolypectomy surveillance is to detect recurrent neoplasia. Patients with large (≥10 mm) or dysplastic sessile serrated polyps or traditional serrated adenomas should undergo colonoscopy in 3 years.

A 1-year surveillance interval is recommended for patients with serrated polyposis syndrome. Serrated polyposis syndrome is a rare condition characterized by multiple or large serrated polyps, including hyperplastic polyps, sessile serrated polyps, traditional serrated adenomas, and possibly also adenomatous polyps. Patients with serrated polyposis syndrome are at increased risk of colorectal cancer.

The recommended postpolypectomy interval for patients with sessile serrated polyps smaller than 10 mm is 5 years. This patient's sessile serrated polyp is larger than 10 mm, so this recommendation is not appropriate.

A 10-year average-risk interval is recommended for patients with small rectosigmoid hyperplastic polyps, but it is not appropriate for this patient because her large sessile serrated polyp carries a higher cancer risk.

> **KEY POINT**
>
> - For patients with large (≥10 mm) or dysplastic sessile serrated polyps or traditional serrated adenomas, the recommended postpolypectomy surveillance colonoscopy interval is 3 years.

Bibliography

Lieberman DA, Rex DK, Winawer SJ, Giardiello FM, Johnson DA, Levin TR; United States Multi-Society Task Force on Colorectal Cancer. Guidelines for colonoscopy surveillance after screening and polypectomy: a consensus update by the US Multi-Society Task Force on Colorectal Cancer. Gastroenterology. 2012 Sep;143(3):844-57. [PMID: 22763141]

Item 25   Answer: D

Educational Objective: Manage asymptomatic cholelithiasis.

The most appropriate management for this patient's gallstones is clinical observation. Her symptoms are consistent with gastroesophageal reflux. Gallstones were incidentally found on her evaluation but are asymptomatic. Biliary colic is the most common clinical presentation in patients with symptomatic gallstones. The usual presentation of biliary colic is episodic, severe abdominal pain typically in the epigastrium and/or right upper quadrant but occasionally in the right lower or mid-abdomen. The pain rapidly intensifies over a 15-minute interval to a steady plateau that lasts as long as 3 hours and resolves slowly. The pain is often associated with nausea or vomiting, and there is no jaundice. Pain may radiate to the interscapular region or right shoulder. An estimated 60% to 80% of gallstones are asymptomatic. Over a 20-year period, 50% of patients remain asymptomatic, 30% have biliary colic, and 20% have more serious complications. Observation is recommended for adult patients with asymptomatic gallstones. The possible exceptions to this recommendation are groups at higher risk for gallbladder carcinoma, such as patients with a calcified (porcelain) gallbladder, certain American Indians, and patients with gallstones larger than 3 cm.

Risks for symptoms or complications from silent gallstones are about 2% per year and cumulative, and risks for complications in the absence of antecedent pain are minimal. Therefore, annual ultrasonography is unlikely to alter management decisions for this patient and she can be treated expectantly, based on the occurrence of symptoms.

Laparoscopic cholecystectomy is the treatment of choice for symptomatic biliary colic and acute cholecystitis. Mortality rates following laparoscopic cholecystectomy are less than 0.7%, and complication rates (including bile duct injuries) do not differ between laparoscopic and open cholecystectomy. However, this patient's pain is inconsistent with

biliary pain, and neither laparoscopic nor open cholecystectomy is indicated.

Oral administration of ursodiol for dissolution of gallstones is rarely used. It can be considered in patients with symptomatic noncalcified gallbladder stones who are at high risk for cholecystectomy.

> **KEY POINT**
>
> - Observation is recommended for adult patients with asymptomatic gallstones.

Bibliography

Gracie WA, Ransohoff DF. The natural history of silent gallstones: the innocent gallstone is not a myth. N Engl J Med. 1982 Sep 3;307(13):798-800. [PMID: 7110244]

Item 26   Answer: C

Educational Objective: Diagnose pyoderma gangrenosum as an extraintestinal manifestation of inflammatory bowel disease.

This patient's ulcerating lesion is characteristic of pyoderma gangrenosum (PG). PG is an uncommon skin disease characterized by intense neutrophilic inflammation and invasion of the skin. Lesions are classically ulcerated, but PG may also present with bullae, pustulonodules, and vegetative plaques. Typical lesions begin as painful pustules that rapidly ulcerate and expand, with an edematous, rolled, or undermined-appearing border that may have a violaceous hue. Annular rings are sometimes noted. As with other neutrophilic dermatoses, when the process is active, approximately 25% of patients will exhibit pathergy or induction of new lesions at sites of trauma, including ostomy, phlebotomy, and intravenous sites. Peristomal PG, occurring around ostomy sites, is common and can be challenging to manage. As PG resolves, it tends to heal with atrophic scarring in a cross-like or cribriform pattern. There are no definitive diagnostic tests, and PG is a diagnosis of exclusion. Skin biopsy may be required to exclude other diseases such as cutaneous Crohn disease but may cause worsening of the PG. Treatment can be challenging, and if there is an associated underlying disease, therapy should be directed at controlling that process. Extraintestinal manifestations such as oral aphthous ulcers, arthralgia, inflammatory eye diseases, and PG are seen in approximately 10% of patients with inflammatory bowel disease.

Acrodermatitis enteropathica (AE) is an inherited or acquired metabolic disorder characterized by perioral and acral (in the extremities) erythematous and vesiculobullous dermatitis and alopecia related to zinc deficiency. AE has been associated with Crohn disease, but this patient's stomal ulcer is not consistent with AE.

Erythema nodosum is the most common cutaneous manifestation of inflammatory bowel disease, occurring in up to 20% of patients, particularly women. The lesions of EN are tender, subcutaneous nodules presenting as barely appreciable convexities on the skin surface, with a reddish hue in the acute phase. EN is frequently bilateral and symmetrical, and it usually occurs on the distal lower extremities, but it may also appear on the trunk, thighs, or upper extremities.

Squamous cell carcinoma (SCC) usually appears as a scaly, crusted, well-demarcated red papule, plaque, or nodule. SCC can develop in patients with Crohn disease, most commonly at sites of chronic, long-standing inflammation such as chronic fistulas. This patient's ulcerative skin lesion with undermined and violaceous borders is not consistent with the appearance of SCC.

KEY POINT

- Pyoderma gangrenosum (PG) is characterized by painful pustules that rapidly ulcerate and expand, with edematous, rolled, or undermined borders that may have a violaceous hue; PG may be an extraintestinal manifestation of Crohn disease.

Bibliography

Larsen S, Bendtzen K, Nielsen OH. Extraintestinal manifestations of inflammatory bowel disease: epidemiology, diagnosis, and management. Ann Med. 2010 Mar;42(2):97-114. [PMID: 20166813]

Item 27   Answer: C

Educational Objective: Evaluate chronic diarrhea.

The most appropriate management is stool testing for ova and parasites. Infectious causes of chronic diarrhea are uncommon in immunocompetent adults in developed countries, except for infection with *Giardia lamblia*. Giardiasis should be considered in patients with exposure to young children or potentially contaminated water such as lakes and streams. Infection is asymptomatic in more than 50% of patients, and the protozoa clear spontaneously. In the remaining patients, symptoms typically occur 1 to 2 weeks after infection and include watery, foul-smelling diarrhea; bloating; flatulence; and belching. Significant weight loss is common because of anorexia and malabsorption, but fever is distinctly unusual. Gastrointestinal symptoms can persist for several weeks to months in the absence of treatment. Patients with hypogammaglobulinemia are at increased risk of developing severe or chronic infection. Given this patient's profession as a day care worker, she is at risk for exposure to a number of infectious causes of diarrhea. The duration of her diarrhea, as well as the associated bloating and weight loss, are more consistent with giardiasis than a bacterial infection. Therefore, an assessment of this patient's stools for ova and parasites would be more appropriate than stool cultures.

A colonoscopy is not indicated at this time because this patient is otherwise healthy and does not have gastrointestinal bleeding or signs suggesting inflammatory bowel disease, such as blood in the stool.

Given the chronic nature of this patient's symptoms and her associated weight loss, avoiding further testing would not be appropriate. Her symptoms warrant evaluation with stool testing.

KEY POINT

- Giardiasis should be considered in patients with chronic diarrhea and exposure to young children or potentially contaminated water such as lakes and streams.

Bibliography

Schiller LR. Definitions, pathophysiology, and evaluation of chronic diarrhoea. Best Pract Res Clin Gastroenterol. 2012 Oct;26(5):551-62. [PMID: 23384801]

Item 28   Answer: C

Educational Objective: Treat autoimmune pancreatitis.

The most appropriate management is prednisone. Type I autoimmune pancreatitis (AIP) typically presents in older men, with a mean age of onset in the fifth decade of life. This patient has evidence of type 1 AIP based on the presence of three diagnostic criteria: imaging features (focal pancreatic enlargement with a featureless rim and a nondilated pancreatic duct), increased serum IgG4 level, and extrapancreatic organ involvement (sclerosing cholangitis or IgG4-associated cholangitis). Almost all patients (>90%) enter clinical remission in response to glucocorticoids, but relapse is common.

There are no data to support antioxidant treatment for AIP; however, some patients may develop nutritional deficiencies, which warrant treatment.

A biliary metal stent is generally reserved for long-term palliation of malignant biliary strictures and is not required for IgG4-associated cholangitis. IgG4-associated cholangitis typically responds to glucocorticoids, but it may not resolve completely and can relapse. Temporary plastic biliary stents may be required in patients presenting with jaundice who have a dominant stricture, which is not present in this patient.

Surgery is not indicated in this patient but should be considered when the diagnosis is uncertain and pancreatic cancer cannot be excluded.

KEY POINT

- Glucocorticoids are the cornerstone of treatment for autoimmune pancreatitis.

Bibliography

Hart PA, Kamisawa T, Brugge WR, et al. Long-term outcomes of autoimmune pancreatitis: a multicentre, international analysis. Gut. 2013 Dec;62(12):1771-6. [PMID: 23232048]

Item 29   Answer: B

Educational Objective: Treat small-bowel bleeding with push enteroscopy.

The most appropriate procedure is push enteroscopy, which will allow for therapeutic intervention. Angiodysplasias are the most common cause of obscure gastrointestinal bleeding. Push enteroscopy will be able to reach the lesion and

H
CONT.

allow for treatment with electrocautery, argon plasma coagulation, injection therapy, mechanical hemostasis (hemoclips or banding), or a combination of these techniques. This patient had a negative upper endoscopy. Capsule endoscopy was helpful in this patient because it identified active bleeding as well as several angiodysplasias, which are causing the bleeding. Enteroscopy should be performed after a negative upper endoscopy and colonoscopy or after a positive capsule endoscopy. Complications of push enteroscopy are rare but include perforation, mucosal avulsion, and bleeding.

Intraoperative endoscopy is reserved for patients with active bleeding from the small bowel in whom both endoscopy and angiography have failed to identify the small-bowel bleeding source.

A repeat upper endoscopy would not be helpful in this situation because it will be unable to reach the lesion in the small bowel.

Technetium-labeled nuclear scans are used in patients with active bleeding (melena or hematochezia) who are transfusion dependent and hospitalized. This is a diagnostic test that will supply no additional information to what has already been provided by the results of the capsule endoscopy, and it does not allow for therapeutic intervention.

KEY POINT

- Enteroscopy should be performed after a negative upper endoscopy and colonoscopy or after a positive capsule endoscopy.

Bibliography

Leighton JA. The role of endoscopic imaging of the small bowel in clinical practice. Am J Gastroenterol. 2011 Jan;106(1):27–36; quiz 37. [PMID: 20978483]

Item 30   Answer: C

Educational Objective: Treat irritable bowel syndrome with constipation that is refractory to standard laxative therapy.

The most appropriate treatment is to start linaclotide. This patient's symptoms have not responded to initial trials of two over-the-counter laxatives for treatment of his irritable bowel syndrome with constipation (IBS-C) symptoms. Linaclotide is a synthetic peptide that acts peripherally in the gut and activates guanylate cyclase-C receptors on the enterocytes lining the small bowel and colon. Activation of the guanylate cyclase-C receptors results in increased production of cyclic guanosine monophosphate (cGMP), which in turn activates the movement of chloride ions into the intestinal lumen and promotes passive movement of sodium ions and water in the intestinal lumen. These secretory effects lead to treatment of constipation symptoms. In a multicenter randomized controlled trial (RCT) involving 804 patients with IBS-C, linaclotide significantly improved abdominal and bowel symptoms associated with IBS-C over 26 weeks of treatment.

Diarrhea was the most common side effect, prompting discontinuation in 4.5% of patients. Linaclotide has an FDA indication for the treatment of adults with IBS-C and chronic constipation. Linaclotide is not a first-line agent in IBS-C, but it is appropriate for patients whose symptoms persist despite the use of fiber and standard laxatives. Lubiprostone, a chloride channel activator that increases intestinal fluid secretion, can also be used as a second-line agent in patients with IBS-C or chronic idiopathic constipation.

Bran has not shown any benefit compared with placebo in the treatment of IBS-C and is likely to worsen symptoms of bloating.

Bisacodyl has not been assessed for use in IBS-C in any RCTs. Furthermore, the side effect of abdominal cramping associated with bisacodyl is likely to exacerbate this patient's baseline abdominal pain.

Rifaximin is a nonabsorbable antibiotic under development for use in IBS with diarrhea and mixed IBS (not FDA approved). There is no established benefit for rifaximin in IBS-C.

KEY POINT

- Linaclotide is FDA approved for the treatment of irritable bowel syndrome with constipation in adults; like lubiprostone, it is second-line therapy for patients whose symptoms have not responded to standard laxative therapy.

Bibliography

Chey WD, Lembo AJ, Lavins BJ, et al. Linaclotide for irritable bowel syndrome with constipation: a 26-week, randomized, double-blind, placebo-controlled trial to evaluate efficacy and safety. Am J Gastroenterol. 2012 Nov;107(11):1702–12. [PMID: 22986437]

Item 31   Answer: C

Educational Objective: Diagnose fat-soluble vitamin deficiency following malabsorptive bariatric surgery.

Vitamin A deficiency is most likely to explain this patient's findings, and the most appropriate and important study is immediate assessment of this patient's vitamin A status with serum retinol measurement. Her ocular symptoms are very serious manifestations of vitamin A deficiency, which may be progressive and may lead to permanent visual impairment if left untreated. Symptoms associated with vitamin A deficiency include decreased vision at night or in dim light, dry eyes, corneal and/or eyelid inflammation, and rough and/or dry skin. The absorption of the fat-soluble vitamins A, D, E, and K can be severely impaired following malabsorptive bariatric surgery, including Roux-en-Y gastric bypass (RYGB) and biliopancreatic diversion with duodenal switch. Vitamin A deficiency has been reported to occur in 11% of patients after gastric bypass despite taking a daily multivitamin. This deficiency can occur within 1 year of surgery; the reported prevalence is 10% to 50% in patients with RYGB and 61% to 69% in those with biliopancreatic diversion. Vitamin A deficiency is believed to arise from multiple factors such as fat malabsorption, decreased intake from reduced overall food consumption, and possible underlying fatty liver disease. Other micronutrient deficiencies (in addition to the previously mentioned fat-soluble vitamins A, D, E, and K) that can develop following RYGB include iron, folic acid, zinc, selenium, copper, magnesium, thiamine (vitamin B_1), cobalamin (vitamin B_{12}), vitamin C, and in rare cases, riboflavin (vitamin B_2) and pyridoxine (vitamin B_6).

Copper deficiency causes a chronic syndrome similar to subacute combined degeneration and is also associated with macrocytic anemia and leukopenia. Therefore, this deficiency can be difficult to differentiate from vitamin B_{12} deficiency. Less common findings include sudden bilateral visual loss.

Although iron deficiency does occur following RYGB, this patient is on iron replacement and has a normal mean corpuscular volume. Patients with iron deficiency are likely to have hypochromic, microcytic anemia and may have brittle or deformed nails, cheilitis, pica, and restless legs syndrome. Visual symptoms are not seen with iron deficiency anemia.

Although vitamin B_{12} deficiency may occur following RYGB, this is unlikely given this patient's normal mean corpuscular volume. Furthermore, a vitamin B_{12} deficiency could lead to peripheral neuropathy and gait disturbance but not the skin or visual disturbances seen in this patient.

KEY POINT

- The absorption of the fat-soluble vitamins A, D, E, and K can be severely impaired following malabsorptive bariatric surgery, including Roux-en-Y gastric bypass and biliopancreatic diversion with duodenal switch.

Bibliography

Strohmayer E, Via MA, Yanagisawa R. Metabolic management following bariatric surgery. Mt Sinai J Med. 2010 Sep-Oct;77(5):431-45. [PMID: 20960547]

Item 32   Answer: D

Educational Objective: Manage advanced liver disease due to nonalcoholic fatty liver disease.

The most appropriate diagnostic test to perform next is ultrasound of the liver and spleen. This patient has a history of nonalcoholic fatty liver disease (NAFLD) and now has abdominal distention suggestive of ascites. Her low platelet count is suggestive of portal hypertension, and liver dysfunction is supported by the slightly elevated serum bilirubin and low albumin levels. The next test should be liver imaging with a test such as ultrasound to assess for changes consistent with portal hypertension. In the United States, many cases of "cryptogenic" liver disease are likely related to advanced NAFLD.

Although this patient has risk factors for cardiac disease, she does not have other signs or symptoms suggestive of heart failure. In addition, cardiac dysfunction, unless very long-standing, would not produce splenomegaly. Therefore, echocardiography is not necessary at this time.

Liver biopsy to diagnose cirrhosis is not necessary in patients with other clear manifestations of liver dysfunction and portal hypertension, such as is seen in this patient.

Simvastatin rarely produces mild liver test abnormalities but does not cause chronic liver injury or portal hypertension. Patients with NAFLD have a high prevalence of coronary artery disease; therefore, risk-factor reduction, including the use of statins where appropriate, is advised.

KEY POINT

- Liver imaging with a test such as ultrasound is useful for assessing changes consistent with portal hypertension.

Bibliography

Chalasani N, Younossi Z, Lavine JE, et al; American Gastroenterological Association; American Association for the Study of Liver Diseases; American College of Gastroenterology. The diagnosis and management of non-alcoholic fatty liver disease: practice guideline by the American Gastroenterological Association, American Association for the Study of Liver Diseases, and American College of Gastroenterology. Gastroenterology. 2012 Jun;142(7):1592-609. Erratum in: Gastroenterology. 2012 Aug;143(2):503. [PMID: 22656328]

Item 33   Answer: D

Educational Objective: Provide surveillance for Barrett esophagus without dysplasia.

The most appropriate next step in management is to repeat upper endoscopy in 3 to 5 years. Although there is no evidence of the benefit of endoscopic screening of the general population, endoscopic assessment for Barrett esophagus (BE) in patients with chronic reflux symptoms may be appropriate in specific patients. It is reasonable to consider screening men older than 50 years with gastroesophageal reflux disease (GERD) symptoms for more than 5 years and additional risk factors (nocturnal reflux symptoms, hiatal hernia, elevated BMI, tobacco use, and intra-abdominal distribution of fat) to detect esophageal adenocarcinoma and BE. This patient is male, older than 50 years, overweight, and is an active smoker; therefore, pursuing screening was reasonable in this patient. His endoscopy revealed BE without evidence of dysplasia. BE is thought to be a complication of GERD resulting in a change in the normal squamous lining of the distal esophagus to a specialized columnar epithelium due to the effect of refluxed gastric secretions. BE is a spectrum ranging from no dysplasia to high-grade dysplasia, and some patients progress to esophageal cancer. Recommended surveillance of patients with newly diagnosed BE is based on the presence and degree of dysplasia on biopsy. In those with no dysplasia, surveillance with upper endoscopy is recommended in 3 to 5 years. In patients with low-grade dysplasia, surveillance is more frequent, usually 6 to 12 months following confirmation by an expert pathologist. High-grade dysplasia requires either more aggressive surveillance or treatment to remove BE (such as with endoscopic ablation or esophagectomy).

Patients with BE with high-grade dysplasia are often treated with endoscopic ablation. This patient has BE with no dysplasia, so this therapy is not appropriate at this time.

Esophagectomy should be reserved for patients in whom endoscopic ablation fails or in those with evidence of esophageal cancer.

Fundoplication is the appropriate treatment for GERD in patients who wish to stop taking medication or in those with a poor response to medical therapy. This patient's symptoms are well controlled on omeprazole, so fundoplication is not appropriate at this time. Fundoplication does not prevent the progression of BE to dysplasia or cancer.

KEY POINT

- In patients with Barrett esophagus and no dysplasia, surveillance with upper endoscopy is recommended in 3 to 5 years.

Bibliography

American Gastroenterological Association, Spechler SJ, Sharma P, Souza RF, Inadomi JM, Shaheen NJ. American Gastroenterological Association medical position statement on the management of Barrett's esophagus. Gastroenterology. 2011 Mar;140(3):1084-91. [PMID: 21376940]

Item 34   Answer: C

Educational Objective: Diagnose primary biliary cirrhosis.

The most likely diagnosis is primary biliary cirrhosis (PBC). PBC is a chronic cholestatic liver disease of unknown cause. PBC mainly affects middle-aged women. Most patients are asymptomatic at presentation but develop symptoms of PBC within 10 years; symptoms include fatigue, dry eyes, dry mouth, and pruritus. Hyperlipidemia is common, but jaundice, cutaneous hyperpigmentation, hepatosplenomegaly, and xanthelasmas are rarely observed at diagnosis. PBC is diagnosed by serum alkaline phosphatase levels greater than 1.5 times the upper limit of normal and typically normal serum total bilirubin levels. Serum aspartate (AST) and alanine (ALT) aminotransferase levels are typically less than five times the upper limit of normal. Serum antimitochondrial antibody is present in 90% to 95% of patients. For patients with undetectable serum antimitochondrial antibody levels, a liver biopsy is required for diagnosis. Treatment with ursodiol slows disease progression and may prevent or delay advanced disease and the need for liver transplantation.

Autoimmune hepatitis is a chronic inflammatory liver disease that is usually seen in women. The disease presentation ranges from asymptomatic to acute liver failure. Autoimmune hepatitis typically causes a predominant elevation of the serum ALT level rather than the serum alkaline phosphatase level, as was seen in this patient.

Cholangiocarcinoma is classified by location as intrahepatic and hilar/extrahepatic. Intrahepatic cholangiocarcinoma is typically asymptomatic until the tumor is advanced, at which time right upper quadrant discomfort, weight loss, and fever may be the only symptoms. An elevated serum alkaline phosphatase level may be noted. Risk factors for cholangiocarcinoma are primary sclerosing cholangitis, biliary atresia, chronic infection with liver flukes, and biliary cysts. This patient has no risk factors for cholangiocarcinoma, and that diagnosis would not explain her positive antimitochondrial antibody test.

Primary sclerosing cholangitis (PSC) is a chronic inflammatory disorder that affects the intra- and extrahepatic bile ducts. Approximately 70% to 80% of patients with PSC have inflammatory bowel disease, usually ulcerative colitis. Serum alkaline phosphatase values are 3 to 10 times the upper limit of normal, and serum ALT and AST levels are two to three times the upper limit of normal. Serum total bilirubin levels may be normal in 60% of patients. PSC is not the most likely diagnosis in this patient because she has a positive antimitochondrial antibody test and does not have ulcerative colitis.

KEY POINT

- The diagnosis of primary biliary cirrhosis is generally made on the basis of a cholestatic liver enzyme profile in the setting of a positive antimitochondrial antibody test.

Bibliography

Lindor KD, Gershwin ME, Poupon R, Kaplan M, Bergasa NV, Heathcote EJ; American Association for Study of Liver Diseases. Primary biliary cirrhosis. Hepatology. 2009 Jul;50(1):291-308. [PMID: 19554543]

Item 35   Answer: B

Educational Objective: Evaluate obscure gastrointestinal bleeding with capsule endoscopy.

Capsule endoscopy is the most appropriate diagnostic test for this patient with obscure gastrointestinal bleeding. Obscure gastrointestinal bleeding refers to recurrent or persistent bleeding from the gastrointestinal tract without an obvious source on endoscopic studies. The evaluation of gastrointestinal bleeding of obscure origin usually begins with repeat endoscopy directed at the most likely site. Approximately 30% to 50% of lesions can be detected using this approach. If repeat endoscopy is unrevealing in a patient who is not actively bleeding, examination should focus on the small intestine, using such tests as capsule endoscopy. Wireless capsule endoscopy allows excellent visualization of the small bowel. Unlike angiography and technetium scans, wireless capsule endoscopy is effective even in the absence of active bleeding. Wireless capsule endoscopy detects the source of occult bleeding in 50% to 75% of patients. In patients with iron deficiency anemia, in whom bleeding can be episodic, capsule endoscopy is another way to investigate potential sources of blood loss after other investigations have been unrevealing. This patient, who is on anticoagulation and has heme-positive stool, is likely to have vascular lesions such as angiodysplasia in the small bowel. Angiodysplasia is the most common cause of small-bowel bleeding in older patients.

Angiography and technetium-labeled nuclear scans are used in patients with active bleeding (melena or hematochezia) who are transfusion dependent and hospitalized. This patient does not meet these criteria.

Intraoperative endoscopy is generally employed only as a last resort for the evaluation of obscure gastrointestinal bleeding. The patient undergoes laparotomy or laparoscopy, and the bowel is evaluated with a colonoscope following surgical enterotomy. This technique should only be used if other less invasive options have been exhausted or if a patient has unexplained, life-threatening bleeding. In addition, the yield is somewhat low (approximately 25%).

KEY POINT

- Capsule endoscopy has become the first-line test in evaluating the small bowel in patients with obscure gastrointestinal bleeding after a negative upper endoscopy and colonoscopy.

Bibliography

Leighton JA. The role of endoscopic imaging of the small bowel in clinical practice. Am J Gastroenterol. 2011;106(1):27-36. [PMID: 20978483]

Item 36   Answer: C

Educational Objective: Treat acute pancreatitis with enteral nutrition.

Enteral feeding is the most appropriate management. Enteral feeding has been shown to reduce infectious complications, multiple organ failure, operative interventions, and mortality compared with feeding by total parenteral nutrition in patients with severe acute pancreatitis. This patient has moderately severe acute pancreatitis based on evidence of pancreatic necrosis and peripancreatic fluid collections. He also has several risk factors for severe disease based on the presence of three of four Systemic Inflammatory Response Syndrome (SIRS) criteria (pulse rate >90/min, leukocyte count >12,000/µL [12×10^9/L], and respiration rate >20/min) and a blood urea nitrogen level greater than 23 mg/dL (8.2 mmol/L). Nasogastric and nasojejunal feeding appear to be comparable in safety and efficacy. The optimal time to start enteral nutrition remains under investigation, but it should commence no later than 72 hours after presentation. In mild acute pancreatitis, oral feeding may start when nausea and vomiting resolve.

Drainage of acute peripancreatic fluid collections (APFCs) is not appropriate at this time because most collections resolve without intervention. Asymptomatic APFCs require no treatment. Symptomatic APFCs can be treated medically with bowel rest, jejunal feeding, pancreatic enzymes, octreotide, and rarely pancreatic duct stenting. Rarely, APFCs persist beyond 4 weeks, when they become encapsulated and are labeled a pancreatic pseudocyst. Pseudocysts are amenable to drainage if clinically indicated based on persistent pain despite medical therapy, infected pseudocyst, or obstruction of the gastric outlet or biliary tract.

Endoscopic retrograde cholangiopancreatography in acute pancreatitis should be used only in the following clinical scenarios: (1) in a patient with ascending cholangitis (fever, right upper quadrant pain, and jaundice) concomitant with acute pancreatitis, or (2) in a patient with gallstone pancreatitis who is not improving clinically and has worsening liver chemistry test results. Patients with gallstone pancreatitis and no complications should have a cholecystectomy prior to discharge.

KEY POINT

- Enteral feeding has been shown to reduce infectious complications, multiple organ failure, operative interventions, and mortality compared with feeding by total parenteral nutrition in patients with severe acute pancreatitis.

Bibliography

Tenner S, Baillie J, DeWitt J, Vege SS; American College of Gastroenterology. American College of Gastroenterology guideline: management of acute pancreatitis. Am J Gastroenterol. 2013 Sep;108(9):1400-15; 1416. [PMID: 23896955]

Item 37   Answer: C

Educational Objective: Manage lower gastrointestinal bleeding caused by an anal fissure.

The most appropriate management is outpatient follow-up. This patient meets four criteria for nonadmission with outpatient follow-up based on the 2008 Scottish Intercollegiate Guidelines Network (SIGN) (www.sign.ac.uk/pdf/sign105.pdf). These criteria include age less than 60 years, no hemodynamic instability, no evidence of gross rectal bleeding, and identification of an obvious anorectal source of bleeding on rectal examination or sigmoidoscopy.

Admission to the hospital for observation is not necessary because this patient's bleeding is attributable to a specific, minor cause of lower gastrointestinal bleeding, namely an anal fissure that is appropriate for outpatient management. The diagnosis is based on physical findings and a compelling clinical history. Anal fissures are tears in the anal skin distal to the dentate line; they may therefore be exquisitely painful, particularly with defecation. They are most often caused by local trauma such as hard stools. Anoscopy or direct visualization typically reveals a small mucosal tear, most often in the posterior midline. Hospitalization should be considered in patients with any of the following five criteria that predict severe bleeding: age 60 years or older, comorbid illnesses (particularly when two or more are present), hemodynamic instability, gross rectal bleeding (or early rebleeding), or exposure to antiplatelet drugs and anticoagulants.

Colonoscopy within 12 to 18 hours is not appropriate because this patient's clinical status does not warrant urgent or emergent investigations based on the SIGN guidelines. Elective colonoscopy or sigmoidoscopy might be performed on an outpatient basis to exclude causes other than chronic constipation, such as proctitis from inflammatory bowel disease or infection (such as herpesvirus or HIV).

Surgery is not necessary because this option is typically offered for chronic rather than acute anal fissures and only after exhausting medical options.

KEY POINT

- Patients with lower gastrointestinal bleeding do not require hospitalization when they meet four criteria (based on the 2008 Scottish Intercollegiate Guidelines Network): age less than 60 years, no hemodynamic instability, no evidence of gross rectal bleeding, and identification of an obvious anorectal source of bleeding on rectal examination or sigmoidoscopy.

Bibliography

Scottish Intercollegiate Guidelines Network. Management of acute upper and lower gastrointestinal bleeding: a national clinical guideline. http://www. sign.ac.uk/pdf/sign105.pdf. September 2008. Accessed March 10, 2015.

Item 38   Answer: B

Educational Objective: Treat a hepatocellular adenoma.

The most appropriate treatment is resection. This 42-year-old woman has a large hepatocellular adenoma, which has been confirmed by biopsy of the mass, and β-catenin activation mutation is positive. Hepatic adenomas can be subclassified based on genotype or immunohistochemistry, which provides information about the risk of transformation to hepatocellular carcinoma (HCC). Hepatic adenomas with positive genotyping for β-catenin activation or that are positive for the correlating immunohistochemistry study for glutamine synthetase have a higher risk of transformation to liver cancer. It is generally best to resect hepatic adenomas that are larger than 5 cm, arise in males (because they carry a higher risk of transformation to HCC), exhibit hemorrhage, or are positive for β-catenin activation/glutamine synthetase antibody. Low-risk hepatocellular adenomas are those smaller than 5 cm that arise in young women on oral contraceptives (reversible cause), as well as steatotic hepatocellular adenomas that are positive for the HNF-1α inactivation mutation. These low-risk hepatocellular adenomas require CT imaging surveillance at 6- to 12-month intervals.

Oral contraceptives are associated with the development and growth of hepatocellular adenomas, and cessation of oral contraceptives may lead to shrinkage and/or resolution. However, stopping oral contraceptives is not by itself sufficient treatment for this patient because her hepatic adenoma is larger than 5 cm and is β-catenin positive.

CT imaging surveillance is not appropriate given the high-risk characteristics of this patient's adenoma.

Transarterial chemoembolization is not an established treatment modality for hepatocellular adenomas. This therapy may be appropriate in a patient with cirrhosis and large or multiple hepatocellular carcinoma lesions that are unresectable.

KEY POINT

- Hepatocellular adenomas that are larger than 5 cm or that exhibit β-catenin nuclear reactivity should be treated with surgical resection.

Bibliography

Shaked O, Siegelman ES, Olthoff K, Reddy KR. Biologic and clinical features of benign solid and cystic lesions of the liver. Clin Gastroenterol Hepatol. 2011 Jul;9(7):547-62.e1-4. [PMID: 21397723]

Item 39   Answer: B

Educational Objective: Treat Candida esophagitis.

The most appropriate treatment is fluconazole. This patient has a clinical presentation and findings characteristic of Candida albicans esophagitis. Infectious esophagitis can be caused by bacterial (uncommon), fungal, viral, and parasitic pathogens. Patients may be asymptomatic, but common symptoms are odynophagia or dysphagia. C. albicans is the most common cause of infectious esophagitis in immunocompromised patients and is often associated with oropharyngeal candidiasis. It often presents with dysphagia, odynophagia, and curdy white esophageal plaques seen on upper endoscopy, which is confirmed with esophageal brushings. This patient's immunocompromised status after liver transplantation puts her at risk for Candida esophagitis; however, Candida infection can occur in immunocompetent patients as well. Candida esophagitis should be treated with fluconazole.

The differential diagnosis also includes possible viral causes. Cytomegalovirus often presents with a single ulcer in the esophagus. The diagnosis is established with biopsies from the ulcer base, and treatment should be with ganciclovir. Herpes simplex virus is also characterized by ulcers, typically multiple, found on upper endoscopy. The diagnosis is established with biopsy of the ulcer edge, and treatment should be with acyclovir.

Swallowed aerosolized glucocorticoids such as fluticasone are often used as a treatment for eosinophilic esophagitis. Patients who respond typically do so quickly, but symptoms often relapse when the treatment is discontinued. Esophageal candidiasis is a side effect of this therapy. Treatment with swallowed aerosolized fluticasone is likely to exacerbate, not improve, this patient's symptoms.

Fluconazole is the first-line therapy for Candida esophagitis and is a more effective therapy than swallowed nystatin.

KEY POINT

- Candida albicans is the most common cause of infectious esophagitis in immunocompromised patients and is often associated with oropharyngeal candidiasis.

Bibliography

Sharma S, Gurakar A, Camci C, Jabbour N. Avoiding pitfalls: what an endoscopist should know in liver transplantation-part II. Dig Dis Sci. 2009 Jul;54(7):1386-402. [PMID: 19085103]

Item 40   Answer: C

Educational Objective: Treat constipation due to dyssynergic defecation with biofeedback therapy.

The most appropriate management is to refer for biofeedback therapy. The cause of this patient's refractory constipation is dyssynergic defecation. Dyssynergic defecation is characterized by the inability to coordinate the relaxation of the puborectalis and external anal sphincter muscles while increasing intraabdominal pressure that results in normal evacuation of stool. Dyssynergic defecation is believed to be an acquired behavioral disorder, resulting from causes such as sexual abuse, obstetric trauma, pelvic/abdominal surgery, or traumatic injury to the pelvis/abdomen. The mechanisms underlying this condition can include some combination of the following factors: inability to contract the abdominal wall musculature, deficient relaxation or paradoxical contraction of the puborectalis muscle, impaired rectal contraction, paradoxical anal contraction, and/or inadequate anal relaxation. These abnormal muscle actions of the pelvic floor and anorectum can be detected by asking the patient to bear down during a digital rectal examination (DRE). The inability to relax the puborectalis and external anal sphincter when instructed or with bearing down is indicative of dyssynergia. The positive predictive value of such findings on DRE is 97%. Dyssynergia generally responds poorly to laxative therapy. Biofeedback therapy, also termed neuromuscular re-education, entails a program of neuromuscular training utilizing visual and verbal feedback to restore coordinated muscle activity involved with defecation and improve rectal sensory function. Biofeedback therapy is commonly provided by a physical therapist with this specialized training. Biofeedback therapy is superior to all forms of laxative therapy because it corrects the underlying pathologic mechanisms responsible for dyssynergic defecation.

This patient's stool is already soft, so further softening with more polyethylene glycol is unlikely to be of any sustained benefit.

Psyllium bulks the stool, which is likely to worsen symptoms in the presence of an underlying problem with stool evacuation.

Enema therapy may promote further dyssynergia by providing an artificial means of emptying the rectal vault, leading to progressive pelvic floor weakness and dysfunction.

KEY POINT

• Biofeedback therapy is superior to all forms of laxative therapy for dyssynergic defecation because it corrects the underlying pathologic mechanisms.

Bibliography

American Gastroenterological Association, Bharucha AE, Dorn SD, Lembo A, Pressman A. American Gastroenterological Association medical position statement on constipation. Gastroenterology. 2013 Jan;144(1):211-7. [PMID: 23261064]

Item 41   Answer: E

Educational Objective: Manage sporadic fundic gland polyps.

The most appropriate next step in management is reassurance. Fundic gland polyps (FGPs) are among the most commonly found gastric polyps and are reported to be diagnosed in up to 5% of patients undergoing upper endoscopy. Sporadic FGPs are usually 1 to 5 mm in size and fewer than 10 in number. Sporadic FGPs have been associated with proton pump inhibitor (PPI) use; the exact mechanism of this association is not known. Sporadic FGPs do not have malignant potential; therefore, this patient does not require PPI cessation, excision of the remaining polyps, or surveillance.

It is important to distinguish sporadic FGPs from those related to a hereditary colon cancer syndrome. Familial adenomatous polyposis (FAP) is an autosomal dominant hereditary colon cancer syndrome caused by an *APC* gene mutation. It is associated with the near-universal presence of gastric fundic gland polyposis, duodenal adenomas, and a personal or family history of early-onset colonic adenomas or colorectal cancer. FAP-related FGPs frequently harbor dysplasia. *APC* gene testing is not warranted because this patient does not have dysplastic FGPs, a personal history of duodenal or colonic adenomas, or a family history of colorectal cancer.

Colonoscopy is recommended in patients with dysplastic FGPs or in those younger than 40 years of age with fundic gland polyposis; neither of these characteristics is present in this patient, so colonoscopy is not necessary at this time.

This patient's esophageal ring is an acid-related complication of gastroesophageal reflux disease that requires esophageal dilation and ongoing use of a PPI. Therefore, stopping PPI therapy is not appropriate at this time.

KEY POINT

• Sporadic fundic gland polyps have been associated with proton pump inhibitor use and do not require excision or surveillance.

Bibliography

Shaib YH, Rugge M, Graham DY, Genta RM. Management of gastric polyps: an endoscopy-based approach. Clin Gastroenterol Hepatol. 2013 Nov;11(11):1374-84. [PMID: 23583466]

Item 42   Answer: B

Educational Objective: Provide long-term prevention of recurrent NSAID-induced peptic ulcer disease.

The most appropriate management is celecoxib and omeprazole. Patients such as this with a history of an NSAID-associated bleeding ulcer have a substantial risk for developing recurrent ulcer bleeding. A series of randomized clinical trials in a Hong Kong population illustrated the relative effectiveness of the various treatment strategies in the secondary prevention of NSAID-induced bleeding ulcer disease. Despite endoscopic documentation of complete ulcer healing, the reinitiation of NSAID therapy without a proton pump inhibitor (PPI) resulted in a recurrent ulcer bleeding rate of nearly 20% over a 6-month time frame. The addition of a PPI along with the NSAID lowered the recurrent ulcer bleeding rate to nearly 5% in the same 6-month time frame. Use of the cyclooxygenase-2 (COX-2) selective NSAID celecoxib resulted in a similar 6-month bleeding rate of nearly 5%. Additionally, co-therapy with sucralfate is ineffective in preventing NSAID- or aspirin-related gastric or duodenal ulceration. The most effective treatment strategy in the prevention of recurrent ulcer bleeding was use of celecoxib plus twice-daily PPI therapy, which had a 12-month rebleeding rate of 0%. Therefore, patients with a previous NSAID-associated bleeding ulcer who must remain on NSAIDs should receive a COX-2 selective NSAID plus PPI therapy to maximize risk reduction for a recurrent ulcer bleed.

KEY POINT

- A series of randomized clinical trials showed that the most effective treatment strategy in the prevention of recurrent ulcer bleeding was the use of celecoxib plus twice-daily proton pump inhibitor therapy.

Bibliography
Lanza FL, Chan FK, Quigley EM; Practice Parameters Committee of the American College of Gastroenterology. Guidelines for prevention of NSAID-related ulcer complications. Am J Gastroenterol. 2009 Mar;104(3):728-38. [PMID: 19240698]

Item 43   Answer: B
Educational Objective: Diagnose Crohn colitis.

The most likely diagnosis is Crohn colitis. This patient has severe, patchy colitis with some large, deep ulcers and rectal sparing, which is consistent with Crohn colitis. In Crohn disease, endoscopic findings vary from superficial aphthous ulcers to discrete, deep ulcers that can be linear, stellate, or serpiginous and that may coalesce into a "cobblestone" appearance. Rectal sparing is typical, as are areas of inflammation separated by normal mucosa (known as skip lesions). The ileum is inspected during colonoscopy to detect ileal inflammation characteristic of Crohn disease. Histology may show patchy submucosal inflammation, but more superficial inflammation does not rule out Crohn disease.

Collagenous colitis is a form of microscopic colitis. Microscopic colitis accounts for 10% to 15% of patients with chronic, watery diarrhea. In contrast to inflammatory bowel disease, microscopic colitis is more common in older persons and does not cause endoscopically visible inflammation, as was seen in this patient.

Ischemic colitis is the most common form of intestinal ischemic injury. Approximately 90% of cases occur in patients older than 60 years. Symptoms include sudden abdominal pain and diarrhea followed by rectal bleeding. Ischemic colitis can result in segmental colitis, but it is typically not patchy and would be unusual in a 28-year-old patient.

In ulcerative colitis, inflammation typically begins in the rectum and extends proximally in a circumferential manner. Mild ulcerative colitis is characterized by mucosal edema, erythema, and loss of the normal vascular pattern. More significant disease produces granularity, friability,

ulceration, and bleeding. Ulcerative colitis would typically feature rectal involvement and continuous colitis rather than patchy colitis, as was seen in this patient.

KEY POINT

- In Crohn disease, endoscopic findings vary from superficial aphthous ulcers to discrete, deep ulcers; rectal sparing is typical, as are areas of inflammation separated by normal mucosa (known as skip lesions).

Bibliography
Baumgart DC, Sandborn WJ. Crohn's disease. Lancet. 2012 Nov 3;380(9853):1590-605. Erratum in: Lancet. 2013 Jan 19;381(9862):204. [PMID: 22914295]

Item 44   Answer: C
Educational Objective: Diagnose chronic mesenteric ischemia.

The most likely diagnosis is chronic mesenteric ischemia and the next diagnostic test should be CT angiography. Chronic mesenteric ischemia is typically a manifestation of mesenteric atherosclerosis and presents as abdominal pain beginning within 60 minutes after eating. The pain is believed to be due to diversion of small-bowel blood flow to the stomach as digestion begins. The blood flow to the small bowel, which is already compromised, then has even more limited oxygen supply, leading to ischemia and subsequent abdominal pain. This typical symptom leads to a fear of eating (sitophobia), which causes the weight loss that is seen in most patients with chronic mesenteric ischemia. Abdominal bruits are present in 50% of patients, and 50% of patients have peripheral vascular or coronary artery disease. The natural history is progression of mild pain with eating to food avoidance, weight loss, and eventually pain without eating. Upper endoscopy is typically normal, and a CT scan may show evidence of diffuse small-bowel dilation, which is suggestive of abnormal small-bowel motility. If progressive and left untreated, chronic mesenteric ischemia can rarely lead to intestinal infarction. Vascular surgical intervention is the treatment of choice. Both magnetic resonance angiography and CT angiography have high sensitivity and specificity for detecting mesenteric stenosis, although MR angiography may not be as good at detecting distal stenosis.

Doppler ultrasound is a useful screening test for chronic mesenteric ischemia. Peak systolic velocities greater than 275 cm/s in the superior mesenteric artery and greater than 200 cm/s in the celiac artery correlate with stenoses of greater than 70% in each vessel. Doppler ultrasound is often of limited use if patients are obese or there is overlying bowel gas. Ultrasonography without Doppler modality to assess blood flow will not help establish the diagnosis in this patient.

Capsule endoscopy is contraindicated in patients with small-bowel obstruction regardless of whether obstruction is due to a mechanical or functional cause (such as dysmotility due to underlying chronic ischemia, as in this patient).

Splanchnic angiography is useful if the results of noninvasive testing are equivocal to confirm the diagnosis and to plan intervention; in particular, it allows for performance of endovascular procedures at the time of diagnosis. However, owing to its invasive nature it is typically not the first diagnostic test for chronic mesenteric ischemia.

KEY POINT

- The typical presentation of chronic mesenteric ischemia consists of abdominal pain within an hour of meals, fear of food ingestion, and weight loss.

Bibliography

Pecoraro F, Rancic Z, Lachat M, et al. Chronic mesenteric ischemia: critical review and guidelines for management. Ann Vasc Surg. 2013 Jan;27(1):113-22. [PMID: 23088809]

Item 45   Answer: A

Educational Objective: Screen for hereditary nonpolyposis colon cancer.

The most appropriate colon cancer screening strategy is colonoscopy beginning now. This patient's family history is consistent with hereditary nonpolyposis colorectal cancer (HNPCC). The Amsterdam II criteria include (1) three or more relatives with an HNPCC–associated cancer (including colorectal, endometrial, ovarian, urothelial, gastric, brain, small bowel, hepatobiliary, or skin), (2) two successive generations of relatives affected, (3) one affected relative a first-degree relative to two other affected relatives, and (4) one cancer diagnosed before age 50 years. Patients with HNPCC should undergo genetic counseling, and an attempt should be made to ascertain the genetic cause of cancer in the patient and family. Surveillance colonoscopy is indicated in patients who meet the clinical criteria for HNPCC, have Lynch syndrome (defined by the presence of a germline genetic mutation), or are at risk for Lynch syndrome and have not had genetic testing. The recommended surveillance interval for colonoscopy screening in patients who have or are at risk for Lynch syndrome is every 1 to 2 years beginning at age 25 years, or 2 to 5 years earlier than the youngest age at diagnosis of colorectal cancer if the affected relative was younger than 25 years old.

Colonoscopy every 5 years beginning at age 40 years (or 10 years before the earliest case in the immediate family) is the surveillance recommendation for a patient with either colorectal cancer or adenomatous polyps in a first-degree relative before age 60 years or colorectal cancer in two or more first-degree relatives at any age.

Colonoscopy every 10 years beginning at age 40 years is the U.S. Multi-Society Task Force on Colorectal Cancer recommendation for a patient with either colorectal cancer or adenomatous polyps in a first-degree relative aged 60 years or older or colorectal cancer in two second-degree relatives with colorectal cancer at any age.

Although the earliest colorectal cancer diagnosis in this patient's family was at age 47 years, she should begin screening now owing to her increased risk related to her family history consistent with HNPCC.

A 5-year interval beginning at age 50 years is not recommended for patients who have or who are at risk for Lynch syndrome; it would be appropriate for low-risk patients diagnosed with one to two tubular adenomas smaller than 10 mm.

KEY POINT

- The recommended surveillance interval for colonoscopy screening in patients who have or are at risk for Lynch syndrome is every 1 to 2 years beginning at age 25 years, or 2 to 5 years earlier than the youngest age at diagnosis of colorectal cancer if the affected relative was younger than 25 years old.

Bibliography

Giardiello FM, Allen JI, Axilbund JE, et al. Guidelines on Genetic Evaluation and Management of Lynch Syndrome: A Consensus Statement by the US Multi-Society Task Force on Colorectal Cancer. Gastroenterology. 2014 Aug;147(2):502-26. [PMID: 25043945]

Item 46   Answer: D

Educational Objective: Manage chronic hepatitis B infection in the inactive carrier state.

The most appropriate management is to perform no further treatment at this time. Hepatitis B virus (HBV) is diagnosed by serologic tests for HBV antigens and antibodies as well as direct HBV DNA assays. Inactive carriers of HBV have a normal alanine aminotransferase level and low levels of HBV DNA (generally less than 10,000 IU/mL) and are at low risk for progression of liver disease; therefore, initiation of medications to treat HBV in these patients is not justified. These patients remain at risk for reactivation of HBV, which may cause subsequent progression of liver disease. Monitoring for the development of chronic active HBV is therefore warranted. This patient's laboratory studies are consistent with HBV infection (positive hepatitis B surface antigen). His negative hepatitis B e antigen, low HBV DNA level, and normal serum alanine aminotransferase (ALT) level indicate that he is in the inactive carrier state. Hepatitis B treatment is not indicated; however, serum ALT levels should be monitored at 6-month intervals to detect potential transitions to other disease phases. Surveillance for hepatocellular carcinoma (HCC) is advised for patients with chronic HBV who have cirrhosis, a family history of HCC, or persistent elevation of ALT and HBV DNA levels. HCC surveillance is also advised in Asian men older than 40 years, Asian women older than 50 years, and African patients older than 20 years.

Treatment with pegylated interferon or entecavir should be considered if the patient has an elevated serum ALT level and HBV DNA level greater than 10,000 IU/mL. These features are not present in this patient, so treatment is not warranted at this time.

Treatment with lamivudine is seldom advised owing to the high rate of resistance with chronic administration.

KEY POINT

- Patients in the inactive carrier phase of hepatitis B virus (HBV) infection, characterized by a normal serum alanine aminotransferase level and a low HBV DNA level, do not require treatment.

Bibliography

Lok AS, McMahon BJ. Chronic hepatitis B: update 2009. Hepatology. 2009 Sep;50(3):661-2. [PMID: 19714720]

Item 47   Answer: E

Educational Objective: Screen for celiac disease in a patient with symptoms of irritable bowel syndrome with diarrhea.

The most appropriate diagnostic test to perform next is tissue transglutaminase serology. This patient fulfills the criteria for irritable bowel syndrome with diarrhea (IBS-D) and has no accompanying alarm features. Therefore, the diagnosis of IBS-D can be confidently made with minimal testing. Such testing should be limited to studies assessing for organic diseases that are more prevalent in patients with IBS-D than in the general population. A meta-analysis and systematic review of 14 studies including 4204 patients (54% meeting criteria for IBS) found that patients with IBS are three to four times more likely to have positive celiac antibodies and are more than four times more likely to have biopsy-proven celiac disease than controls. Therefore, screening for celiac disease with tissue transglutaminase testing is warranted.

This patient has no alarm features to warrant a colonoscopy or sigmoidoscopy. Furthermore, a study of more than 900 adults (466 with IBS and 451 controls undergoing screening colonoscopy) found the prevalence of structural abnormalities on colonoscopy, including polyps, colorectal cancer, and inflammatory bowel disease, to be no greater in patients with IBS than in controls.

Lactose hydrogen breath testing would be a consideration only if there was a reported connection between the ingestion of milk and bowel symptoms. This patient reported no change when eliminating milk from her diet.

The prevalence of abnormal thyroid-stimulating hormone (TSH) findings is no greater in patients with IBS than in the general population. Furthermore, there is no established causality between abnormal TSH results and the symptoms reported in IBS.

KEY POINT

- Patients with irritable bowel syndrome with diarrhea (IBS-D) should undergo screening for celiac disease with serum tissue transglutaminase testing, as celiac disease has greater prevalence in patients with IBS-D than in the general population.

Bibliography

Ford AC, Chey WD, Talley NJ, Malhotra A, Spiegel BM, Moayyedi P. Yield of diagnostic tests for celiac disease in individuals with symptoms suggestive of irritable bowel syndrome: systematic review and meta-analysis. Arch Intern Med. 2009;169(7):651-8. [PMID: 19364994]

Item 48   Answer: E

Educational Objective: Diagnose the cause of obscure gastrointestinal bleeding with repeat upper endoscopy.

The most appropriate diagnostic test is a repeat upper endoscopy. The underlying cause of obscure gastrointestinal bleeding can often be found by repeating upper endoscopy or colonoscopy. Approximately 30% to 50% of lesions can be detected using this approach. Bleeding sources found by these modalities include Cameron ulcerations in a hiatal hernia, bleeding colonic diverticula, and vascular lesions. This patient had an initial upper endoscopy that showed a hiatal hernia and old blood in the stomach. She also reported dark stools, which suggests an upper gastrointestinal bleeding source. She subsequently had a colonoscopy with normal results. Her large hiatal hernia and old blood in the stomach are clues that she may have chronic bleeding from within the hiatal hernia. Cameron ulcerations are linear gastric erosions found within a hiatal hernia. These erosions have been associated with both iron deficiency anemia and acute and chronic blood loss. Repeating the upper endoscopy will allow re-evaluation of the hiatal hernia and the possible diagnosis of Cameron erosions.

Push enteroscopy and balloon enteroscopy are used for evaluating and treating a small-bowel source of bleeding. The clues of a hiatal hernia and blood in the stomach support upper endoscopy as a higher-yield test to perform next.

Intraoperative endoscopy is generally employed only as a last resort for the evaluation of obscure gastrointestinal bleeding. The patient undergoes laparotomy or laparoscopy, and the bowel is evaluated with a colonoscope following surgical enterotomy. This technique should only be used if other less invasive options have been exhausted or if a patient has unexplained, life-threatening bleeding. In addition, the yield is somewhat low (approximately 25%).

A repeat colonoscopy would not be as helpful as a repeat upper endoscopy because this patient has clues to an upper gastrointestinal bleeding source (hiatal hernia, blood in the stomach, and dark stools).

KEY POINT

- After an initial negative evaluation, the underlying cause of obscure gastrointestinal bleeding can often be found by repeating either upper endoscopy or colonoscopy depending on presenting features.

Bibliography

Raju GS, Gerson L, Das A, Lewis B; American Gastroenterological Association. American Gastroenterological Association (AGA) Institute technical review on obscure gastrointestinal bleeding. Gastroenterology. 2007 Nov;133(5):1697-717. [PMID: 17983812]

Item 49   Answer: C

Educational Objective: Evaluate chest pain with an exercise stress test in a patient with suspected gastro-esophageal reflux disease.

The most appropriate next step in management is an exercise stress test. Chest pain caused by esophageal disorders can be difficult to distinguish from cardiac chest pain because of the anatomic proximity and common innervation of the esophagus and the heart. Esophageal chest pain is often prolonged, nonexertional, and associated with other esophageal symptoms such as dysphagia, odynophagia, or reflux. The most common cause of noncardiac chest pain is untreated gastroesophageal reflux disease (GERD), followed by motility disorders. Owing to the potentially life-threatening consequences of untreated cardiac chest pain, a cardiac evaluation must be performed and cardiac causes must be ruled out before attributing chest pain to an esophageal cause. In addition, the rationale for evaluating this patient for coronary artery disease is particularly compelling. She has atypical chest pain. Atypical chest pain meets two of the three diagnostic criteria for typical chest pain: substernal in location, provoked by exertion or emotional distress, relieved by rest or nitroglycerin. Taking into account the description of the chest pain, sex, and age, this patient has a 51% pretest probability of coronary artery disease and should be further evaluated with an exercise stress test. If this patient's cardiac evaluation is negative, she should receive an empiric trial of a proton pump inhibitor. If symptoms resolve, this confirms the diagnosis of GERD.

Ambulatory pH testing is used to identify patients with GERD. Esophageal manometry testing will identify an underlying motility disorder of the esophagus. Lastly, upper endoscopy is used to identify mucosal inflammation in the upper gastrointestinal tract. These tests should be performed only after a cardiac condition has been ruled out as the cause of this patient's chest pain.

KEY POINT

- Although gastroesophageal reflux disease (GERD) is the most common cause of noncardiac chest pain, a cardiac evaluation should be considered to rule out cardiac causes before initiating treatment for GERD.

Bibliography

Katz PO, Gerson LB, Vela MF. Guidelines for the diagnosis and management of gastroesophageal reflux disease. Am J Gastroenterol. 2013 Mar; 108(3):308-28; quiz 329. Erratum in: Am J Gastroenterol. 2013 Oct;108(10): 1672. [PMID: 23419381]

Item 50   Answer: E

Educational Objective: Treat chronic hepatitis C virus infection.

The most appropriate management is to initiate treatment for hepatitis C virus (HCV) infection. Testing for HCV consists of detecting antibody to HCV and has a very high positive predictive value in patients with elevated liver test results and risk factors for HCV infection. HCV RNA by polymerase chain reaction confirms HCV infection. HCV genotyping should be performed at the time of diagnosis to help choose a treatment regimen. This patient has HCV genotype 2 with significant fibrosis on liver biopsy. Effective antiviral treatment of HCV infection can prevent or delay the development of cirrhosis and hepatocellular carcinoma. Patients with HCV genotype 2 have a very high likelihood of sustained virologic response with sofosbuvir and ribavirin, and therefore treatment should be initiated with these agents.

This patient's positive IgG antibody to hepatitis A virus test is a marker of previous infection; therefore, hepatitis A vaccination will not be useful or necessary.

Likewise, this patient has immunity to hepatitis B based on her positive hepatitis B surface antibody test, and therefore hepatitis B vaccination is not necessary.

Although this patient has a normal alanine aminotransferase level, she has evidence of active inflammation with fibrosis on liver biopsy, and antiviral treatment is indicated despite her normal aminotransferase level. The need for treatment in individuals with HCV infection and normal liver enzyme levels is generally assessed similarly to those with abnormal liver enzyme levels.

Testing for IgM antibody to hepatitis A virus is helpful in the diagnosis of acute hepatitis A; however, this patient has no clinical features of acute hepatitis.

KEY POINT

- Effective antiviral treatment of hepatitis C virus infection can prevent or delay the development of cirrhosis and hepatocellular carcinoma.

Bibliography

Ghany MG, Strader DB, Thomas DL, Seeff LB; American Association for the Study of Liver Diseases. Diagnosis, management, and treatment of hepatitis C: an update. Hepatology. 2009 Apr;49(4):1335-74. [PMID: 19330875]

Item 51   Answer: A

Educational Objective: Perform ambulatory pH impedance monitoring for gastroesophageal reflux disease in a patient whose symptoms did not respond to proton pump inhibitor therapy.

The most appropriate next step in management is ambulatory pH impedance monitoring. This patient has features of refractory gastroesophageal reflux disease (GERD). The first step in treating refractory GERD is to optimize proton pump inhibitor (PPI) therapy by verifying correct administration (30-60 minutes before meals) or increasing to twice-daily dosing. Despite increasing this patient's PPI therapy to twice daily, symptoms have persisted. Upper endoscopy has been performed, and the normal results have ruled out an alternative cause of symptoms such as eosinophilic esophagitis or erosive esophagitis. Ambulatory pH impedance monitoring is usually performed in patients who do not respond to antireflux medications and who have a negative upper endoscopy to make a definitive diagnosis. Ambulatory pH impedance testing while not taking a PPI is useful in patients who have atypical symptoms to determine if reflux is the cause of the symptoms. If pH testing is done with impedance, the PPI can be continued, as impedance can measure nonacid reflux. Testing is also helpful in patients who have had a partial response to treatment to determine if there is continued acid exposure despite the use of a PPI. The finding of continued acid exposure despite the proper dose and use of a PPI is most helpful in patients considering GERD surgery (fundoplication). Ambulatory pH impedance monitoring can be done with a pH catheter over 24 hours or with an endoscopically placed wireless transmitter over 48 hours.

A barium esophagogram would be the appropriate test for evaluation of dysphagia. Barium radiographs have low sensitivity in the evaluation of GERD and should not be performed.

Esophageal manometry measures the pressure levels in the esophagus and is useful in evaluating esophageal motility disorders such as achalasia. This patient does not have dysphagia or signs of a motility disorder, so manometry is not needed.

Fundoplication may be considered for patients with refractory GERD; however, a pH monitoring study is needed to help determine if antireflux surgery is appropriate.

KEY POINT

- Ambulatory pH impedance testing while not taking a proton pump inhibitor is useful in patients who have atypical symptoms of gastroesophageal reflux to determine if reflux is the cause of the symptoms; it is also useful in patients who are symptomatic while on a proton pump inhibitor to determine if there is continued acid exposure.

Bibliography
Katz PO, Gerson LB, Vela MF. Guidelines for the diagnosis and management of gastroesophageal reflux disease. Am J Gastroenterol. 2013 Mar; 108(3):308-28; quiz 329. Erratum in: Am J Gastroenterol. 2013 Oct;108(10): 1672. [PMID: 23419381]

Item 52   Answer: D
Educational Objective: Diagnose lymphocytic colitis.

The most likely diagnosis is lymphocytic colitis, a form of microscopic colitis. Microscopic colitis (MC) accounts for 10% to 15% of patients with chronic, watery diarrhea. In contrast to inflammatory bowel disease, MC is more common in older persons and does not cause endoscopically visible inflammation. The symptoms of MC are similar to other chronic causes of nonbloody diarrhea, such as celiac disease and irritable bowel syndrome; therefore, colonic mucosal biopsies are required for diagnosis. Lymphocytic and collagenous colitis are the two subtypes of MC, and they are distinguishable only by histology. The diagnosis of MC is made by histologic evaluation of colonic biopsies; the classic finding is intraepithelial lymphocytosis (>20 intraepithelial lymphocytes per 100 epithelial cells).

In collagenous colitis, the increase in intraepithelial lymphocytes may be less pronounced than in lymphocytic colitis, and the main histologic feature is thickening of the subepithelial collagen band (usually >10 µm). This patient's histologic findings are pathognomonic of lymphocytic colitis. Microscopic colitis often is idiopathic, but in a small subset of patients it may be a side effect of medications. A diagnosis of microscopic colitis should prompt a careful review of prescription and over-the-counter medications such as NSAIDs, aspirin, proton pump inhibitors, and others. Celiac disease should also be considered, as it can be associated with microscopic colitis.

The hallmark of *Clostridium difficile* colitis is watery diarrhea that is frequently associated with fever and abdominal pain or cramps. Diarrhea may be absent in patients with significant ileus or toxic megacolon, leading to a delay in diagnosis. Grossly bloody stools are rare. Risk factors for *C. difficile* infection include use of antibiotics or chemotherapeutic agents in the 8 weeks preceding infection because this causes alterations in enteric flora that allow bacterial overgrowth and toxin production. Typical symptoms of ischemic colitis are the acute onset of mild, crampy abdominal pain with tenderness on examination over the affected region of colon. Bleeding may not occur early but often occurs within a few days of pain onset. This patient does not have clinical features or colonoscopic findings of either *C. difficile* colitis or ischemic colitis.

KEY POINT

- Microscopic colitis is characterized by histologic inflammation in endoscopically normal-appearing colonic mucosa; patients lack signs of systemic inflammation and present with painless watery diarrhea without bleeding.

Bibliography
Pardi DS, Kelly CP. Microscopic colitis. Gastroenterology. 2011 Apr;140(4): 1155-65. [PMID: 21303675]

Item 53   Answer: C
Educational Objective: Diagnose nonocclusive mesenteric ischemia.

Nonocclusive mesenteric ischemia is the most likely cause of this patient's jejunal wall thickening and dilation, ongoing hypotension, fever, and abdominal pain. Nonocclusive mesenteric ischemia is caused by decreased mesenteric perfusion in low-flow states such as heart failure, sepsis, profound hypotension, or hypovolemia. It may also occur with use of vasoactive medications such as vasopressors, ergots, triptans, cocaine, and digitalis. This patient most likely developed sepsis following induction chemotherapy. The severe and sustained hypotension from sepsis in addition to the use of vasopressor medications results in decreased mesenteric perfusion.

Although this patient has thrombocytopenia, which can predispose to bowel-wall hemorrhage and CT scan findings of wall thickening, bowel-wall hemorrhage would not be associated with the clinical picture of sepsis and fever.

Ischemic colitis is the most common form of ischemic injury to the gastrointestinal tract. Although the vast majority of cases occur in patients older than 60 years of age, it can be seen in this setting owing to altered arterial flow secondary to hypotension and vasopressor medications. This patient has predisposing factors for ischemic colitis with systemic alterations in blood flow, and the typical clinical features of the disease with left lower abdominal pain and diarrhea. However, the lack of rectal bleeding and absence of left colon inflammatory changes on CT do not support ischemic colitis as the cause for this patient's life-threatening clinical scenario.

Mesenteric artery emboli account for 50% of cases of acute mesenteric ischemia. They are usually of cardiac origin owing to atrial fibrillation or left ventricle thrombus. This patient has no evidence of atrial fibrillation, and the clinical picture of severe, unresponsive hypotension before the onset of the gastrointestinal symptoms makes nonocclusive mesenteric ischemia a more likely diagnosis than mesenteric artery embolism.

KEY POINT

- Nonocclusive mesenteric ischemia is caused by decreased mesenteric perfusion in low-flow states such as heart failure, sepsis, profound hypotension, or hypovolemia.

Bibliography

Brandt LJ, Boley SJ. AGA technical review on intestinal ischemia. American Gastrointestinal Association. Gastroenterology. 2000 May;118(5):954-68. [PMID: 10784596]

Item 54   Answer: B

Educational Objective: Manage decompensated cirrhosis with referral for liver transplantation.

The most appropriate next step in management is an evaluation for liver transplantation. This patient has decompensated cirrhosis as manifested by ascites and has a moderately elevated Model for End-Stage Liver Disease (MELD) score. The MELD score is an equation that incorporates the bilirubin, INR, and creatinine levels and was derived initially as a way to accurately predict 3-month and 1-year survival in patients undergoing a transjugular intrahepatic portosystemic shunt (TIPS) procedure. The MELD score has also been validated as a tool for accurately predicting 3-month survival in patients with cirrhosis. This score is the basis for considering referral for liver transplantation (MELD ≥15) and organ allocation. Patients with cirrhotic-stage liver disease and a MELD score of 15 or greater have better survival with liver transplantation than without.

Diuretics have been unsuccessful in this patient owing to the development of kidney dysfunction. Further administration of diuretics may precipitate the development of hepatorenal syndrome; therefore, diuretics should be discontinued.

Patients with MELD scores greater than 10 are at risk of hepatic decompensation and mortality from any surgery, and especially with higher-risk surgeries such as a surgical portosystemic shunt. Therefore, surgical portosystemic shunt should not be performed in this patient, who has a MELD score of 21.

A TIPS can be an attractive option for patients whose ascites does not improve with medical management with a low-sodium diet (<2 g/d) and the usual diuretics (spironolactone and furosemide). However, a TIPS is contraindicated in patients with MELD scores greater than 15 to 18 or serum bilirubin levels greater than 4 mg/dL (68.4 µmol/L), owing to high risk of mortality.

KEY POINT

- Patients with cirrhotic-stage liver disease and a Model for End-Stage Liver Disease (MELD) score of 15 or greater have better survival with liver transplantation than without.

Bibliography

Boyer TD, Haskal ZJ; American Association for the Study of Liver Diseases. The Role of Transjugular Intrahepatic Portosystemic Shunt (TIPS) in the Management of Portal Hypertension: update 2009. Hepatology. 2010 Jan;51(1):306. [PMID: 19902484]

Item 55   Answer: C

Educational Objective: Manage gallstone disease during pregnancy with surgery.

The most appropriate management is laparoscopic cholecystectomy prior to hospital discharge. This patient has uncomplicated gallstone pancreatitis in her second trimester. This is very likely her second symptomatic episode of gallstone disease, and cholecystectomy should be performed. Her risk of recurrent pancreatitis over the next 90 days is about 20%. Laparoscopic cholecystectomy can be safely performed during pregnancy, particularly in the second trimester.

Bile acid dissolution therapy for gallstones has not gained widespread acceptance because most patients, such as this one, are candidates for laparoscopic cholecystectomy and few are candidates for bile acid dissolution therapy. Bile acid dissolution therapy is expensive, requires long-term multiple daily dosing, necessitates repeated ultrasonography, and has a potential long-term risk for cancer in the remaining gallbladder. Finally, most nonsurgical therapies for gallstones are contraindicated in pregnant patients. The safety of bile acid therapy in pregnant women is largely unknown.

In a study of pregnant women who had complications related to gallstones during pregnancy, recurrent biliary symptoms, repeated visits to the emergency department, and recurrent hospitalizations were significantly more common in patients who received conservative treatment as compared with women who underwent laparoscopic cholecystectomy or endoscopic retrograde cholangiopancreatography (ERCP). Waiting until after delivery is not the best option for this patient.

CONT.

ERCP with sphincterotomy could be used, but it should be performed only if this patient had contraindications to cholecystectomy or if there was high clinical suspicion of a persistent common bile duct stone. Neither of these conditions is present in this patient.

Extracorporeal shock-wave lithotripsy (ESWL) is reserved for patients with symptomatic gallstones who are poor candidates for surgery and in those patients with bile duct stones that are refractory to removal at ERCP owing to large size. After ESWL, the gallbladder remains in place and stones recur in about 50% of patients. This patient does not have an indication for ESWL.

KEY POINT

- Laparoscopic cholecystectomy can be safely performed during pregnancy, particularly in the second trimester.

Bibliography

Othman MO, Stone E, Hashimi M, Parasher G. Conservative management of cholelithiasis and its complications in pregnancy is associated with recurrent symptoms and more emergency department visits. Gastrointest Endosc. 2012 Sep;76(3):564-9. [PMID: 22732875]

Item 56   Answer: D

Educational Objective: Diagnose peptic ulcer disease as the cause of upper gastrointestinal bleeding.

The most likely cause of this patient's gastrointestinal bleeding (GIB) is peptic ulcer disease. This patient has upper GIB, which is predicted based on four aspects of his presentation: hematemesis, melena detected on physical examination, absence of blood clots in the stool, and an elevated blood urea nitrogen to creatinine ratio (>30). The most common causes of upper GIB are peptic ulcer disease (34%), esophageal varices (33%), esophagitis (8%), and Mallory-Weiss tear (6%). Peptic ulcer disease (PUD) can cause severe upper GIB in the absence of coagulopathy. PUD is asymptomatic in 4% to 20% of patients and is commonly diagnosed because of complications such as bleeding.

Duodenal angiodysplasia is not the most likely cause of bleeding because severe GIB is rare in the absence of a bleeding diathesis or use of medications that affect hemostasis, including NSAIDs, aspirin, and anticoagulants.

Erosive gastritis is not likely in this patient because it would not cause severe GIB; the injury does not extend deeper than the mucosa, which lacks arteries and veins.

Variceal bleeding can be responsible for severe GIB that should not be overlooked because the mortality rate is high. Variceal bleeding may be the first presentation of cirrhosis, and therefore a high index of suspicion is needed. This patient has no history or biochemical evidence of cirrhosis, making variceal bleeding unlikely.

Portal gastropathy is unlikely because it is a mucosal cause of chronic, slow GIB. It can rarely cause acute but not severe GIB. In addition, this patient has no risk factors for chronic liver disease that would raise suspicion for this condition.

KEY POINT

- Peptic ulcer disease is the most common cause of upper gastrointestinal bleeding.

Bibliography

Kim JJ, Sheibani S, Park S, Buxbaum J, Laine L. Causes of bleeding and outcomes in patients hospitalized with upper gastrointestinal bleeding. J Clin Gastroenterol. 2014 Feb;48(2):113-8. [PMID: 23685847]

Item 57   Answer: D

Educational Objective: Manage a curable malignant polyp.

The most appropriate management is to repeat colonoscopy in 3 months. A malignant polyp was discovered during this patient's colonoscopy and was endoscopically resected. Invasive adenocarcinoma arising in a pedunculated polyp may be considered adequately treated by endoscopic en bloc polypectomy alone if the lesion is confined to the submucosa and possesses no adverse histologic features such as poor differentiation, lymphatic or vascular invasion, or involved margins. National recommendations for postpolypectomy surveillance intervals are as short as 3 to 6 months in patients with large (>2 cm) adenomas or adenomas with invasive cancer and favorable prognostic features. These shorter surveillance intervals help to ensure that no residual polyp tissue remains.

If any adverse histologic features are noted, the risk of lymph node involvement is increased substantially and surgical resection of the involved colon is required. Surgical resection should also be considered if the lesion is removed piecemeal and the adequacy of resection cannot be confirmed.

Since this tumor is endoscopically cured, neither radiation therapy nor CT scan of the abdomen or pelvis is necessary.

KEY POINT

- National recommendations for postpolypectomy surveillance intervals are as short as 3 to 6 months in patients with large (>2 cm) adenomas or adenomas with invasive cancer and favorable prognostic features.

Bibliography

ASGE Standards of Practice Committee, Fisher DA, Shergill AK, Early DS, et al. Role of endoscopy in the staging and management of colorectal cancer. Gastrointest Endosc. 2013 Jul;78(1):8-12. Erratum in: Gastrointest Endosc. 2013 Sep;78(3):559. [PMID: 23664162]

Item 58   Answer: A

Educational Objective: Diagnose and treat small-bowel bleeding with angiography.

The most appropriate test to perform next is angiography, which will allow for bleeding localization and embolization of the bleeding source. Angiography should only be performed in patients with active overt bleeding, as it requires a bleeding rate greater than 0.5 mL/min. Complications such as acute kidney injury, organ necrosis, and vascular dissection/aneurysm can occur.

Balloon enteroscopy is used to visualize the small bowel. Latex balloons are mounted on an overtube that can deliver the enteroscope into the small bowel by successive inflation and deflation. Balloon enteroscopy can deliver the enteroscope orally or rectally (retrograde) and can be used for diagnosis and therapy. Complications of balloon enteroscopy are perforation and bleeding via avulsion of the bowel. Contraindications are radiation enteritis, severe ulceration, and recent bowel surgery. Retrograde balloon enteroscopy is not necessary because blood was seen in the colon; balloon enteroscopy is reserved for evaluation of the small intestine, which is not needed in this patient.

Repeat colonoscopy could be attempted, but visualization would be limited because the colon lumen would be filled with blood.

Technetium-labeled nuclear scans are used in patients with active bleeding (melena or hematochezia) who are transfusion dependent and hospitalized. This a diagnostic test and does not allow for therapeutic intervention.

> **KEY POINT**
>
> - In patients with gastrointestinal bleeding, angiography can identify bleeding and allows for therapeutic intervention with embolization.

Bibliography
Feinman M, Haut ER. Lower gastrointestinal bleeding. Surg Clin North Am. 2014 Feb;94(1):55-63. [PMID: 24267497]

Item 59   Answer: E
Educational Objective: Manage acalculous cholecystitis.

The most appropriate management is percutaneous cholecystostomy. This ill patient presents with symptoms, signs, and imaging studies consistent with cholecystitis. Hospitalized patients can have acute cholecystitis without gallstones. This is known as acalculous cholecystitis and is thought to reflect either bacterial seeding of the gallbladder wall or gallbladder wall ischemia. Fever accompanying abdominal pain in a critically ill patient should prompt an assessment for cholecystitis. Diagnosis is usually made with ultrasound findings of acute cholecystitis or a radionuclide biliary scan that fails to visualize the gallbladder. Approximately 50% of these high-risk patients will develop cholangitis, empyema, gangrene, or gallbladder perforation during their hospitalization. Supportive treatment with intravenous antibiotic coverage of anaerobic and gram-negative bacteria is required. Definitive therapy with cholecystectomy is preferred but may be contraindicated in severely ill patients. Therapeutic decompression can be achieved with image-guided percutaneous cholecystostomy tube placement. The mortality rate for acute acalculous cholecystitis is between 10% and 50%.

An abdominal CT with contrast will add little useful information to this patient's clinical picture, and it might worsen his kidney disease.

Endoscopic retrograde cholangiopancreatography with sphincterotomy would be a consideration if this patient had gallbladder stones and/or a common bile duct stone. However, his normal liver chemistry studies and absence of biliary dilatation on ultrasound make a common bile duct stone unlikely.

Magnetic resonance cholangiopancreatography, similarly to CT, would not add important clinical information and would be difficult to perform in this ill, ventilated patient.

> **KEY POINT**
>
> - Fever accompanying abdominal pain in a critically ill patient should prompt an assessment for acalculous cholecystitis (acute cholecystitis without gallstones).

Bibliography
Simorov A, Ranade A, Parcells J, et al. Emergent cholecystostomy is superior to open cholecystectomy in extremely ill patients with acalculous cholecystitis: a large multicenter outcome study. Am J Surg. 2013 Dec;206(6):935-40; discussion 940-1. [PMID: 24112675]

Item 60   Answer: D
Educational Objective: Manage upper gastrointestinal bleeding caused by a low-risk gastric ulcer.

The most appropriate next step in management is to switch the intravenous proton pump inhibitor (PPI) to an oral PPI because this patient's low-risk ulcer does not require prolonged intravenous treatment or observation. Low-risk gastric ulcers are clean-based or have a nonprotuberant pigmented spot and should be treated with oral PPI therapy, initiation of refeeding within 24 hours, and early hospital discharge.

Blood transfusion should be performed in patients with (1) hemodynamic instability and ongoing bleeding or susceptibility to complications from oxygen deprivation (for example, ischemic heart disease) and (2) a hemoglobin level less than 7 g/dL (70 g/L) if hemodynamically stable with no active or massive bleeding. This patient does not meet these criteria.

Endoscopic treatment of the ulcer is not appropriate because clean-based ulcers are at low risk for rebleeding and the risks of endoscopic therapy outweigh any potential benefits in this patient.

Octreotide is not a routine treatment, even for acute active bleeding, unless variceal bleeding is suspected. This patient has a low-risk ulcer and no evidence of esophageal varices, so octreotide is not indicated.

> **KEY POINT**
>
> - Low-risk gastric ulcers are clean-based or have a nonprotuberant pigmented spot; they should be treated with oral proton pump inhibitor therapy, initiation of refeeding within 24 hours, and early hospital discharge.

Bibliography

Barkun AN, Bardou M, Kuipers EJ, et al; International Consensus Upper Gastrointestinal Bleeding Conference Group. International consensus recommendations on the management of patients with nonvariceal upper gastrointestinal bleeding. Ann Intern Med. 2010 Jan 19;152(2):101-13. [PMID: 20083829]

Item 61   Answer: B

Educational Objective: Manage hepatocellular carcinoma in a patient who meets the Milan criteria.

The most appropriate next step in management is to refer this patient for liver transplantation evaluation. A diagnosis of hepatocellular carcinoma can be made in a patient with cirrhosis in the presence of lesions larger than 1 cm that enhance in the arterial phase and have washout of contrast in the venous phase. Patients who meet the Milan criteria (up to three hepatocellular carcinoma tumors ≤3 cm or one tumor ≤5 cm) have excellent 5-year survival rates after liver transplantation. Patients who meet Milan criteria and have a tumor 2 cm or larger with arterial enhancement and venous washout on CT or MRI are eligible to receive Model for End-Stage Liver Disease (MELD) exception points, placing them at a higher priority for liver transplantation.

This patient does not require a biopsy of the liver masses because the radiographic characteristics of his liver tumors meet criteria for a diagnosis of hepatocellular carcinoma. The vast majority of hepatocellular carcinomas in the context of cirrhosis can be diagnosed with radiologic criteria alone. There is also a small risk (1%-3%) of seeding the needle track with tumor cells with percutaneous biopsy of hepatocellular carcinoma.

Sorafenib, a compound that targets growth signaling and angiogenesis, should be reserved for patients with Child-Turcotte-Pugh class A or B cirrhosis, good performance status, and vascular, lymphatic, or extrahepatic spread of the tumor. This patient has no evidence of angiolymphatic or extrahepatic involvement, and the tumor sizes are within Milan criteria; therefore, he should be evaluated for liver transplantation rather than started on sorafenib.

Surgical resection is not an appropriate option in this patient with evidence of hyperbilirubinemia and portal hypertension; he would be at high risk for postsurgical hepatic decompensation.

Transarterial chemoembolization (TACE) should not be performed before referral to a transplant center. Ultimately, patients who are expected to be on the waiting list for longer than 6 months are recommended to receive locoregional therapy such as TACE to control the tumor while awaiting a transplant. However, TACE should only be performed after the liver transplant evaluation is completed.

KEY POINT

- Patients with cirrhosis who meet the Milan criteria (up to three hepatocellular carcinoma tumors ≤3 cm or one tumor ≤5 cm) are best treated with liver transplantation and have excellent 5-year survival rates.

Bibliography

Mazzaferro V, Regalia E, Doci R, et al. Liver transplantation for the treatment of small hepatocellular carcinomas in patients with cirrhosis. N Engl J Med. 1996;334(11):693-9. [PMID: 8594428]

Item 62   Answer: E

Educational Objective: Evaluate a patient with a positive hepatitis C virus (HCV) antibody test and a negative HCV RNA test.

Patients who are hepatitis C virus (HCV) antibody positive but HCV RNA negative do not have HCV infection and require no further testing. Repeating HCV RNA testing can be considered if there are risk factors for recent HCV infection or if there is other clinical evidence of liver disease, but neither of these is present in this patient. A 2013 guideline from the U.S. Preventive Services Task Force recommended screening for hepatitis C once in all persons born between 1945 and 1965, as well as targeted screening of persons with risk factors such as illicit drug use, receipt of blood products, hemodialysis, and multiple sex partners. Screening is accomplished by testing for antibody to HCV (anti-HCV). If antibody testing is positive, the next step is to perform HCV RNA testing, which is often done by "reflex" testing in many laboratories. The test results are interpreted in the following ways: Positive anti-HCV with negative HCV RNA indicates either false-positive anti-HCV or cleared infection, and positive anti-HCV with positive HCV RNA indicates active infection. Rarely, in instances of acute HCV infection or in an immunosuppressed patient, HCV RNA may be positive despite a negative anti-HCV.

Liver ultrasound and serial alanine aminotransferase monitoring are not necessary in the absence of clinical evidence of liver disease.

KEY POINT

- Patients with a positive antibody to hepatitis C virus (HCV) but negative HCV RNA do not have HCV infection, and no further testing is required.

Bibliography

Centers for Disease Control and Prevention (CDC). Testing for HCV infection: an update of guidance for clinicians and laboratorians. MMWR Morb Mortal Wkly Rep. 2013 May 10;62(18):362-5. [PMID: 23657112]

Item 63   Answer: D

Educational Objective: Perform genetic testing to evaluate the inheritance pattern of *MYH*-associated polyposis.

The most important person to receive genetic testing is the patient's wife. *MYH*-associated polyposis (MAP) is the only known autosomal recessive hereditary colorectal cancer syndrome. MAP should be considered as a cause for multiple colorectal adenomas (>10) in patients with an apparent autosomal recessive inheritance of colorectal polyposis or cancer. MAP is caused by biallelic mutations in the base excision repair gene *MYH*. Because the disorder is autosomal recessive, both parents must be carriers of an *MYH* mutation in order for a child to inherit the syndrome. Therefore, testing the patient's wife would provide the knowledge required to make a risk assessment for the children. If the patient's wife is negative for the *MYH* mutation, the children will not be biallelic mutation carriers and do not need genetic testing. If the patient's wife has a genetic mutation in the *MYH* gene, each child has a 25% chance of inheriting both *MYH* gene mutations (and would have the disease), a 50% chance of inheriting at least one *MYH* gene mutation (and would be a carrier), and a 25% chance of inheriting no *MYH* gene mutations. In that circumstance, the children should each undergo genetic testing.

Performing genetic testing on the patient's father or mother would not provide any useful information at this time. The patient has already been diagnosed with the two mutations; therefore, both his mother and father must be positive for the mutation.

If the patient's wife was unavailable for genetic testing, it would be appropriate to perform genetic testing on the children. Genetic testing is usually done at the age at which high-risk colorectal cancer screening would begin, which is 18 years in MAP and attenuated familial adenomatous polyposis and 12 to 15 years in classic FAP.

KEY POINT

- Because *MYH*-associated polyposis is an autosomal recessive disorder, both parents must be carriers of an *MYH* mutation in order for a child to inherit the syndrome.

Bibliography

Hegde M, Ferber M, Mao R, Samowitz W, Ganguly A; a Working Group of the American College of Medical Genetics and Genomics (ACMG) Laboratory Quality Assurance Committee. ACMG technical standards and guidelines for genetic testing for inherited colorectal cancer (Lynch syndrome, familial adenomatous polyposis, and MYH-associated polyposis). Genet Med. 2013 Dec 5. [PMID: 24310308]

Item 64   Answer: A

Educational Objective: Provide antibiotic prophylaxis for variceal hemorrhage in a patient with cirrhosis but without ascites.

The most appropriate next step in management is administration of antibiotics. This patient has decompensated cirrhosis as evidenced by previous ascites and jaundice, and she has developed hematemesis, which is most suggestive of a variceal hemorrhage. Patients with cirrhosis, especially those with decompensated cirrhosis, are at high risk for developing bacterial infections during an episode of variceal hemorrhage. A common misperception is that antibiotic prophylaxis need only be provided for patients with variceal hemorrhage and ascites (at risk for spontaneous bacterial peritonitis). A Cochrane systematic review confirmed that antibiotic prophylaxis during variceal bleeding not only helps prevent spontaneous bacterial peritonitis but also helps reduces the risk of bacteremia, pneumonia,

and urinary tract infection and reduces mortality. Therefore, prophylactic antibiotics should be provided for patients with cirrhosis and variceal hemorrhage, regardless of the presence or absence of ascites. An oral fluoroquinolone such as norfloxacin or intravenous ciprofloxacin (when oral intake is not possible) are the acceptable choices. Intravenous ceftriaxone may be more effective for patients with Child-Turcotte-Pugh class B and C cirrhosis. The maximum duration of antibiotic administration is 7 days.

A nonselective β-blocker is recommended as secondary prophylaxis after recovery from a variceal bleed, but it would not be warranted in the acute setting in this patient with hypotension.

Evidence regarding the early placement (within 72 hours) of a transjugular intrahepatic portosystemic shunt (TIPS) for patients with variceal hemorrhage is evolving. Despite some evidence of improved mortality for early TIPS placement after endoscopic and pharmacologic control of variceal hemorrhage, this is not the current standard of care. In addition, variceal hemorrhage has not yet been confirmed in this patient, so this intervention is not appropriate at this time.

An upper endoscopy should be performed in this patient with presumed variceal hemorrhage within 12 hours, but only after she has been treated with standard pharmacotherapy (octreotide and antibiotics) and appropriately resuscitated to enable safe endoscopy. A blood pressure of 72/54 mm Hg is too low to be able to proceed immediately with a safe endoscopy.

KEY POINT

- Patients with variceal hemorrhage and cirrhosis are at high risk for infection and require antibiotic prophylaxis, regardless of the presence or absence of ascites.

Bibliography

Chavez-Tapia NC, Barrientos-Gutierrez T, Tellez-Avila F, et al. Meta-analysis: antibiotic prophylaxis for cirrhotic patients with upper gastrointestinal bleeding - an updated Cochrane review. Aliment Pharmacol Ther. 2011 Sep;34(5):509-18. [PMID: 21707680]

Item 65   Answer: B

Educational Objective: Diagnose celiac disease in a patient with abnormal liver chemistry studies.

The most likely diagnosis is celiac disease. This patient has the combination of loose stools, unintentional weight loss, elevated liver chemistry test results, and iron deficiency anemia without an obvious source of blood loss. Minor elevations of serum aminotransferase levels are found in up to 50% of patients with celiac disease and may be the only presenting feature in approximately 9% of patients. Serum aspartate aminotransferase (AST) is usually less than 80 U/L, and alanine aminotransferase (ALT) is usually less than 130 U/L. Patients with celiac disease can also have coexisting liver disease such as autoimmune hepatitis, primary sclerosing cholangitis, or primary biliary cirrhosis. Improvements in liver chemistry studies that are related to celiac disease occur when such patients are treated with a gluten-free diet.

Alcohol-induced liver disease (ALD) is diagnosed by a history of significant alcohol intake and clinical evidence of liver disease. Serum AST level is typically elevated two to six times the upper limit of normal in severe alcoholic hepatitis. AST levels above 500 U/L and ALT levels above 200 U/L are uncommon. An AST/ALT ratio above 2 to 3 is typical for ALD. This patient does not have significant alcohol intake or an aminotransferase profile typical of alcohol-induced liver disease.

Chronic viral hepatitis can result in modest elevations in the aminotransferase levels; typically ALT is greater than AST. The alkaline phosphatase level may be normal or slightly elevated. A diagnosis of chronic hepatitis would not account for the patient's diarrhea or iron deficiency anemia.

Primary biliary cirrhosis (PBC) is a chronic cholestatic liver disease of unknown cause. PBC is diagnosed by serum alkaline phosphatase levels greater than 1.5 times the upper limit of normal and typically normal serum total bilirubin levels. Increases in serum AST and ALT levels less than five times the upper limit of normal may be seen as well. PBC is not associated with diarrhea or iron deficiency anemia.

KEY POINT

- Celiac disease is identified in 9% of patients with otherwise unexplained elevated serum aminotransferase levels.

Bibliography

Rubio-Tapia A, Murray JA. The liver in celiac disease. Hepatology. 2007 Nov;46(5):1650-8. [PMID: 17969053]

Item 66   Answer: D

Educational Objective: Diagnose a common bile duct stone.

The most likely diagnosis is choledocholithiasis. This patient's pain is consistent with biliary pain, and the presence of a transient elevation of serum alanine aminotransferase and the dilated bile ducts on ultrasound are consistent with intermittent biliary obstruction due to a common bile duct stone. Up to 20% of patients with symptomatic gallbladder stones will have a common bile duct stone. Although complications are more common than with symptomatic gallstones, less than 50% of patients with choledocholithiasis develop symptoms, and 20% spontaneously pass stones from the common bile duct. Assessment of the bile duct preoperatively with endoscopic ultrasound or magnetic resonance cholangiopancreatography is recommended if the clinical suspicion is high.

Acute pancreatitis could be a complication of a common bile duct stone, but the pain would not be intermittent and it would result in an elevated serum amylase level, which was not present in this patient.

A bile leak would present earlier, within a day or two after surgery. It would cause more continuous pain and

would result in signs of peritonitis on examination. In addition, the bile ducts would not be dilated.

Fever suggests the development of cholangitis, which is potentially life threatening. Additional findings of cholangitis include jaundice and pain in the right upper quadrant (Charcot triad). Most patients will have cholelithiasis, elevated aminotransferase levels, and hyperbilirubinemia. Ultrasonography may show a dilated common bile duct.

Sphincter of Oddi dysfunction would produce the same symptoms as are found in this patient; however, this condition is typically diagnosed in patients with biliary-type pain without an alternative explanation. This patient's recent history of cholelithiasis, cholecystectomy, and dilated intrahepatic and extrahepatic bile ducts strongly suggests choledocholithiasis, not sphincter of Oddi dysfunction.

KEY POINT

- Biliary pain associated with dilated bile ducts on ultrasound is consistent with the diagnosis of choledocholithiasis.

Bibliography

ASGE Standards of Practice Committee, Maple JT, Ben-Menachem T, Anderson MA, et al. The role of endoscopy in the evaluation of suspected choledocholithiasis. Gastrointest Endosc. 2010 Jan;71(1):1-9. [PMID: 20105473]

Item 67   Answer: B

Educational Objective: Manage gastroparesis.

The most appropriate management is to discontinue metoclopramide and begin promethazine. Replacing the metoclopramide with a scheduled antiemetic is the safest and most cost-effective next step in management. The initial treatment of diabetic gastroparesis should include a dietary management plan consisting of frequent small-volume meals that are low in fat and soluble fiber. Equally important is tight glycemic control because acute hyperglycemia can impair gastric emptying, often resulting in nausea, vomiting, and abdominal pain. When these initial treatment modalities are ineffective, the use of the prokinetic agent metoclopramide is indicated. Metoclopramide is the only drug approved by the FDA for the treatment of gastroparesis. Metoclopramide crosses the blood-brain barrier and potentially causes side effects such as hyperprolactinemia, galactorrhea, and a variety of neurologic symptoms such as tardive dyskinesia. The risks of neurologic side effects are increased with chronic therapy (greater than 3 months) and with use in the elderly and in women. Drug-induced movement disorders are the most concerning neurologic symptoms. Patients taking metoclopramide should receive counseling about these potential adverse effects and should notify the prescriber immediately if these symptoms develop. Symptoms are likely to progress in severity and may become permanent with continued therapy. Although metoclopramide was effective at relieving this patient's gastroparesis symptoms, her neurologic symptoms mandate its prompt discontinuation. Simply decreasing the dose of metoclopramide is unlikely to resolve the neurologic symptoms. Although antiemetic therapy will not improve gastric emptying, it can be very effective for symptoms of nausea and vomiting.

Gastric electrical stimulation with a gastric pacemaker may be considered for compassionate treatment in patients with refractory symptoms of nausea and vomiting in whom all other forms of more conservative therapy have failed.

Given the lack of superiority to placebo in randomized clinical trials, intrapyloric injection of botulinum toxin cannot be recommended for patients with gastroparesis.

KEY POINT

- Metoclopramide is the only drug approved by the FDA for the treatment of gastroparesis; however, metoclopramide is associated with side effects such as hyperprolactinemia, galactorrhea, and tardive dyskinesia that require discontinuation of the drug.

Bibliography

Camilleri M, Parkman HP, Shafi MA, Abell TL, Gerson L; American College of Gastroenterology. Clinical guideline: management of gastroparesis. Am J Gastroenterol. 2013 Jan;108(1):18-37; quiz 38. [PMID: 23147521]

Item 68   Answer: C

Educational Objective: Treat non–acetaminophen-related acute liver failure with *N*-acetylcysteine.

The most appropriate treatment is intravenous *N*-acetylcysteine (NAC). This patient has features of acute liver failure (ALF). ALF is defined by the absence of previous liver disease accompanied by new-onset hepatic encephalopathy and coagulopathy, usually in the presence of jaundice. The cause of ALF is most likely amoxicillin-clavulanate, which is the most common cause of drug-induced liver injury. Intravenous NAC was shown to be effective for non–acetaminophen-related ALF in a randomized, placebo-controlled trial (N=173). The transplant-free survival was 40% in the NAC-treated patients compared with 27% in the placebo group, and this survival benefit was seen only in early-grade (grade I to II) hepatic encephalopathy. This patient has grade II hepatic encephalopathy as evidenced by the presence of asterixis.

Intravenous acyclovir would be an appropriate treatment for herpes hepatitis. Herpes hepatitis classically presents with serum aminotransferase values in the multiple thousands and a disproportionately low serum bilirubin level, which is not the case for this patient.

Intravenous glucocorticoids are not appropriate because they are not proved to be effective in ALF related to drug-induced liver injury.

Oral pentoxifylline is a second-line treatment for alcoholic hepatitis. This patient has a non–alcohol-related cause of ALF; her drinking history does not suggest that alcoholic hepatitis is likely.

KEY POINT

- *N*-acetylcysteine has been shown in a randomized controlled trial to improve transplant-free survival in non–acetaminophen-related acute liver failure in patients with grade I or II hepatic encephalopathy.

Bibliography

Lee WM, Hynan LS, Rossaro L, et al; Acute Liver Failure Study Group. Intravenous N-acetylcysteine improves transplant-free survival in early stage non-acetaminophen acute liver failure. Gastroenterology. 2009 Sep;137(3):856-64, 864.e1. Erratum in: Gastroenterology. 2013 Sep;145(3):695. [PMID: 19524577]

Item 69   Answer: D

Educational Objective: Diagnose eosinophilic esophagitis.

The most likely diagnosis is eosinophilic esophagitis (EoE). This patient has the classic presentation of EoE, which occurs in a young man with solid-food dysphagia that requires endoscopy for removal. EoE is the result of eosinophil cell infiltration of the esophageal squamous mucosa. The incidence of EoE is thought to be increasing, and it seems to parallel the increasing incidence of allergic disease and asthma. Asthma and systemic and seasonal allergies have significant prevalence in adults with EoE. EoE is diagnosed by the finding of greater than 15 eosinophils/hpf on esophageal endoscopic biopsy and by exclusion of GERD. GERD must be excluded because it can also cause esophageal eosinophilic infiltration. This can be done with a therapeutic trial of a proton pump inhibitor (PPI) for 8 weeks. Clinical response to PPI therapy should be assessed based on improvement of clinical symptoms and even repeating the upper endoscopy with biopsies to demonstrate mucosal healing. Endoscopy often reveals characteristic findings of EoE such as rings, longitudinal furrows, and sometimes strictures. Medical therapy consists of swallowed aerosolized topical glucocorticoids (fluticasone or budesonide).

Achalasia is also characterized by dysphagia; however, endoscopic findings of achalasia would include a dilated esophagus with a tight gastroesophageal junction, where the lower esophageal sphincter is located. These endoscopic findings are not present in this patient.

Barrett esophagus (BE) is the result of chronic acid reflux, but it is usually not associated with dysphagia, especially in a young person. The diagnosis of BE is suggested by endoscopic findings of salmon-colored mucosa at the gastroesophageal junction compared with the normal pearl-colored squamous mucosa and is confirmed histologically by the presence of specialized intestinal metaplasia with acid-mucin–containing goblet cells.

Diffuse esophageal spasm is usually characterized by dysphagia or chest pain but not food impaction. Manometry shows intermittent, high-amplitude, simultaneous, nonperistaltic contractions in response to swallowing. Findings of a "corkscrew esophagus" (caused by multiple simultaneous contractions) on barium swallow are typical of diffuse esophageal spasm. Longitudinal rings or furrows are not seen on endoscopic examination.

> **KEY POINT**
> - The classic presentation of eosinophilic esophagitis is a young man with solid-food dysphagia that requires endoscopy for removal.

Bibliography

Dellon ES, Gonsalves N, Hirano I, Furuta GT, Liacouras CA, Katzka DA; American College of Gastroenterology. ACG clinical guideline: Evidenced based approach to the diagnosis and management of esophageal eosinophilia and eosinophilic esophagitis (EoE). Am J Gastroenterol. 2013 May;108(5):679-92; quiz 693. [PMID: 23567357]

Item 70   Answer: D

Educational Objective: Recommend surveillance upper endoscopy in a patient with familial adenomatous polyposis.

The most appropriate recommendation for surveillance of a familial adenomatous polyposis (FAP)–related cancer is upper endoscopy. Once the colon is removed in a patient with FAP, duodenal and periampullary cancers are the second leading causes of cancer deaths. The cumulative lifetime risk of duodenal cancer is based on the size, number, and pathology of duodenal polyps and ranges from 2.5% for stage I to 30% for stage IV duodenal polyposis. Gastric fundic gland polyps and duodenal adenomas are almost always present in patients with FAP. Upper endoscopy is recommended for surveillance of duodenal cancer every 1 to 5 years in all patients with FAP; the exact interval is based on the stage of duodenal polyposis.

CT of the abdomen and pelvis is not a standard recommendation for patients with FAP, but it may be useful for surveillance of patients with FAP-related intra-abdominal desmoid tumors.

A phenotypic variant of FAP called Gardner syndrome is associated with extraintestinal manifestations of FAP, which include congenital hypertrophy of the retinal pigment epithelium (CHRPE). CHRPE may be an indication of underlying FAP, but it has no attendant health risks for patients with FAP and does not require ongoing surveillance if detected.

Small-bowel capsule endoscopy is not a standard surveillance recommendation for a patient with FAP because the risk for small-bowel cancer beyond the duodenum is small.

> **KEY POINT**
> - Upper endoscopy is recommended for surveillance of duodenal cancer every 1 to 5 years in all patients with familial adenomatous polyposis.

Bibliography

Vasen HF, Möslein G, Alonso A, et al. Guidelines for the clinical management of familial adenomatous polyposis (FAP). Gut. 2008 May;57(5):704-13. [PMID: 18194984]

Item 71   Answer: D

Educational Objective: Manage acute hepatitis B.

The most appropriate management is serial monitoring of liver enzymes. This patient has acute hepatitis B without evidence of marked liver dysfunction (such as markedly increased INR or hepatic encephalopathy). Typical clinical symptoms include malaise, fatigue, nausea, and right upper quadrant discomfort. Jaundice and cholestasis can develop 1 to 2 weeks after the onset of symptoms. Acute hepatitis B infection will resolve (defined as clearance of hepatitis B surface antigen within 6 months) in 90% of adult patients. Serial monitoring of liver enzymes and markers of liver synthetic function is the most appropriate management strategy.

Given this patient's essentially unremarkable ultrasound and laboratory tests consistent with acute hepatitis B, abdominal CT is not necessary at this time.

Patients with fulminant acute hepatitis B or severe protracted acute hepatitis B may be offered antiviral therapy with agents such as lamivudine, entecavir, or tenofovir. This patient does not have marked liver dysfunction, so these agents are not appropriate at this time.

Pegylated interferon is contraindicated in acute hepatitis B owing to the risk of exacerbating liver inflammation and is therefore not appropriate for this patient.

> **KEY POINT**
> - Acute hepatitis B infection will resolve (defined as clearance of hepatitis B surface antigen within 6 months) in 90% of adult patients.

Bibliography

Jindal A, Kumar M, Sarin SK. Management of acute hepatitis B and reactivation of hepatitis B. Liver Int. 2013 Feb;33 Suppl 1:164-75. [PMID: 23286861]

Item 72   Answer: D

Educational Objective: Manage pain in chronic pancreatitis using a gabapentinoid.

The most appropriate additional treatment is pregabalin, a gabapentinoid. Pain can be difficult to treat in patients with chronic pancreatitis. In the absence of a local anatomic cause of pain, a stepwise approach to analgesia is appropriate starting with simple analgesics such as NSAIDs or acetaminophen. Non–enteric-coated pancreatic enzymes, which theoretically limit stimulation of the pancreas by inhibiting the cholecystokinin feedback loop, can be tried for pain control. They seem to be most effective in patients with idiopathic pancreatitis. For patients with persistent pain despite the use of simple analgesics, initiating opioids is a reasonable consideration while developing a pain management program that includes adjunctive agents to minimize chronic narcotic use, which can create addiction and gastrointestinal side effects. Most experts begin with tramadol, a nonopioid with opioid actions that provides analgesia comparable to other opioid analgesics in patients with chronic pancreatitis but causes fewer gastrointestinal side effects. Pregabalin (or a low-dose tricyclic antidepressant) may be offered adjunctively, as part of a step-up approach to pain management, after an initial trial of acetaminophen, ibuprofen, and/or tramadol. According to a recent randomized controlled trial, the gabapentinoid pregabalin used as adjuvant treatment reduced constant pain in chronic pancreatitis but has an unclear durability of action and may cause central nervous system side effects in up to 30% of patients.

Celiac plexus blockade (using glucocorticoids) or neurolysis (using ethanol) can be performed percutaneously or via endoscopic ultrasonography, but any relief from this procedure tends to be short lived and is associated with risks of diarrhea, postural hypotension, and rarely paraplegia. Adding pregabalin as adjuvant therapy is a more reasonable and less invasive next therapeutic step for this patient.

Extracorporeal shock wave lithotripsy can be used to break up stones obstructing pancreatic ducts and improve ductal drainage and relieve pain. Extracorporeal shock wave lithotripsy is not appropriate for this patient because she does not have an intraductal pancreatic duct stone and dilated main pancreatic duct.

Surgical management of chronic pancreatitis is reserved for patients in whom conventional medical management is unsuccessful. Surgical management is categorized into operative resection (pancreaticoduodenectomy or distal pancreatectomy) and drainage procedures (lateral pancreaticojejunostomy), and the choice of surgery is dependent on the clinical situation.

KEY POINT

- For patients with persistent pain due to chronic pancreatitis, pregabalin (or a low-dose tricyclic antidepressant) may be offered adjunctively, as part of a step-up approach to pain management, after an initial trial of acetaminophen, ibuprofen, and/or tramadol.

Bibliography
Forsmark CE. Management of chronic pancreatitis. Gastroenterology. 2013 Jun;144(6):1282-91.e3. [PMID: 23622138]

Item 73   Answer: B

Educational Objective: Treat gastroesophageal reflux disease in a patient with an incomplete response to once-daily proton pump inhibitor therapy.

The most appropriate next step in management is to increase the pantoprazole to twice daily. This patient has classic symptoms of gastroesophageal reflux disease (GERD), with heartburn and a sour taste in his mouth. Once-daily proton pump inhibitor (PPI) therapy has significantly improved his symptoms, but he still has breakthrough symptoms at night. Patients with no alarm symptoms (dysphagia, unintentional weight loss, hematemesis, or melena) and a partial response to PPI therapy should have their dose increased to twice daily. Genetic variation in rates of drug metabolism, including PPIs, may decrease effectiveness in some populations (especially

white patients), providing a rationale for twice-daily dosing for some patients. Before drug dose escalation, adherence and correct administration (30 to 60 minutes before a meal) should be confirmed. When adequate symptom relief is obtained, it is reasonable to decrease to the lowest effective dose or even stop therapy.

Prokinetic medications such as metoclopramide have no role in the therapy of GERD. Tardive dyskinesia is a serious complication of metoclopramide therapy, is more common in women, occurs with increased frequency with prolonged use, and may be irreversible.

This patient's symptoms are improving with medical therapy, so upper endoscopy is not necessary at this point. Upper endoscopy would be warranted if this patient's symptoms do not improve with twice-daily PPI therapy.

There are no convincing data to suggest that one PPI is superior to another in the treatment of uncomplicated GERD. Increasing the dose of the current PPI is more likely to be beneficial than is switching to another PPI such as omeprazole.

KEY POINT

- Patients with gastroesophageal reflux disease with no alarm symptoms who have a partial response to once-daily proton pump inhibitor therapy should have their dose increased to twice daily.

Bibliography
Katz PO, Gerson LB, Vela MF. Guidelines for the diagnosis and management of gastroesophageal reflux disease. Am J Gastroenterol. 2013 Mar; 108(3):308-28; quiz 329. Erratum in: Am J Gastroenterol. 2013 Oct; 108(10):1672. [PMID: 23419381]

Item 74   Answer: B

Educational Objective: Treat refractory ulcerative colitis with an anti-tumor necrosis factor agent.

The most appropriate treatment is to initiate an anti–tumor necrosis factor (anti-TNF) agent such as adalimumab. This patient has moderate to severe ulcerative colitis that is not responding to 60 mg/d of prednisone. Moderate to severe ulcerative colitis is often treated with oral glucocorticoids such as prednisone, 40 to 60 mg/d. Patients whose disease does not respond to oral glucocorticoids should be hospitalized and given intravenous glucocorticoids or should be treated with an anti-TNF agent. Randomized controlled clinical trials have shown three anti-TNF antibodies (infliximab, adalimumab, and golimumab) to be effective for inducing and maintaining remission in patients such as this with ulcerative colitis. Indications for hospital admission include dehydration, inability to tolerate oral intake, fever, significant abdominal tenderness, and abdominal distention.

A meta-analysis of clinical trials showed that using doses of prednisone above 60 mg/d provides little if any additional efficacy and produces more side effects.

Ciprofloxacin and metronidazole should be used in patients with severe colitis associated with high fever, significant leukocytosis, peritoneal signs, or toxic megacolon.

However, antibiotics are not indicated in a patient such as this with colitis without signs of systemic toxicity.

Patients with mild to moderate ulcerative colitis respond well to 5-aminosalicylate agents. Patients with proctitis or left-sided colitis should receive topical therapy with a 5-aminosalicylate or hydrocortisone suppositories or enemas. If patients require repeated courses of glucocorticoids or become glucocorticoid dependent, thiopurines (6-mercaptopurine or azathioprine) or an anti-TNF agent should be initiated (methotrexate has not been shown to be effective in ulcerative colitis). Anti-TNF agents should be used in patients who do not maintain remission with thiopurines or patients whose disease is refractory to glucocorticoids. It is unlikely that 5-aminosalicylates would be beneficial in this patient with more severe disease that is refractory to prednisone.

KEY POINT

- Patients with moderate to severe ulcerative colitis whose disease does not respond to oral glucocorticoids should be treated with either intravenous glucocorticoids or an anti–tumor necrosis factor agent.

Bibliography
Talley NJ, Abreu MT, Achkar JP, et al; American College of Gastroenterology IBD Task Force. An evidence-based systematic review on medical therapies for inflammatory bowel disease. Am J Gastroenterol. 2011 Apr;106 Suppl 1:S2-25; quiz S26. [PMID: 21472012]

Item 75   Answer: C

Educational Objective: Manage upper gastrointestinal bleeding in a patient with cardiovascular disease.

The most appropriate postendoscopic management is to resume aspirin before discharge. This patient has upper gastrointestinal bleeding due to a low-risk (clean-based) ulcer. Aspirin should be resumed within 3 to 5 days for patients such as this with established cardiovascular disease. Aspirin reduces all-cause mortality (attributable primarily to cardiovascular, cerebrovascular, or gastrointestinal complications) tenfold over 30 days while increasing rebleeding rates only twofold. Long-term, daily proton pump inhibitor therapy should be offered to aspirin users who are *Helicobacter pylori* negative or those who use concomitant NSAIDs, anticoagulants, glucocorticoids, or other antiplatelet drugs.

This patient has no indication for changing his antiplatelet therapy from aspirin to clopidogrel. Although the relative risk for gastrointestinal bleeding is slightly lower with clopidogrel than aspirin, the absolute risk reduction from making the change is low enough that this patient's medication should not be switched; he has a low-risk ulcer and no other cardiovascular indication for clopidogrel (such as a recent drug-eluting stent). In addition, clopidogrel carries a high risk of bothersome side effects such as rash and diarrhea. It is also more expensive than aspirin.

KEY POINT

- In patients with upper gastrointestinal bleeding due to peptic ulcer disease and concomitant cardiovascular disease, aspirin should be resumed within 3 to 5 days; aspirin reduces mortality tenfold over 30 days while increasing rebleeding rates only twofold.

Bibliography
Barkun AN, Bardou M, Kuipers EJ, et al; International Consensus Upper Gastrointestinal Bleeding Conference Group. International consensus recommendations on the management of patients with nonvariceal upper gastrointestinal bleeding. Ann Intern Med. 2010 Jan 19;152(2):101-13. [PMID: 20083829]

Item 76   Answer: D

Educational Objective: Diagnose serrated polyposis syndrome.

The most likely diagnosis is serrated polyposis syndrome. Serrated polyposis syndrome (SPS) is a familial polyposis syndrome without a known genetic cause. It is diagnosed by the World Health Organization criteria of (1) five or more serrated polyps proximal to the sigmoid colon, two or more of which are 10 mm in diameter or greater, (2) any number of serrated polyps proximal to the sigmoid colon in an individual with a first-degree relative who has SPS, or (3) more than 20 serrated polyps distributed throughout the colon. This patient has had six serrated polyps, two of which are larger than 10 mm; therefore, she meets criteria for SPS. SPS is associated with an increased risk of colorectal but not extraintestinal cancer. The mean age of colon cancer diagnosis is 56 years, and metachronous colon cancer occurs in 7% of patients at 5 years of follow-up. Because of this, patients with SPS should undergo colonoscopy yearly. Serrated polyps are a common finding on screening colonoscopy. It is important to recognize that hyperplastic polyps are the most common type of serrated polyp and, when small and located in the rectosigmoid colon, are believed to impart no risk to the patient. However, the other two forms of serrated polyps, sessile serrated polyps and traditional serrated adenomas, are precancerous lesions that occur in 3% and less than 1%, respectively, of individuals undergoing screening colonoscopy. Approximately 30% of colon cancers develop from sessile serrated polyps. Patients with neoplastic serrated polyps should undergo colonoscopy at an interval based on the size and pathology of the lesion.

Familial adenomatous polyposis (FAP) is characterized by tens to thousands of adenomatous colorectal polyps. This patient has no adenomatous polyps and, therefore, FAP is not the most likely diagnosis.

Lynch syndrome is a hereditary colon cancer syndrome caused by a germline mutation in a mismatch repair gene. Colorectal cancers in Lynch syndrome arise from adenomatous polyps. Although patients with Lynch syndrome can have numerous adenomatous polyps, it does not appear typically as a polyposis syndrome.

Peutz-Jeghers syndrome (PJS) is an autosomal dominant hamartomatous polyposis syndrome. The intestinal polyps in PJS are hamartomatous rather than serrated, as was seen in this patient.

KEY POINT

- Serrated polyposis syndrome is associated with an increased risk of colorectal but not extraintestinal cancer; patients with serrated polyposis syndrome should undergo colonoscopy yearly.

Bibliography

Rex DK, Ahnen DJ, Baron JA, et al. Serrated lesions of the colorectum: review and recommendations from an expert panel. Am J Gastroenterol. 2012 Sep;107(9):1315-29; quiz 1314, 1330. [PMID: 22710576]

Item 77 Answer: B

Educational Objective: Evaluate recurrent symptoms with a dietary history in a patient with celiac disease.

The most appropriate management is a careful dietary review. Celiac disease is an immunologic response to dietary gliadins in patients who are genetically at risk as deemed by the presence of *HLA-DQ2* or *HLA-DQ8*. All patients with celiac disease should adhere to a gluten-free diet by avoiding wheat, barley, and rye. Because of cross-contamination with other cereal grains, oats should be avoided for the first year and should only be introduced if the patient is doing well clinically. In patients whose symptoms are recurrent or do not respond to a gluten-free diet, gluten ingestion (either surreptitious or inadvertent) is the most likely explanation. In many cases, patients believe they are being compliant with a strict gluten-free diet, but careful review by an experienced dietitian reveals inadvertent gluten ingestion. Associated conditions that may account for recurrent diarrhea are microscopic colitis (70-fold increased risk), lactose malabsorption, small intestinal bacterial overgrowth, pancreatic insufficiency, inflammatory bowel disease, refractory celiac disease, or enteropathy-associated T-cell lymphoma. A careful review of diet and potential nondietary sources of gluten exposure (such as medications, lipstick, and toothpaste) should be explored before performing additional testing.

A CT scan would be helpful to exclude enteropathy-associated lymphoma or adenocarcinoma; however, these diagnoses are extremely uncommon, even in patients with celiac disease. Dietary indiscretion is a much more likely cause.

Colonoscopy with biopsies would be useful to exclude microscopic colitis, which is associated with celiac disease, but a second diagnosis should be pursued only after ruling out gluten ingestion.

Upper endoscopy with small-bowel biopsies would be helpful to evaluate for active celiac disease, but it would not determine whether gluten ingestion is the cause of this patient's symptoms.

KEY POINT

- Assessment for intentional or unintentional gluten ingestion is the first step in evaluating recurrent symptoms in a patient with celiac disease.

Bibliography

Rubio-Tapia A, Murray JA. Classification and management of refractory coeliac disease. Gut. 2010 Apr;59(4):547-57. [PMID: 20332526]

Item 78 Answer: C

Educational Objective: Treat *Helicobacter pylori* infection after initial treatment failure.

The most appropriate treatment for this patient is a 10-day course of levofloxacin, amoxicillin, and omeprazole. *Helicobacter pylori* infection is closely linked with recurrent peptic ulcer disease, chronic metaplastic gastritis, gastric mucosa-associated lymphoid tissue (MALT) lymphoma, gastric adenocarcinoma, iron deficiency anemia, and primary immune thrombocytopenia. Therefore, an effort should be made to successfully eradicate the infection once it is identified. Initial treatment regimens are effective in *H. pylori* eradication in only 70% to 80% of patients. The most common reason for treatment failure is antibiotic resistance. In the United States, *H. pylori* resistance prevalence is 37% for metronidazole and 13% for clarithromycin. Clarithromycin resistance is absolute and cannot be overcome by increasing the dose or re-treating with a longer course of therapy. Conversely, metronidazole resistance can be overcome by increasing the dose or by using metronidazole in an alternative medication regimen. If *H. pylori* infection is not eradicated with primary therapy, as in this patient, a second-line salvage therapy should contain an alternative antibiotic to clarithromycin, and the treatment should be at least 10 days in duration to maximize the likelihood of treatment success. Two universally recommended second-line therapies are (1) a 10- to 14-day course of bismuth subsalicylate, metronidazole, tetracycline, and a proton pump inhibitor (PPI), or (2) a 10-day course of levofloxacin, amoxicillin, and a PPI.

KEY POINT

- If *Helicobacter pylori* infection is not eradicated with primary therapy, a second-line salvage therapy should contain an alternative antibiotic to clarithromycin, and the treatment should be at least 10 days in duration to maximize the likelihood of treatment success.

Bibliography

Luther J, Chey WD, Saad RJ. A clinician's guide to salvage therapy for persistent Helicobacter pylori infection. Hosp Pract (1995). 2011 Feb;39(1):133-40. [PMID: 21441768]

Item 79 Answer: D

Educational Objective: Diagnose Gilbert syndrome.

This patient requires no further tests for his scleral icterus. He has an indirect hyperbilirubinemia with normal liver enzyme levels, reticulocyte count, and blood smear. These findings are consistent with Gilbert syndrome, and no further tests are necessary. Gilbert syndrome is a benign condition characterized by mild unconjugated hyperbilirubinemia, which is caused by a congenital decrease in hepatic uridine diphosphate glucuronyl transferase. Patients with Gilbert syndrome have a defect in the ability to conjugate bilirubin, resulting in unconjugated hyperbilirubinemia. The bilirubin level tends to be highest when the patient is fasting or ill but is usually less than 3 mg/dL (51.3 μmol/L).

Patients with warm autoimmune hemolytic anemia (WAIHA) may present with rapid or more insidious symptoms of anemia or jaundice; mild splenomegaly is often present. Spherocytes are seen on the peripheral blood smear. The direct antiglobulin (Coombs) test is used to diagnose WAIHA and is typically positive for IgG and negative or only weakly positive for complement (C3). Hemolytic anemia is associated with a low hemoglobin level, a high reticulocyte count, and an abnormal blood smear. Because these features are not present in this patient, there is no need for further hematologic evaluation with a direct antiglobulin (Coombs) test.

Hepatitis is associated with hepatocyte inflammation and injury typically manifested as elevations of serum aspartate aminotransferase (AST) and alanine aminotransferase (ALT). This patient's laboratory abnormality is limited to unconjugated hyperbilirubinemia, which is not consistent with either hepatitis B or C; serologic screening for these conditions is unnecessary.

Primary sclerosing cholangitis (PSC) is a chronic inflammatory disorder that affects the intra- and extrahepatic bile ducts. Serum alkaline phosphatase values are 3 to 10 times the upper limit of normal, and serum ALT and AST levels are two to three times the upper limit of normal. The diagnosis is made by cholangiography. This patient's solitary finding of unconjugated hyperbilirubinemia is not compatible with the diagnosis of PSC.

KEY POINT

- The finding of predominantly unconjugated hyperbilirubinemia indicates non–liver-disease states such as hemolysis or Gilbert syndrome, which is characterized by benign defects in bilirubin conjugation.

Bibliography

Ehmer U, Kalthoff S, Fakundiny B, et al. Gilbert syndrome redefined: a complex genetic haplotype influences the regulation of glucuronidation. Hepatology. 2012 Jun;55(6):1912–21. [PMID: 22213127]

Item 80   Answer: C

Educational Objective: Provide colonoscopy surveillance in a patient with a history of colorectal cancer.

The most appropriate time to repeat colonoscopy is in 5 years. Patients who undergo curative surgical resection for colon cancer should have a complete perioperative colonoscopy to remove all synchronous neoplasia. A subsequent surveillance colonoscopy is recommended within 1 year. If results of that colonoscopy are normal, repeat colonoscopy is recommended at 3 years, and, if normal, every 5 years thereafter. If colorectal polyps are detected, the surveillance interval should be based upon the number, size, and pathology of the polyps. This patient has received his 1- and 3-year follow-up colonoscopies and has had normal results; therefore, colonoscopy can now be repeated every 5 years.

A 10-year colonoscopy interval is appropriate for patients with a family history of adenoma or colorectal cancer in one first-degree relative or two second-degree relatives older than age 60 years. It is not recommended for this patient because his history of colorectal cancer requires more frequent surveillance.

KEY POINT

- Screening recommendations for patients with a history of colorectal cancer consist of follow-up colonoscopy at 1 year and 3 years after curative surgical resection; if results of these colonoscopies are normal, the surveillance interval can be extended to 5 years.

Bibliography

Levin B, Lieberman DA, McFarland B, et al; American Cancer Society Colorectal Cancer Advisory Group; US Multi-Society Task Force; American College of Radiology Colon Cancer Committee. Screening and surveillance for the early detection of colorectal cancer and adenomatous polyps, 2008: a joint guideline from the American Cancer Society, the US Multi-Society Task Force on Colorectal Cancer, and the American College of Radiology. CA Cancer J Clin. 2008 May-Jun;58(3):130-60. [PMID: 18322143]

Item 81   Answer: C

Educational Objective: Manage gastroesophageal reflux disease with an empiric trial of a proton pump inhibitor.

The most appropriate next step in management is a trial of a proton pump inhibitor (PPI). This patient has classic symptoms of gastroesophageal reflux disease (GERD) in the form of heartburn. Symptoms of heartburn and regurgitation are strong predictors for the clinical diagnosis of GERD. The most appropriate next step in a patient without alarm symptoms (dysphagia, unintentional weight loss, hematemesis, or melena) is an empiric trial of a PPI.

Although ambulatory esophageal pH monitoring is the most accurate technique to diagnose GERD, it is expensive and invasive and is therefore only indicated in patients whose symptoms have not responded to medication. This patient has never taken a PPI previously to control his symptoms, so pH testing is not needed at this point in management.

Esophageal manometry measures the pressure levels in the esophagus and is useful in evaluating esophageal motility disorders such as achalasia. However, this patient has not had dysphagia to solids and liquids, which makes an esophageal motility disorder unlikely.

This patient has not had any alarm symptoms such as difficulty swallowing or weight loss that would warrant an upper endoscopy at this time. An upper endoscopy would be necessary if this patient had alarm symptoms or if his symptoms did not respond to the empiric trial of a PPI.

KEY POINT

- In a patient without alarm features (dysphagia, unintentional weight loss, hematemesis, or melena), symptom relief with an empiric trial of a proton pump inhibitor confirms the diagnosis of gastroesophageal reflux disease.

Bibliography

Katz PO, Gerson LB, Vela MF. Guidelines for the diagnosis and management of gastroesophageal reflux disease. Am J Gastroenterol. 2013 Mar; 108(3):308-28; quiz 329. Erratum in: Am J Gastroenterol. 2013 Oct;108(10): 1672. [PMID: 23419381]

Item 82   Answer: D

Educational Objective: Diagnose ischemic colitis as a cause of lower gastrointestinal bleeding.

The most likely diagnosis is ischemic colitis. The most common causes of acute, severe lower gastrointestinal (LGI) bleeding are colonic diverticula, angiodysplasia, colitis (due to inflammatory bowel disease, infection, ischemia, or radiation therapy), and colonic neoplasia. Other than colitis, LGI bleeding is typically painless. Ischemic colitis is due to a temporary interruption in mesenteric blood flow and typically occurs in older individuals with significant cardiac and peripheral vascular disease. Typical symptoms are the acute onset of mild, crampy abdominal pain with tenderness on examination over the affected region of the colon. Bleeding may occur early but often occurs within a few days of pain onset.

Angiodysplasia is most common among the elderly and usually presents as chronic or occult blood loss, but it can also cause acute painless, hemodynamically significant bleeding.

Colonic neoplasms may present with bleeding but it is typically of small volume and is not associated with abdominal pain.

Bleeding from a colonic diverticulum typically is acute and painless. Bleeding stops spontaneously in approximately 80% of patients but recurs in 10% to 40%.

Patients with ulcerative colitis almost always have a sense of bowel urgency due to rectal inflammation. Frequent watery bowel movements are typical, and bleeding occurs with more severe inflammation. The onset of ulcerative colitis is typically acute, and patients often remember when symptoms first started. Severe abdominal pain is an unusual manifestation of ulcerative colitis and suggests a complication such as toxic megacolon or perforation. Most patients with toxic megacolon related to ulcerative colitis have at least 1 week of bloody diarrhea symptoms.

KEY POINT

- The presence of abdominal pain in a patient with lower gastrointestinal bleeding raises the possibility of colitis from ischemia, inflammatory bowel disease, infection, or radiation.

Bibliography

Ghassemi KA, Jensen DM. Lower GI bleeding: epidemiology and management. Curr Gastroenterol Rep. 2013 Jul;15(7):333. [PMID: 23737154]

Item 83   Answer: C

Educational Objective: Provide colonoscopy surveillance following a diagnosis of adenomatous polyps.

Colonoscopy should be repeated in 3 years. Patients with adenomas are at increased risk for colon cancer. They can be stratified into low- and high-risk groups for metachronous neoplasia based on the polyp size, number, and pathology. This risk stratification has a strong evidence base and guides when the next colonoscopy should be performed. Patients with (1) an adenoma 10 mm or larger, (2) three to ten adenomas, (3) an adenoma with a villous component (such as a tubulovillous or villous adenoma), or (4) an adenoma with high-grade dysplasia are considered high risk and should undergo their next colonoscopy in 3 years. Diminutive (<5 mm) rectosigmoid (hyperplastic) polyps are not a known risk factor for colorectal cancer and do not warrant more than average-risk colorectal cancer screening.

Patients with polyps larger than 20 mm or polyps removed in pieces should undergo their next colonoscopy in 3 to 6 months to ensure that no residual polyp tissue remains.

Patients with colon cancer, not adenomas, should have their first postoperative colonoscopy examination within 1 year of the clearing colonoscopy.

Patients with one to two tubular adenomas smaller than 10 mm are considered low risk and should undergo their next colonoscopy in 5 years.

KEY POINT

- Patients with (1) an adenoma 10 mm or larger, (2) three to ten adenomas, (3) an adenoma with a villous component (such as a tubulovillous or villous adenoma), or (4) an adenoma with high-grade dysplasia are considered high risk for colon cancer and should undergo their next colonoscopy in 3 years.

Bibliography

Lieberman DA, Rex DK, Winawer SJ, Giardiello FM, Johnson DA, Levin TR; United States Multi-Society Task Force on Colorectal Cancer. Guidelines for colonoscopy surveillance after screening and polypectomy: a consensus update by the US Multi-Society Task Force on Colorectal Cancer. Gastroenterology. 2012 Sep;143(3):844-57. [PMID: 22763141]

Item 84   Answer: D

Educational Objective: Diagnose esophageal cancer with upper endoscopy.

The most appropriate next step in management is upper endoscopy. Progressive solid-food dysphagia is the most common presenting symptom of esophageal cancer. Associated weight loss (as a consequence of reduced oral intake), anorexia, and anemia (from gastrointestinal bleeding) may be present as well. Despite the association of gastroesophageal reflux disease (GERD) with adenocarcinoma, many patients do not have frequent or severe reflux symptoms. This may be because of decreased perception of acid reflux in these patients. Endoscopy is usually diagnostic. Upper endoscopy is the preferred test to assess for esophageal cancer, as it allows for tissue biopsy. Squamous cell carcinoma usually affects the proximal esophagus, whereas adenocarcinoma usually affects the distal esophagus. Risk factors for squamous cell carcinoma include long-term exposure to alcohol and tobacco, nitrosamine exposure, corrosive injury to the esophagus, dietary deficiencies (zinc, selenium), achalasia, tylosis (keratosis of the palms and soles), and human papillomavirus infection. In addition to GERD, risk factors for the development of adenocarcinoma include tobacco use, obesity (especially central obesity), and Barrett esophagus. Staging of the tumor is critical in determining therapy and prognosis. Staging is typically done with CT (to detect distant metastases), endoscopic ultrasound (for locoregional staging), and PET (to follow up on indeterminate lesions found with other staging modalities).

A CT of the chest could be used later to assess locoregional spread of esophageal cancer (such as lymph node involvement), but upper endoscopy should be performed first to assess for esophageal cancer.

Esophageal manometry is the test of choice to evaluate an underlying motility disorder. In this patient, the concern is for an esophageal mass, which does not require manometry.

A pH study would be useful to evaluate a patient with acid reflux whose symptoms are not responding to medical therapy. This test would not be appropriate to evaluate this patient's solid-food dysphagia, and his GERD symptoms have been controlled with omeprazole.

KEY POINT

- Upper endoscopy with biopsy is the preferred initial diagnostic test for suspected esophageal cancer.

Bibliography
Varghese TK Jr, Hofstetter WL, Rizk NP, et al. The society of thoracic surgeons guidelines on the diagnosis and staging of patients with esophageal cancer. Ann Thorac Surg. 2013 Jul;96(1):346-56. [PMID: 23752201]

Item 85 Answer: D

Educational Objective: Manage a gastric neuroendocrine tumor.

The most appropriate management is observation. This patient has a gastric neuroendocrine tumor (NET) that has developed in the presence of chronic autoimmune gastritis, which is characterized by pernicious anemia and hypergastrinemia due to achlorhydria or hypochlorhydria. Endoscopic polypectomy is considered curative treatment for this patient's NET. Gastric NETs are classified into three subtypes: type I, II, and III. This classification distinguishes the underlying pathogenesis and guides the appropriate management of the NET.

Type I NETs account for the majority of gastric NETs, have an increased prevalence in older women, and are associated with autoimmune atrophic gastritis and hypergastrinemia. Type I gastric NETs are not associated with multiple endocrine neoplasia or Zollinger-Ellison syndrome (unlike type II gastric NETs) and rarely metastasize. Curative treatment of type I NETs is achieved with endoscopic removal of these lesions when they are small (<1 cm) and few lesions are present (<5), as is the case in this patient.

Tumor staging for type I gastric NETs (using CT of the abdomen and pelvis or radiolabeled somatostatin receptor scintigraphy) is not indicated because type I NETs rarely metastasize.

Surgical intervention is not indicated for this patient's small, type I NET that has been completely eradicated. Partial gastrectomy would be indicated if this patient's tumor was larger than 2 cm because of a risk of metastasis.

KEY POINT

- Curative treatment of type I gastric neuroendocrine tumors is achieved with endoscopic removal of these lesions when they are small (<1 cm) and few lesions are present (<5).

Bibliography
Crosby DA, Donohoe CL, Fitzgerald L, et al. Gastric neuroendocrine tumours. Dig Surg. 2012;29(4):331-48. [PMID: 23075625]

Item 86 Answer: A

Educational Objective: Diagnose achalasia.

The most likely diagnosis is achalasia. This patient has dysphagia to both solids and liquids, suggesting a motility disorder. This patient's diagnostic evaluation and associated findings represent the classic presentation of achalasia, which is characterized by dysphagia to solids and liquids, regurgitation, and possibly weight loss, chest pain, and heartburn. Barium radiography shows a dilated esophagus with narrowing at the lower esophageal sphincter, described as a "bird's beak." Upper endoscopy was performed to rule out mechanical obstruction in the region of the lower esophageal sphincter as a cause of dysphagia. If obstruction is caused by a malignant lesion, the disorder is designated "pseudoachalasia." Manometry is required to confirm the diagnosis of achalasia.

Diffuse esophageal spasm is a rare hypertonic motility disorder that presents with chest pain or dysphagia. Clinical manifestations are similar to those of angina pectoris. On esophageal manometry, simultaneous high-amplitude (>30 mm Hg) esophageal contractions are seen with intermittent aperistaltic contractions. The barium esophagogram finding of a "corkscrew" esophagus is typical of diffuse esophageal spasm. This patient's manometric and barium radiography findings are not consistent with diffuse esophageal spasm.

Esophageal hypomotility disorders can involve a hypotense lower esophageal sphincter, aperistaltic contractions, or both. In most patients, the cause of the hypotensive esophageal disorder is unknown. However, secondary causes include smooth-muscle relaxants, anticholinergic agents, estrogen, progesterone, connective tissue disorders (such as systemic sclerosis), and pregnancy. Esophageal hypomotility disorders are characterized by low-amplitude contractions on manometry with a hypotensive lower esophageal sphincter; this differs from achalasia, which is characterized by incomplete relaxation of the lower esophageal sphincter. These manometric findings are the opposite of what was found on this patient's manometry, which was consistent with achalasia.

Nutcracker esophagus is a hypertonic motility disorder that is characterized by high-amplitude peristaltic contractions of greater than 220 mm Hg. This patient does not have these manometric findings.

KEY POINT

- The primary screening test for achalasia is a barium esophagogram, which demonstrates dilation of the esophagus and narrowing at the gastroesophageal junction, described as a "bird's beak."

Bibliography
Vaezi MF, Pandolfino JE, Vela MF. ACG clinical guideline: diagnosis and management of achalasia. Am J Gastroenterol. 2013 Aug;108(8):1238-49; quiz 1250. [PMID: 23877351]

Item 87   Answer: B

Educational Objective: Manage small intestinal bacterial overgrowth in a patient with Roux-en-Y gastric bypass.

The most appropriate management is empiric treatment for small intestinal bacterial overgrowth (SIBO) with antibiotics. Digestive enzymes and intestinal motility normally limit the growth of excessive bacteria, but SIBO can occur in conditions in which these functions are disrupted, such as the creation of a blind loop. Bacterial metabolism of carbohydrates prior to small-bowel absorption results in symptoms of SIBO (diarrhea, bloating, flatulence, and weight loss). This patient's symptoms of diarrhea, increased gas, bloating, and abdominal discomfort can collectively be explained by the bacterial fermentation of simple carbohydrates in the small bowel from SIBO. Given her presentation, the pretest probability is high enough to justify empiric therapy for SIBO and monitoring of symptoms for a response.

Because SIBO is a very plausible explanation for this patient's diarrhea, performing a colonoscopy would be premature at this time.

A potent antisecretory agent such as omeprazole is indicated for acid-related disorders, and the symptoms reported by this patient are not suggestive of an acid-related disorder. Furthermore, there is some evidence to suggest that the use of a proton pump inhibitor may promote bacterial overgrowth in the small bowel. Therefore, a trial of omeprazole is unlikely to improve this patient's symptoms.

The nature of this patient's abdominal pain is atypical for a biliary source, as it is not meal related or located in

the right upper quadrant. Furthermore, this patient's liver chemistry studies were unremarkable and the gallbladder was resected during her gastric bypass surgery. Therefore, the yield of a right upper quadrant ultrasound would be low in this setting.

Stool cultures are generally not helpful in assessing a patient with chronic diarrhea, except if *Giardia* infection is suspected. In addition, stool cultures are not capable of making the diagnosis of bacterial overgrowth because the bacteria in the blind loop resemble the normal flora of the large bowel. Because this patient's surgical history supports bacterial overgrowth as the cause of diarrhea, an empiric trial of antibiotics is warranted.

KEY POINT

- Small intestinal bacterial overgrowth is common following Roux-en-Y gastric bypass; patients with typical symptoms (diarrhea, bloating, flatulence, and weight loss) should receive empiric antibiotic treatment.

Bibliography
Machado JD, Campos CS, Lopes Dah Silva C, et al. Intestinal bacterial overgrowth after Roux-en-Y gastric bypass. Obes Surg. 2008 Jan;18(1):139-43. [PMID: 18080824]

Item 88   Answer: D

Educational Objective: Manage acute diarrhea.

The most appropriate management is supportive care. Most cases of acute diarrhea in developed countries are self-limited and due to a viral infection. In this otherwise healthy young woman with no alarm features (gastrointestinal bleeding, dehydration, fever, significant abdominal tenderness, recent antibiotic use), further testing is not indicated. Supportive measures, such as ensuring adequate oral fluid intake and using acetaminophen for muscle aches, are the only necessary intervention for most patients. Antimotility agents such as loperamide may be useful for patients with mild diarrhea, but they should not be used in patients with fever, significant abdominal pain, or bloody stools because they may worsen inflammatory diarrhea and increase the risk of complications such as toxic megacolon. Diarrhea in an otherwise healthy person lasting for more than 7 days suggests a parasitic or noninfectious origin and evaluation is appropriate.

Given this patient's age, absence of bleeding, and acute onset of symptoms, a colonoscopy is not indicated. A colonoscopy would be warranted if features of inflammatory bowel disease, such as blood in the stool, were present.

The diagnostic yield of bacterial stool culture for acute diarrhea is low (less than 3%); however, identification of a pathogen has important treatment and public health implications and may be useful in identifying and tracking a food-borne outbreak. Because most cases of community-acquired diarrhea are self-limited, stool cultures are not required in most patients; cultures may be indicated for symptoms lasting longer than 72 hours, particularly in patients with associated fever, tenesmus, or bloody stools.

Parasitic infection should be considered as a potential cause of diarrhea lasting for more than 7 days. *Giardia lamblia* and *Cryptosporidium parvum* are the most commonly identified parasitic agents definitively known to cause diarrhea in the United States. Amebiasis is relatively uncommon in the United States but can cause hemorrhagic colitis in travelers and may occur several years after return from an endemic area. Because this patient does not have a travel history and her symptoms are of short duration, stool testing for ova and parasites is not necessary at this time.

KEY POINT

- Because most cases of community-acquired diarrhea are self-limited, stool cultures or evaluation for ova and parasites are not required in most patients; studies may be indicated for symptoms lasting longer than 72 hours, particularly in patients with associated fever, tenesmus, or bloody stools.

Bibliography
Sweetser S. Evaluating the patient with diarrhea: a case-based approach. Mayo Clin Proc. 2012 Jun;87(6):596-602. [PMID: 22677080]

Item 89   Answer: E
Educational Objective: Manage a sporadic juvenile polyp.

The most appropriate management is reassurance. Solitary juvenile polyps are one of the most commonly found polyps, particularly in children under the age of 10 years; they confer no future health risk once the polyp is removed, and follow-up surveillance colonoscopy is not required. It is important to distinguish between a sporadic, nonsyndromic juvenile polyp and juvenile polyposis syndrome (JPS) because management of JPS is substantially different. The clinical criteria for diagnosis of JPS include (1) more than three juvenile polyps of the colon, (2) juvenile polyps throughout the gastrointestinal tract, or (3) one or more juvenile polyps combined with a family history of JPS. Patients with JPS have an increased risk for colon cancer (39%), gastric cancer (25%), and more rarely small-bowel and pancreatic cancer.

Patients with JPS should undergo genetic counseling and testing for the mutations known to cause the disease (*SMAD4* and *BMPR1A* genes). Surveillance guidelines for patients with JPS recommend colonoscopy and upper endoscopy every 2 to 3 years beginning at age 15 years or sooner if symptoms are present. Because this patient does not meet criteria for JPS, these interventions are not appropriate at this time.

KEY POINT

- Solitary juvenile polyps are one of the most commonly found polyps; they confer no future health risk once the polyp is removed and do not require surveillance endoscopy.

Bibliography
Zbuk KM, Eng C. Hamartomatous polyposis syndromes. Nat Clin Pract Gastroenterol Hepatol. 2007 Sep;4(9):492-502. [PMID: 17768394]

Item 90   Answer: D
Educational Objective: Evaluate oropharyngeal dysphagia with videofluoroscopy.

The most appropriate diagnostic test to evaluate this patient's dysphagia is videofluoroscopy. Dysphagia is classified as either oropharyngeal dysphagia (also called transfer dysphagia) or esophageal dysphagia. Each of the two kinds of dysphagia has distinct epidemiology, pathophysiology, and management implications. Oropharyngeal dysphagia usually occurs immediately with deglutition. Causes of oropharyngeal dysphagia may be either neuromuscular or anatomic. Patients may have associated symptoms that provide clues, such as neurologic symptoms like dysphonia, diplopia, and muscular weakness. When this patient starts to eat he coughs, which indicates oropharyngeal impairment of the swallowing mechanism rather than an esophageal cause. Patients with oropharyngeal dysphagia typically describe coughing, choking, and nasal regurgitation. Choking occurs owing to failure to clear food from the epiglottis and may lead to aspiration. The initial test of choice for evaluation of oropharyngeal dysphagia is videofluoroscopy (also known as a modified barium swallow) in which the oropharyngeal phase of swallowing is assessed with foods of different consistencies. Oropharyngeal forms of dysphagia are often managed with dietary adjustment and incorporation of swallowing exercises with the assistance of a speech pathologist.

Barium swallow may be useful in the evaluation of esophageal dysphagia following a normal upper endoscopy when a mechanical obstruction is still suspected. For example, upper endoscopy may miss lower esophageal rings or extrinsic compression of the esophagus. A barium swallow will not be as helpful as videofluoroscopy in a patient with oropharyngeal dysphagia.

Esophageal dysphagia tends to occur after the initiation of the swallow. Esophageal manometry is useful to diagnose an esophageal motility disorder such as achalasia. However, it is not the best test in a patient with symptoms of oropharyngeal dysphagia.

Esophageal dysphagia often has an intraluminal cause, such as strictures, Schatzki rings, or masses. The diagnostic test of choice for esophageal dysphagia is upper endoscopy, which can be both diagnostic (allowing biopsy and visualization of the mucosa) and therapeutic (allowing dilation to be performed if indicated).

KEY POINT

- The initial test of choice for evaluation of oropharyngeal dysphagia is videofluoroscopy.

Bibliography
Logemann JA, Larsen K. Oropharyngeal dysphagia: pathophysiology and diagnosis for the anniversary issue of Diseases of the Esophagus. Dis Esophagus. 2012 May;25(4):299-304. [PMID: 21595782]

Item 91   Answer: B

Educational Objective: Treat ulcerative colitis with the appropriate maintenance therapy.

The most appropriate maintenance therapy is infliximab. This patient's ulcerative colitis symptoms were refractory to mesalamine but have responded to prednisone, and he is doing well after the dose was tapered to 20 mg/d. Glucocorticoids are not effective for maintaining remission in ulcerative colitis. Therefore, in patients whose disease responds to glucocorticoids, the dose should be tapered while transitioning to a maintenance medication (azathioprine, 6-mercaptopurine, or an anti-tumor necrosis factor agent). Randomized controlled clinical trials have shown infliximab to be an effective maintenance therapy in patients such as this one.

Immunosuppression with azathioprine or 6-mercaptopurine is often used to maintain glucocorticoid-induced remission, but the data supporting this practice are scant. Moreover, this patient has a low thiopurine methyltransferase (TPMT) level, which indicates a high likelihood of severe bone marrow toxicity if exposed to azathioprine or 6-mercaptopurine. Azathioprine is converted in the body to 6-mercaptopurine, which is then either inactivated (by xanthine oxidase or TPMT) or activated to 6-thioguanine nucleotide. The level of TPMT should be checked before starting azathioprine or 6-mercaptopurine; 1 in 300 patients (0.3%) lack enzyme activity and are at high risk of toxicity. Azathioprine and 6-mercaptopurine should not be used in these patients.

Methotrexate may be used in the treatment of Crohn disease; however, there is no evidence for efficacy of methotrexate in ulcerative colitis.

Prednisone is not effective for maintenance of ulcerative colitis. In addition, long-term glucocorticoid use carries significant risk of side effects.

KEY POINT

- Glucocorticoids are not effective for maintaining remission in ulcerative colitis; the glucocorticoid dose should be tapered while transitioning to a maintenance medication (azathioprine, 6-mercaptopurine, or an anti-tumor necrosis factor agent).

Bibliography

Talley NJ, Abreu MT, Achkar JP, et al; American College of Gastroenterology IBD Task Force. An evidence-based systematic review on medical therapies for inflammatory bowel disease. Am J Gastroenterol. 2011 Apr;106 Suppl 1:S2-25; quiz S26. [PMID: 21472012]

Item 92   Answer: E

Educational Objective: Provide surveillance for hepatocellular carcinoma in a patient with chronic hepatitis B infection.

The most appropriate management is ultrasound imaging of the liver every 6 months. This patient from Africa has evidence of chronic hepatitis B virus (HBV) infection. In approximately 50% of untreated patients with chronic HBV

infection in the United States, HBV will contribute to the cause of death (from hepatocellular carcinoma [HCC] or other complications of end-stage liver disease, such as cirrhosis). HCC surveillance is advised in African patients over the age of 20 years with chronic HBV infection. Screening and surveillance for HCC consist of cross-sectional imaging with ultrasound, CT, or MRI. Ultrasound is the most widely available and least expensive imaging modality and is preferred. For patients with normal imaging at diagnosis, the recommended interval for surveillance imaging is 6 months. Serum α-fetoprotein measurement does not have sufficient diagnostic accuracy alone to be a valuable tool for early detection. The combination of ultrasonography and α-fetoprotein measurement increases cancer detection rates, but this comes at the expense of increased false-positive findings. Other indications for HCC surveillance in patients with chronic HBV infection are (1) patients with cirrhosis, (2) Asian men older than 40 years, (3) Asian women older than 50 years, (4) patients with a family history of HCC, and (5) patients with persistent hepatocellular inflammation (defined as elevated alanine aminotransferase [ALT] level and HBV DNA level greater than 10,000 IU/mL).

This patient has already been infected with HBV, so vaccination at this point will not be effective.

This patient's HBV infection is in the inactive carrier/immune control state, as evidenced by his normal ALT level and HBV DNA level below 10,000 IU/mL. Treatment with antiviral agents such as pegylated interferon or tenofovir is not necessary for patients in the inactive carrier state. However, surveillance for HCC is still indicated.

KEY POINT

- Screening and surveillance for hepatocellular carcinoma consist of cross-sectional imaging with ultrasound, CT, or MRI.

Bibliography

Bruix J, Sherman M; American Association for the Study of Liver Diseases. Management of hepatocellular carcinoma: an update. Hepatology. 2011 Mar;53(3):1020-2. [PMID: 21374666]

Item 93   Answer: C

Educational Objective: Manage peptic ulcer bleeding.

The most appropriate management is prompt discharge on oral proton pump inhibitor (PPI) therapy. In addition, NSAIDs should be discontinued. Upper endoscopy identified several small gastric ulcers as this patient's bleeding source. Patients with low-risk stigmata (a clean-based ulcer [rebleeding risk with medical therapy 3%-5%] or a nonprotuberant pigmented spot in an ulcer bed [rebleeding risk with medical therapy 5%-10%]) can be fed within 24 hours, should receive oral PPI therapy, and can undergo early hospital discharge. This patient's ulcers did not require endoscopic therapy and are at low risk for rebleeding, especially with the daily use of an oral PPI and discontinuation of NSAIDs. Other clinical predictors that justify prompt discharge are

CONT.

this patient's stable vital signs, stable hemoglobin level, and absence of serious comorbidities.

Several studies have demonstrated similar outcomes in patients with low-risk ulcers who were discharged on the first hospital day compared with those hospitalized for longer periods of time. There is no benefit to another day of hospitalization for observation.

With a low-risk ulcer, feeding can be initiated and PPI therapy can be promptly switched from continuous intravenous infusion to an oral formulation. An additional 24 hours of an intravenous PPI therapy is unnecessary and needlessly expensive.

More than 90% of uncomplicated NSAID-induced gastric ulcers will heal with standard-dose PPI therapy if NSAID therapy is discontinued. This patient could be considered for upper endoscopy in 2 to 3 months to document healing of his gastric ulcers if dyspeptic symptoms persist despite therapy, the initial endoscopy was not complete in evaluating the stomach, gastric biopsies were not obtained on initial endoscopy, or the appearance of the gastric ulcer was suspicious for malignancy. If NSAID therapy is reinitiated in the future, co-therapy with a PPI should be employed to prevent a recurrent peptic ulcer. Misoprostol at 800 µg total daily dosing is an alternative to PPI therapy, but gastrointestinal side effects at this dose may be limiting. Twice-daily H_2-blocker therapy offers some benefit, but protection is inferior to that of PPI therapy. There is no need to routinely perform second-look endoscopy during hospitalization for an acute peptic ulcer bleed. Indications for repeat endoscopy in the hospital setting would include concern for ongoing gastrointestinal bleeding or an incomplete endoscopic evaluation with concern for missing a bleeding source.

KEY POINT

- Peptic ulcers at low risk for bleeding (clean based or with a nonprotuberant pigmented spot) can be managed with oral proton pump inhibitor therapy and early hospital discharge.

Bibliography
Laine L, Jensen DM. Management of patients with ulcer bleeding. Am J Gastroenterol. 2012 Mar;107(3):345-60; quiz 361. [PMID: 22310222]

Item 94   Answer: A

Educational Objective: Treat Barrett esophagus with high-grade dysplasia with endoscopic ablation.

The most appropriate next step in management is endoscopic ablation. Barrett esophagus (BE) is a precancerous condition that can progress to esophageal cancer. Risk factors associated with BE are older age, male gender, white ethnicity, gastroesophageal reflux disease (GERD), hiatal hernia, high BMI, smoking, and an abdominal distribution of fat. This patient has high-grade dysplasia, a high-risk feature of the condition. Treatment to remove BE is recommended for patients with confirmed high-grade dysplasia and can be done with endoscopic therapies such as radiofrequency ablation,

photodynamic therapy, or endoscopic mucosal resection. Choice of treatment may be influenced by local expertise and patient preference.

Esophagectomy is the treatment of choice for esophageal cancer if the patient is a surgical candidate. Esophagectomy may be required in patients with BE and high-grade dysplasia if ablation has failed or progression to cancer occurred during endoscopic treatment. Endoscopic treatment should be attempted for this patient before surgery would be appropriate.

Fundoplication would be indicated in a patient with refractory GERD. Fundoplication has not been shown to reduce the risk of progression of BE with high-grade dysplasia to cancer and is therefore not an appropriate choice.

A repeat surveillance upper endoscopy in 3 to 5 years would be appropriate in a patient with BE with no dysplasia. Because this patient has high-grade dysplasia, more aggressive management is necessary.

KEY POINT

- Treatment to remove Barrett esophagus is recommended for patients with confirmed high-grade dysplasia and can be done with endoscopic therapies that include radiofrequency ablation, photodynamic therapy, or endoscopic mucosal resection.

Bibliography
Spechler SJ, Sharma P, Souza RF, Inadomi JM, Shaheen NJ; American Gastroenterological Association. American Gastroenterological Association technical review on the management of Barrett's esophagus. Gastroenterology. 2011 Mar;140(3):e18-52; quiz e13. [PMID: 21376939]

Item 95   Answer: B

Educational Objective: Diagnose an insulinoma with endoscopic ultrasound.

The most appropriate diagnostic test is endoscopic ultrasound. Hypoglycemia is best diagnosed when three conditions coexist (Whipple triad): (1) hypoglycemic symptoms are present, (2) the plasma glucose level is low, and (3) resolution of symptoms occurs promptly after glucose ingestion. When Whipple triad is observed, further evaluation for the cause of pathologic hypoglycemia should include an inpatient 72-hour fast with regular measurement of simultaneous plasma glucose, insulin, and C-peptide (a measure of endogenous insulin secretion). If the results are consistent with insulinoma, only then should CT imaging of the pancreas be performed to localize the tumor and direct its surgical resection. Because insulinomas are often small, further testing (with, for example, endoscopic ultrasonography) may be necessary for localization, as is required in this patient.

Endoscopic retrograde cholangiopancreatography (ERCP) is an endoscopic test that allows for visualization and therapeutic interventions of the bile and pancreatic ducts. It is an invasive procedure that will not identify small solid tumors of the pancreas such as an insulinoma.

Insulinomas almost always have inadequate expression of somatostatin receptors to be detected by octreotide scanning; therefore, this is not a useful diagnostic test for insulinomas.

Although abdominal ultrasonography is noninvasive, it does not have the resolution to identify small pancreatic tumors, particularly tumors not detected by a higher-resolution imaging procedure such as CT scanning.

KEY POINT

- Endoscopic ultrasound is sensitive for detecting insulinomas, which are typically small and solitary and may not be detected by CT cross-sectional imaging.

Bibliography
Burns WR, Edil BH. Neuroendocrine pancreatic tumors: guidelines for management and update. Curr Treat Options Oncol. 2012 Mar;13(1):24-34. [PMID: 22198808]

Item 96   Answer: A

Educational Objective: **Treat microscopic colitis.**

The most appropriate treatment is budesonide. Collagenous colitis, a form of microscopic colitis, is most often idiopathic, but in a small subset of patients it may be a side effect of medications. Drugs that have been highly associated with microscopic colitis include aspirin, acarbose, lansoprazole, NSAIDs, ranitidine, sertraline, and ticlopidine. Celiac disease is also associated with microscopic colitis. Treatment may be as simple as drug withdrawal or treatment of celiac disease. In mild persistent disease, antidiarrheal therapy such as loperamide or diphenoxylate can be used. In moderate disease, bismuth subsalicylate may be beneficial. This patient has collagenous colitis that has not responded to antidiarrheal therapy with diphenoxylate, loperamide, or bismuth subsalicylate. In patients with severe disease or in those that do not respond to antidiarrheal agents or bismuth, budesonide is the treatment of choice. It is highly effective (response rates of ≥80%). However, the risk of relapse is high once budesonide is stopped (70%-80%). Many patients require long-term maintenance therapy with low-dose budesonide or an immunomodulator such as azathioprine.

There is no evidence of benefit from antibiotics in collagenous colitis; therefore, ciprofloxacin is not appropriate for this patient.

In severe microscopic colitis, treatment with an anti-tumor necrosis factor agent such as infliximab may be effective. However, this expensive, potent immune-suppressing medication should be used only if budesonide is unsuccessful.

Open-label reports of mesalamine suggested a possible small benefit in microscopic colitis; however, a randomized trial showed no benefit compared with placebo.

KEY POINT

- Therapy for microscopic colitis is based on symptom severity and may consist of withdrawal of an offending drug or administration of loperamide or diphenoxylate for mild persistent disease, bismuth subsalicylate for moderate disease, or budesonide for severe disease.

Bibliography
Pardi DS, Kelly CP. Microscopic colitis. Gastroenterology. 2011 Apr;140(4):1155-65. [PMID: 21303675]

Index